Biomechanical Evaluation of
Movement in Sport and Exercise

Biomechanical Evaluation of Movement in Sport and Exercise

Editor: Robert Day

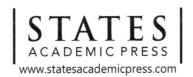

STATES
ACADEMIC PRESS
www.statesacademicpress.com

States Academic Press,
109 South 5th Street,
Brooklyn, NY 11249, USA

Visit us on the World Wide Web at:
www.statesacademicpress.com

ISBN: 978-1-63989-079-8 (Hardback)

Trademark Notice: Registered trademark of products or corporate names are used only for explanation and identification without intent to infringe.

Cataloging-in-Publication Data

Biomechanical evaluation of movement in sport and exercise / edited by Robert Day.
   p. cm.
Includes bibliographical references and index.
ISBN 978-1-63989-079-8
1. Human mechanics. 2. Sports--Physiological aspects. 3. Exercise--Physiological aspects.
I. Day, Robert.
QP303 .B56 2022
612.76--dc23

Table of Contents

Preface

This book aims to highlight the current researches and provides a platform to further the scope of innovations in this area. This book is a product of the combined efforts of many researchers and scientists, after going through thorough studies and analysis from different parts of the world. The objective of this book is to provide the readers with the latest information of the field.

Biomechanics refers to the examination of the structure, function and movement associated with mechanical aspects of the biological system. In order to study the human movement in sports and exercise, the laws and principles of mechanical physics as well as the elements of gait analysis, mechanical engineering, clinical neurophysiology, and computer science are applied. Movement for sports and exercise involves muscular, skeletal and joint actions. The biomechanical evaluation of such aspects serves to understand the factors contributing to sport performance, sport mastery, injury prevention, and rehabilitation. This book is compiled in such a manner, that it will provide in-depth knowledge about the theories and principles of biomechanics. It includes some of the vital pieces of work being conducted across the world, on various topics related to sports biomechanics. With state-of-the-art inputs by acclaimed experts of this field, this book targets students and professionals.

I would like to express my sincere thanks to the authors for their dedicated efforts in the completion of this book. I acknowledge the efforts of the publisher for providing constant support. Lastly, I would like to thank my family for their support in all academic endeavors.

Editor

Improving psychological component, priority training of children and junior player in basketball

Ghețu Roberta Georgiana, Călinescu Brăbiescu Luminița, Burcea George Bogdan

University of Craiova

Abstract. This study aims to highlight of influence of the mental capacity in training by using preparation means, carefully selected. The principle of acting was the systematic use of a set of resources based on adversity and competition. Final test results allowed us to conclude that repeated use of the proposal means have produce modification in the results . (number of execution, number of throws). Those have been superior to the most players. Apart from increase the level of performance we observed during the training, were recorded higher performance in official games.

Key words: training, performanc , psychological component.

Introduction

Individual and collective sports results achieved during last decade special values representing the specialists performance. Dynamics evolution of sports performance, basketball in our case, assume knowledge of development trends, game design features and elements of progress or limiting is an essential requirement in the design and orientation training. In essence the training as the main factor of performance capacity, is a systematic process to drive to improve its components (including psychological preparation). (1)

Choice of the theme has firstly related by the motivation of my professional concern to discover, understand and resolve problems in sport based on scientific and methodological knowledge .

Directly observation of the training develop to the different levels and ages and also the exchange of views with coaches and specialists who working at these levels, regarding the weight given psychological training highlights necessity for same studies .(2)

The observation , the behavioral analysis of players in basketball competition have highlighted significant differences in the mod of expression of players from a game to another.

This fact led me to reflect on causes searching explanation in two directions.

1.The assumption that are structural factors of performance capacity (skills and attitude) which limits the performance .

2.The second supposition is related to the quality in different stages .

Hypotheses .

The approach of the psychological component training based on a methodology agreed upon , increase the chances manifestation of somatic and motor abilities , which will result in influence the behavior performance in training and competition

Materials and methods .

Achievement of a training process at a high level is compatible only with existence of human material able browse through, according the assessment of the athletes under the aspect framing in a performance model is a necessity .

Evolution in time of a mental capacity depends of the one part by the maturity and self-education , and the other part demands education and competitive solicitation.

Preparation of self-mental capacity realize psychological states and behavior of training and competition.(3)

Training will need to develop adaptive capacity of the players through intelligent action directed, it will be able to adopt, cope or to salve the most critical situation in an effort through emotional mastery, motivation combativeness .

After the way of organizing the activities , the study is presented like an experiment, aiming, the analyzing role of psychological preparation in the performance activity at the junior II level (team of C.S.S.U. Craiova) .

This study aim to highlights the existence of some differences which can be appear in performance behavior when mental preparation .

Is a priority to a basketball team who presents homogeneity of tactical and technical knowledge .

Experimental group: was a team who`s participate in the National Junior Championship (age±16).

Control group: was a team of same age.

The experiment consisted in using a 4 means sets executed as a competition, appreciated to be with a very emotionally charged and placed in training for a period of six months .

The means used

P1 – free throwing - wins who enroll first 10 baskets , if you miss throw , the other .

P2 – shooting in dribbling , with active adversity in pair .(attacker , defender) dribble from the center and throw to basket , is applied a rating scale :
  - very good – 9-10 points
  - well – 7-8- points
  - sufficient – 5-6 points
  - weak 3-4 points

P3 – dribble suicide (small marathon).(4)
  Rating scale :
  - excellent – 21 sec .
  - very good – 21-22,5 sec
  - sufficient – 24-25,5 sec
  - weak – over 25,5 sec .

P4 – passing the ball in two, with throw in the running to each panel (4, 6, 8 ,) points.

Final test results allowed us to conclude that repeated use of the proposal means have produce modification in the results . (number of execution, number of throws). Those have been superior to the most players .

Apart from increase the level of performance we observed during the training, were recorded higher performance in official games.

Increased the number of wins achieved, decreased the difference in value between the team and ranked team.

We notice also increase safety in resolving situation of adversity .

Presentation and interpretation

Table no. 1

	T1	T2
Arithmetic average	5,14	6,29
Standard deviation	1,791	1,858
Coefficient of variation		2,02

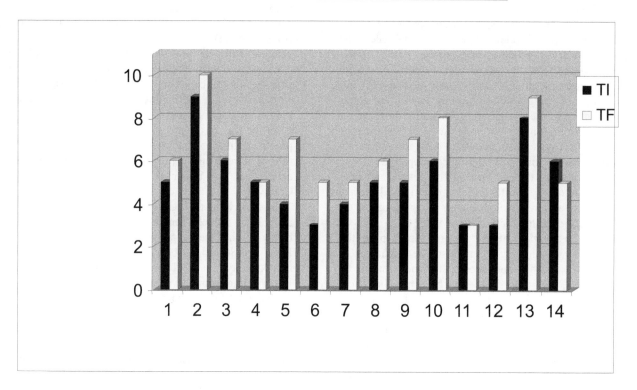

Interpretation.

To initial testing were obtained an average of 5,14% with standard deviation of 1,79% and a coefficient of variation of 2,02% which proves a large degree of homogeneity.

The final testing show an average of 6,29% with a standard deviation of 1,858% which demonstrated a degree of dispersal very small .

Rate of progress between T1 –T2 is 1,15% , appreciated as good.

Table no. 2 Dribble throws

	T1	T2
Arithmetic average	1,83	1,50
Standard deviation	1,119	0,540

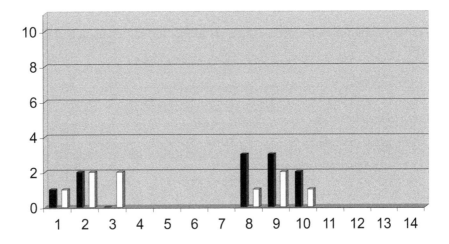

To the initial testing was obtained an average value of 0.0083% wich shows that,there is group homogeneity.After using actions systems to the final testing and obtain value of standard deviation of 0,540% wich indicates low degree of dispersion with value around media.We appreciate headway between T1-T2 for the value of performance parameters.

Table no.3 Dribbling suido small marathon

	T1	T2
Arithmetic average	22,86	22,29
Standard deviation	1,318	1,271
Coefficient of variation		1,54

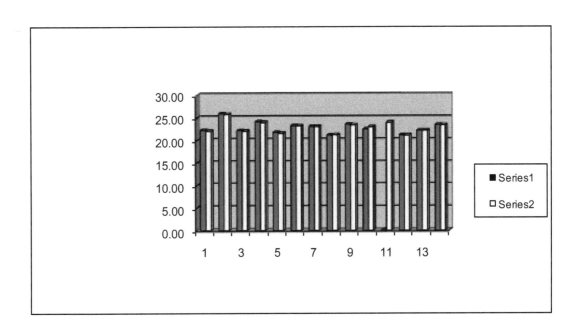

Interpretation
Analysis value obtaining from this text is part of the trend of increase in execution accordingly appreciate influenting favorable means used.

Table no.4 Simple throw

	T1	T2
Arithmetic average	5,43	5,79
Standard deviation	1,785	2,225
Coefficient of variation		3,231

Interpretation.
Initial test achieved a media of 5.49% and a standard deviation of 1.775 and a 3.235 value for coefficient of variation wich shows a difference of value.In final testing actioned after the training intervention werw obtained an average value of 5.791with a standard deviation of 2.225 coresponding values in wich the degree of scatter around the average.
We consider that .because evidence was relevant in media influence.

Conclusion:
1.This study highlights the importance nedeed to acorde to the psychological factor and the weightand working permanently with junior players ,stage in wich must put foundation of performance activity.

2.Following a correct position of a specialists in this field awarded to the psychological training.
3.Through a correctly approach to the mental preparedness training,performance behavior,is adecisively influencing the child.

Reference
1.Dragnea A.,Mate- Teodorescu S.,*Teoria Sportului*,Publishing House Fest, Bucureşti,2002,p.155
2. Horghidan V. - *Metode de psihodiagnostic*, Publishing House EDR,Bucureşti,1999,P. 51
3. Epuran M., Holdevici,I.,Tonita,F.,*Psihologia sportului de performanţă:teorie şi practică*, Publishing House Fest, Bucureşti,2001,p.59
4. Roman Gh.,*Evaluarea în jocul de baschet*,Publishing House Star,Cluj Napoca,2003,p.80

Comparative study on anthropometric indices related to improvement and development of motor skills to secondary education level pupils attending football special program school and —Decebal‖ School from Craiova

Stoica Doru, Barbu Dumitru, Barbu Mihai Constantin Răzvan, Ciocanescu Daniel

University of Craiova – Faculty of Physical Education and Sport

Abstract: The present research represents a comparative study concerning the differences of anthropometric indices related to the growth and the development of motor skills registered by two groups of pupils attending the 7th form, one belonging to a school having football as a major area of study and the other to a general school. As well, the present paper aims at indicating the level of physical and motor improvement and development to pupils attending the secondary cycle within the two school units.

Key words: *football, anthropometric indices, motor skills, performance.*

***Introduction*:** Considering different aspects, the current age requires the individual to continuously adapt to changes related to the dynamics of phenomenon and social actions.(1,2)

During the modern age, the importance of physical education and sport becomes obvious, therefore, in most of the schools all over the world, they belong to the category of instructive-educational activities. Being a developmental-type activity, the physical education perfectly fits with the new tendencies of the modern school, which promotes the formation of social integration skills and abilities to pupils. (3, 4). Therefore, the physical exercise represents an important means of adjustment to changes and new conditions to which the rhythm of the modern social development submits us.

Material and methods

Research Hypothesis

a) it is assumed that pupils attending the secondary school having a special football program register superior anthropometric indices as compared to those registered by the pupils attending ―Decebal" secondary school;

b) considering the fact that pupils attending the secondary school having football as a major area of study have been selected from a number of over 250 pupils, and that they perform a double number of training sessions, the results they achieve during the motor trials will reveal higher indices than those registered by the pupils from "Decebal" secondary school.

Applied Research Methods

a) method of the bibliographical study;
b) observation method;
c) experiment;
d) method of recording and tests;
e) statistical-mathematical method.

Research purpose consists in setting certain ways of improving the instructive-educational process, at the level of the secondary education focused on sport discipline, namely, football, oriented towards the increase and the development of motor skills and towards a balanced physical growth of pupils.

Research structure: The anthropometric indices, as well as those associated to motor skills development, have been sampled during the school year 2011-2012. The experiment continued for a period of nine months, during which, pupils being tested at the beginning, namely, on the 27th-28th of September 2011 for the initial testing and at the end of the school year for the final testing, on the 27th-28th of June 2012, the final experiment data belonging to the two groups being compared. The anthropometric indices registered by the two groups were collected by the staff of the Medical Clinic for sportsmen Dolj county, and the motor skills were observed by the research authors.

The research subjects were 7th grade pupils attending the two secondary school units. From ―Decebal" secondary school only the pupils from A, B and D classes were evaluated, due to the fact that in one class there was a reduced number of boys. From the classes submitted to the evaluation, 5 pupils were excluded for having abandoned the endurance trial, therefore, it remained a number of 25 pupils for each school unit. We should mention the fact that the pupils attending the football secondary school performed a number of five training sessions per week, each session including 100 minutes, while the pupils attending "Decebal" school performed only two sessions per week, of 100 minutes each. The training session content being the same during the whole experiment. Pupils from the football secondary school repeated on Tuesday the training session performed on Monday, and on Thursday the one performed on Wednesday. In addition, every week, for 11 stages during the autumn and 11 stages during the spring, they took part to the County Junior Championship and performed a 60 minute game. As well, pupils from ―Decebal" secondary school, regularly, took part to Football and Handball School Championship which counted 10, respectively, 8 stages only during the spring.

Research results and their interpretation

Processing the experiment data, we have achieved the following results:

➢ the anthropometric data reveal almost the same values, the differences between these data being insignificant to this level;

➢ the two groups register significant differences when dealing with the vital ability and the thoracic elasticity, the pupils attending the football secondary school achieving favorable results;

➢ concerning the indices illustrating the motor skills development, we confirm the existence of significant differences, see table no 1.

For all situations, we may notice a good and very good homogeneity ($C_v < 15\%$). As well the average error of the arithmetic mean is placed below 3%, which indicates the fact that the arithmetic means can be considered.

Applying the —Sudent" significance test, we have achieved significant differences between the two groups of pupils (p<0.01) for all indices of motor skills development. The training programs conceived for the pupils attending the football secondary school provided them a balanced physical development and led them to the achievement of good results during the championships. Comparing the results to the control trials, both groups registered values which were superior to those achieved to the initial testing.

Further on, we present the results achieved to the final test (see table no 1), as well as the charts with the values of quality indices of the two groups, at the end of the experiment (see charts 1-12).

Table with the results of somatic and psychomotor indices achieved by the two groups to the final testing n=25

Table no 1

No	Trials	Secondary School	X	S	C_v (%)	E_m (%)	T	P
1.	Waist / (cm)	Decebal	163.44	5.1	3.12	0.624	0.168	p>0.01
		Sports School	165.52	6.18	3.781	0.752		
2.	Weight / (kg)	Decebal	56.32	5.56	9.872	1.574	1.148	p>0.01
		Sports School	49.84	4.93	9.872	1.578		
3.	Thoracic perimeter / (cm)	Decebal	75.55	3.75	4.583	0.597	1.647	p>0.01
		Sports School	81.53	3.45	4.532	0.546		
4.	Thoracic elasticity / (cm)	Decebal	7.39	0.93	12.602	2.52	2.631	p<0.01
		Sports School	9.87	0.88	8.516	1.783		
5.	Biacromial diameter /(cm)	Decebal	36.52	1.7	4.655	0.531	0.459	p>0.01
		Sports School	37.52	1.96	5.252	1.05		
6.	Bitrochanteric diameter(cm)	Decebal	27.45	1.29	4.699	0.94	2.51	p<0.01
		Sports School	30.88	1.29	4.08	0.816		
7.	Vital ability/ (cm^3)	Decebal	3222	286.32	8.886	1.777	2.654	p<0.01
		Sports School	3996	276.14	6.91	1.582		
8.	Speed / (sec)	Decebal	8.12	278.14	6.91	1.582	2.663	p<0.01
		Sports School	7.5	0.18	6.91	0.48		
9.	Endurance	Decebal	208.84	11.8	5.65	1.13	2.734	p<0.01
		Sports School	176.44	5.38	3.055	0.611		
10.	Standing long jump / (cm)	Decebal	182.4	10.21	5.598	1.12	2.595	p<0.01
		Sports School	209.33	9.33	4.457	0.891		
11.	Left side force / (Kgf)	Decebal	25.53	3.21	12.573	2.515	2.773	p<0.01
		Sports School	34.58	2.96	8.56	1.712		
12.	Right side force / b(Kgf)	Decebal	27.24	3.18	11.674	2.535	2.528	p<0.01
		Sports School	35.72	2.73	7.643	1.589		

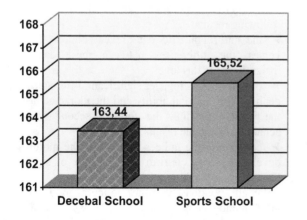

Graphic No. 1
WAIST (cm)

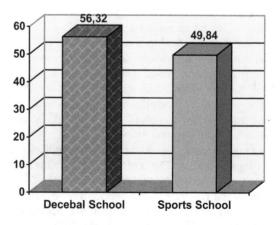

Graphic No. 2
WEIGHT (kg)

Graphic No. 3
Thoracic perimeter (cm)

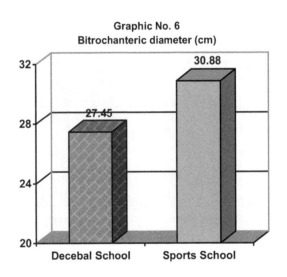

Graphic No. 4
Thoracic elasticity (cm)

Graphic No. 5
Biacromial diameter (cm)

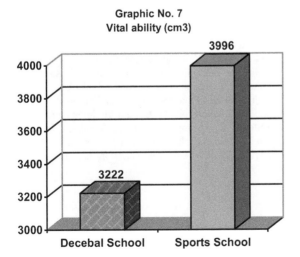

Graphic No. 6
Bitrochanteric diameter (cm)

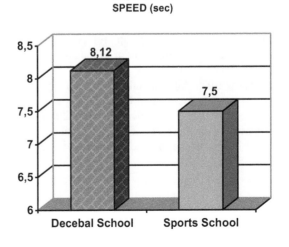

Graphic No. 7
Vital ability (cm3)

Graphic No. 8
SPEED (sec)

Graphic No. 9
Endurance (sec)

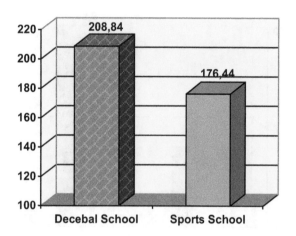

Graphic No. 10
Standing long jump (cm)

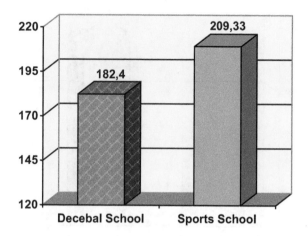

Graphic No. 11
Left side force (kfg)

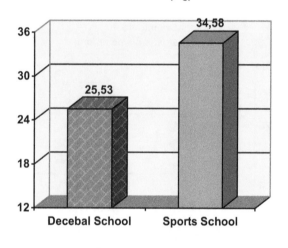

Graphic No. 12
Right side force (kgf)

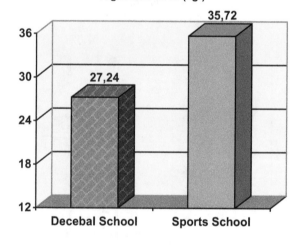

Conclusions:

1. The results to the control trials, the initial as well as the final ones, proved an obvious correlation between the anthropometric growth indices and the motor skills improvement and development indices.

2. The indices attesting the level of psychomotor training, to the experiment group, for all the cases, indicate values statistically superior to the significance threshold $P<0.05$; $P<0.01$.

3. Analyzing the high results achieved by the experiment group, as compared to those register by the control group, we may consider that this situation is due to the educational content of the analytical syllabus conceived by us, to the applied methods, focused on the somatic, physiological and motor skills development.

Reference:

1. Hahn Erwin., (1996), Sports Training to Children. Sport for Children and Juniors) no 104 Bucharest
2. Jarkov, D.M., Kiena A.I., (1996), Indices in Expiration and Inspiration, Indices of Training Level: No 83 Bucharest
3. Lagosa A.L., (2000) Increase of Outlook Value for Indices of Physical and Functional Level of Training to Teenagers and Juniors. Sport for Children and Juniors tome XVIII
4. Todorov T., Lazarov N., (2000), Standards for Physical Development Evaluation and Selection of Young Individuals for Different Sports Disciplines, Bucharest

Dance therapy vs conventional exercise recovery in physical therapy hours

Babolea Oana Bianca[1,2]

[1] *Scoala Gimnazială Specială „Sf. Vasile",Craiova, Romania,*
[2] *Universitatea de Educație Fizică și Sport București - Școala Doctorală I.O.S.U.D*

Abstract. Dance-movement therapy, (DMT) or dance therapy is the psychotherapeutic use of movement and dance for emotional, cognitive, social, behavioral and physical conditions. As a form of expressive therapy, DMT assumes that movement and emotion are directly related. The purpose of DMT is to find a healthy balance and sense of wholeness. Few experiences engages sow good the person in its entirely, as does dance: body, emotions and intellect. Dance is the euphoria that not everyone feels, just the one that invests passion in injoing to move in rhythms of music. Those who do not hear these rhythms they simply live them, they feel vibrating in their bodies, their minds, trying to develop through movements artistic talent. This talent helps to highlight the beauty of the soul, through dance. They share their own need to the world, to be appreciated, to be admired, the cultivation of skills that seem to someone incredible, even impossible. I aplied a questionnaire on the satisfaction survey of children with special educational needs in times of physical therapy.

Key words: *dance therapy, hearing loss, physical therapy*

Introduction

Dance-movement therapy, (DMT) or dance therapy is the psychotherapeutic use of movement and dance for emotional, cognitive, social, behavioral and physical conditions [1]. As a form of expressive therapy, DMT assumes that movement and emotion are directly related.[2] The purpose of DMT is to find a healthy balance and sense of wholeness [3].

Since its origins in the 1950s, DMT has gained popularity and its practices have developed. However, its principles have remained the same. A typical DMT session has four main stages: preparation, incubation, illumination, and evaluation [4]. DMT is practiced in places such as mental health rehabilitation centers, medical and educational settings, nursing homes, day care facilities, and other health promotion programs[5]. This form of therapy which is taught in a wide array of locations goes farther than just centering the body. Specialized treatments of DMT can help cure and aid many types of diseases and disabilities. Other common names for DMT include movement psychotherapy and dance therapy [6].

Dance has been used therapeutically for thousands of years. Traditionally, dance was linked to healing and was used to influence fertility, birth, sickness, or death. Dance has been used as a healing ritual since earliest human history, but the establishment of dance therapy as a profession occurred in the 1950's [7].

Although dance has been a method of expression for centuries, it wasn't until the past half century that it was characterized as a form of therapy.

The theory of DMT is based upon the idea that "the body and mind are inseparable" [8]. DMT rests on certain theoretical principles, which are that body and mind interact, so that a change in movement affects total functioning; that movement reflects personality; that the therapeutic relationship is mediated partly non-verbally.

Through the unity of the body, mind, and spirit, DMT provides a sense of wholeness to all individuals.[9]

Dance styles used

A variety of dance styles are used in DMT, including: various culturally-based dances

- Turkish dance
- ballroom dance
- tango
- waltz
- foxtrot
- aerobic dance
- body psychotherapy [10]

Specialized treatments

DMT can be used to heal serious disorders and diseases. Although DMT is promoted to reduce stress and center the body, this therapy is very effective in helping to heal other disabilities and diseases. Examples of these include:

- Autism: therapists connect on a sensory-motor level, provides a sense of acceptance and expands skills and cognitive abilities, increases maturity;
- Learning Disabilities: develops better organizational skills, learns/experiences control and choice, higher self confidence, new inspirations to learn;
- Mental Retardation: improves body image, social skills, coordination, and motor skills, promotes communication;
- Deaf and Hearing Impaired: reduces feelings of isolation, provides inspiration for relationships;
- Blind and Visually Impaired: improves body image, motor skills, and personal awareness;
- Physically Handicapped: improves motor skills and body image, provides a way to communicate and express emotions;
- Elderly: provides social interaction, expression, and exercise, alleviates fears of loneliness and isolation;
- Eating Disorders: alters distorted body images which helps end destructive behaviors, discovers symbolic meanings behind disorder/food [11];
- PTSD: weaves together past and present through symbolism in a —safe place" to confront painful memories;
- Parkinson's Disease: uses rhythm to help reduce body dysfunctions which improves motor abilities, balance, and use of limbs ;
- Holistic Birth Preparation: implores relaxation techniques to reduce anxiety, learn breathing techniques and release energy, builds confidence to

help cope with labor, birth and early parenting;
• Dementia: improvement in articulacy, oral and body language communication and increased pleasure/enjoyment of activities as well as an increase in involvement of activities [13]
• Depression: reduces stress, anxiety, number of visits to the doctor, medication intake; help build and strengthen bonds and relationships[14]

Effectiveness

Dance therapy has been deemed effective in the treatment of those with developmental, medical, social, physical, and psychological impairments. It has been used as treat people with mental and psychological problems and reduction of stress and anxiety for those with chronic diseases and/or cancer. Dance therapy effectiveness also is seen in enhancement of range of movement (ROM), freedom of total body movement,and improvement of mood, body image, and self-esteem.[15]

Few experiences engages sow good the person in its entirely, as does dance: body, emotions and intellect.

Dance is the euphoria that not everyone feels, just the one that invests passion in injoing to move in rhythms of music.

Those who do not hear these rhythms they simply live them, they feel vibrating in their bodies, their minds, trying to develop through movements artistic talent. This talent helps to highlight the beauty of the soul, through dance. They share their own need to the world, to be appreciated, to be admired, the cultivation of skills that seem to someone incredible, even impossible.

Movement together with others at the same rhythm, usually helps to build relationships. Because communication through movement, the child becomes more aware of themselves and more able to interact with others.

Leventhal (1981) argues that movement and dance therapy for children with special educational needs begins with sensorio-motor and perceptual development, and integration of this information, and then continues with the formation and development of the concept of body schema itself.

Body scheme is one of the fundamental concepts in human development. Schilder (1950) defines body schema as a three-dimensional image of our own body which we form in mind, the way we perceive our body. No body scheme, physical structures necessary symbolic representation of other things can not form as long as they depend on previous purchases.

Schilder (1950) highlights the correlation between exercise and body scheme, arguing that movement leads to a better orientation in relation to our own bodies. You do not know much about your body if you do not move, and movement is a unifying factor between different parts of the body.

Chace writes that dance therapy, using a primary form of communication provides an individual relationship with the environment and with others when it is limited by a disability.

A major ego has body awareness for the organization and internalization impulse control. Children need to understand their own bodies and their ability to move forward to meet the demands of the external environment.

Using mirror reflection is a method (but not to imitate the movements of others) that provide an understanding of a child's experiences at body level. This method not only provides important information about the child, or undiscovered, but also send the message that the child is seen and accepted as it is.

This acceptance, in most cases, moves the child's attention from internal to environmental stimulus, which then will increase interactions. The therapist should not be placed in front of the mirror when is not in control of his behavior, or when the action does not allow for positive change. As adults know the children will be able to detect early state of agitation and can structure classes so as to avoid loss of control.

With the mirror reflection, will occur the eye contact, touch, vocalization, rhythmic activities, music, different ways to support a variety of sensory-motor activities. All these contribute to build a relationship and also the body schema. Dance therapy at children with special needs involves sensory awareness, awareness of body parts, dynamic movement, and possibly more expressive movements.

Dance therapy in children with special educational needs, involves sensory awareness, awareness of body parts, dynamic movement, and possibly more expressive movements.

Promoting and supporting children with hearing loss is a unique experience, a struggle against the refusal and rejection. These children despite weaknesses that have demonstrated that they can provide a successful path in life.

Material and methods

I aplied a questionnaire on the satisfaction survey of children with special educational needs in times of physical therapy(Table 1).

Name...............................
Surname..........................

Nr. crt.	Question	Answer	
1.	Choose what deficiency do you suffer.	Slight hearing loss	
		Averege hearing loss	
		Severe hearing loss	
2.	Gender	Female	
		Male	

3.	Age	6-9 years	
		9-12 years	
		12-15 years	
4.	Do you like physical therapy hours?	Yes	
		No	
5.	What do you like most in physical therapy hours?	Recovery gymnastic exercises	
		Dance therapy	
6.	How many times a week you want to do physical therapy?	Once / week	
		Twice / week	
		More than twice / week	

Table no. 1 Questionnaire on the satisfaction survey of children with special educational needs in times of physical therapy

The group I applied this questionnaire consists of 30 children with special educational needs from Gimnazial Special School "Sf. Vasile" from Craiova, with the average age of 12 years old, 17 female and 13 male.

Results

After the evaluation and interpretation of questionnaires showed that 25 of the children prefer dance therapy classes in physical therapy hours.

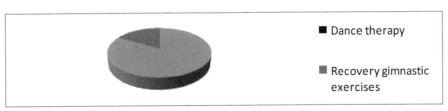

Chart. No. 1

Discussions and conclusions

Movement is a universal mean of communication. All children move in one way or another, and those with disabilities are no exception. Some of them have not developed adequate verbal language, but have a true language of movement, so that non-verbal communication is an effective way of contact.

In conclusion, children with special educational needs prefer dance therapy instead of conventional exercise recovery within hours of physical therapy.

References :

1. "Who We Are," American Dance Therapy Association, <http://www.adta.org/about/who.cfm>.
2. Payne, Helen, Dance Movement Therapy: Theory, Research, and Practice, (Hove, East Sussex: Routledge, 2006).
3. Levy, Fran J., Dance Movement Therapy: A Healing Art, (Reston, VA: The American Alliance for Health, Physical Education, Recreation, and Dance, 1988).
4. Meekums, Bonnie, Dance Movement Therapy, (Thousand Oaks, CA: SAGE Publications Inc.).
5. "Who was Marian Chace?," American Dance Therapy Association, <http://www.adta.org/resources/chace_bio.cfm>.
6. "Who We Are," American Dance Therapy Association, <http://www.adta.org/about/who.cfm>.
7. Strassel, Juliane; Daniel Cherkin, Lotte Steuten, Karen Sherman, Hubertus Vrijhoef (May/June 2011). "A Systematic Review of the Evidence for the Effectiveness of Dance Therapy". *Alternative Therapies* **17** (3): 50.
8. "Who was Marian Chace?," American Dance Therapy Association, <http://www.adta.org/resources/chace_bio.cfm>.
9. "Dance Therapy," American Cancer Society. <http://cancer.org/doctoor/MIT/content/MIT_2_3X_Dance_Therapy.asp>.
10. Strassel, Juliane; Daniel Cherkin, Lotte Steuten, Karen Sherman, Hubertus Vrijhoef (May/June 2011). "A Systematic Review of the Evidence for the Effectiveness of Dance Therapy". *Alternative Therapies* **17** (3): 53.
11. Levy, Fran J., Dance Movement Therapy: A Healing Art, (Reston, VA: The American Alliance for Health, Physical Education, Recreation, and Dance, 1988).
12. Payne, Helen, Dance Movement Therapy Theory, Research, and Practice, (Hove, East Sussex: Routledge, 2006).
13. Rylatt, Paula. "The Benefits of Creative Therapy for People with Dementia". *Nursing Standard*. Academic Search Complete.
14. "Change in the Moving Bodymind: Quantitative Results from a Pilot Study on the Use of the Bodymind Approach (BMA) to Psychotherapeutic Group Work with Patients with Medically Unexplained Symptoms". *Counseling and Psychotherapy Research*. Academic Search Complete.
15. Strassel, Juliane; Daniel Cherkin, Lotte Steuten, Karen Sherman, Hubertus Vrijhoef (May/June 2011). "A Systematic Review of the Evidence for the Effectiveness of Dance Therapy". *Alternative Therapies* **17** (3): 50.
16. Anca, M. (2001). Psihologia deficienților de auz, Cluj-Napoca: Editura Presa Universitară Clujeană.

Gait analysis – a normative plantar pressure study

Ionescu George[1], Avramescu Elena Taina[1], Luminita Georgescu[2], Marius Cristian Neamtu[3]

[1]University of Craiova, Faculty of Physical Education and Sport, Department of Sport Medicine and Kinesitherapy, [2]University of Pitesti, Faculty of Science, [3]University of Medicine and Pharmacy, Craiova

Abstract. The purpose of this study was to establish a dataset for gait parameters, *recte* the variation of plantar pressure, measured in different sub-areas during the roll-over of the foot during walking for a normal population. Also we wanted to appreciate the predictive factors for trauma risk by analysis of recorded parameters using footscan balance and gait curves . The study was conducted on 82 physical education students that had no history of lower limb pathology at the time of the study. The subjects walked at over a 10 meter long walking path, having a built-in pressure platform (Footscan ®, RsScan International Footscan Scientific Version, RSscan International, Olen, Belgia, performing measurments at 500 Hz frequency in 2D mode, measurment surface 0,5m x 0,4m) mounted on an AMTI force platform. We measures different variables as initial contact, final contact, time to peak pressure and the duration of contact. The investigated subareas of the foot were the lateral and medial heel, I to V metatarsal heads and the hallux (8 regions from the maximum accesible 10). These findings provide a reference dataset for temporal characteristics in plantar pressure during walking of young adults. We estimate that our research can be relevant in the evaluation of gait patterns with application in pathology and rehabilitation.

Keywords: *Plantar pressures; Gait; Rehabilitation*

Introduction. Walking is a complex movement and inspired a large number of researchers to study and analyze locomotor function. In recent years remarkable progress has been made in research, involving some border areas and developing interdisciplinary research. The main guidelines for biomedical research today is directed at improvement, generation, standardization, acquisition and analysis of data obtained by non-invasive technologies (1,2)

The complexity of the interactions of the various components of human gait has been researched and documented for many years. The study included the measurement and analysis of different parameters, followed by the interpretation of the date and different applications (3,4). Gait analysis can range from simple measures of timing (temporal analysis) to mechanical analysis using sophisticated instrumentation and computer models

In last years introduction of new devices, such as pressure plates designed to quantify the local loads underneath the foot took place. Plantar pressure measurements provide direct and objective information on how various foot structures interact with the ground and give an opportunity to characterise functional aspects of the ankle-foot complex during the foot-floor or foot-shoe interaction during gait. By application pf the foot on the platform local pressure is measured during the total period of contact with the ground at a high frequency (5). Operational substrate is represented by measuring total impact force applied to the sensor array on a known surface.

Data from plantar pressure measurement can be also used in evaluating and treating patients with neurological and musculoskeletal pathology (6,7). Operational motivation for this method is that the new generation of scanning and pressure measurement systems are able to record and analyze load distribution in foot sub-areas with high accuracy, thus having the potential to achieve rapid movement characteristics prediction of foot and ankle.

These aspects allow prediction of effective therapies by developing and validating an algorithm for gait analysis with applications in orthopedic pathology, in order to achieve a quick and objective interpretations and the exclusion of human subjectivity (8,9).

Using a force platform RSScan, we can make a static analysis of gait but also a dynamic gait analysis in terms of ground reaction force and developed pressure during walking. These determinations allow the complex study of lower limb behavior while walking with or without assistive means. Data analysis includes: information on plantar pressure distribution level versus time, force-time distribution in each plantar sub-area, determine the load on each region, the contact surface which is on direct contact with the surface of the platform produces stimulation of the platform sensors), foot axis and subtalar angle, foot balance in anterior-posterior and frontal plane n pressure center position (10,11).

Gait analysis can be achieved by analysis of the images included into specific screens or appropriate numerical correspondence by studying synthetic numerical data included in tables, graphics showing evolution of parameters and the distribution of forces (dynamic screen, balance screen, gait screen). After the measurement is registered, the software will process the information. Another important feature is the ability to calculate the average of several measurements, to allow comparison of medial and lateral areas for the same foot, left-right comparisons, comparing measurements made at different time intervals.

The purpose of this study was to establish a reference dataset for gait parameters describing the behavior of anatomical plantar pressure sub-areas in the foot roll-over during walking and also to appreciate the predictive factors for trauma risk by analysis of recorded parameters using footscan balance and gait curves.

Material and methods.

The study was conducted on 82 physical education

students who had given informed consent. Their characteristics are given in Table 1 and none had a

history of lower limb pathology at the time of the study or in the preceding six months.

Table 1. Distribution of subject according to age, height and weight

	Age (years)	Height (cm)	Weight (kg)
Men (55)	21.1 ±0,9	179.5 ±5.9	69.0 ±7.2
Women (27)	20.4 ±0.8	166.9 ±5.6	59.3 ±7.1

The subjects walked at over a 10 meter long walking path, having a built-in pressure platform (Footscan ®, RsScan International Footscan Scientific Version, RSscan International, Olen, Belgia, performing measurments at 500 Hz frequency in 2D mode, measurment surface 0,5m x 0,4m) mounted on an

AMTI force platform. The track was covered with rubcor (5mm).

In order to give a direct representation of how the pressure under the foot can be subscribed to relevant anatomical landmarks, the foot can be divided in 10 sub areas. (Figure 1).

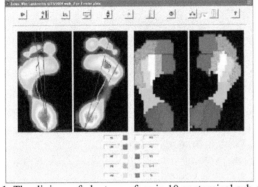

HL: Heel Lateral
HM: Heel Medial
MF: Mid Foot
M5: Metatarsal 5
M4: Metatarsal 4
M3: Metatarsal 3
M2: Metatarsal 2
M1: Metatarsal 1
T2-T5: Toe 2 to Toe 5

Fig.1. The divison of plantar surface in 10 anatomical sub-areas*(Footscan software 6.3.4mst, RsScan Int.)*

In our study we used eight anatomical pressure sub-areas that were semi-automatically identified on the peak pressure footprint. The sub-areas were medial heel (HM), lateral heel (HL), metatarsal joints I to V (Mi, M2, M3, M4 and M5) and the hallux (Ti) (heel areas.

The participants were asked to walk at a convenient speed. After familiarisation, a trial was considered as valid when the following criteria were met: (1) a heel-strike pattern, (2) a prescribed running speed and (3) no adjustment of gait pattern to contact the plate. A minimum of three valid trials from each side leg was analysed.

The recorded variables were:

Start time: the first contact in msec for a specific region under the foot

End time: the last contact in msec for aspecific region under the foot

% Contact: % of contact time compared to the complete stance phase

Max F/P: maximum force (load) measured for the area

Time Max F/P: Actual time where the peak force was recorded

Load rate:–LR(N/cm.s)- the speed of loading in the specific region

Impulse: - I(Ns/cm)- total loading for the specific region under the foot

Contact area: $CA(cm^2)$ cm² for the specified zone

Active contact area: area within the contact area where load is applied

Max peak sensor value: maximum measured pressure within each zone.

Another aspect we wanted to undeline was the use of the footscan balance and gait curves related to reflect

the proportions between certain zones in the foot. Based on the software dedicated to this equipment it is possible to assess the balance by comparing the medial to the lateral side of the foot and the loading values of these areas (for instance comparing the medial with the lateral side of the rear, mid and forefoot with T1 or M1), and assessment of symmetry by comparing the recorded values for the 2 plants

All the curves are standardised by dividing the calculations by the average of the total measured reaction force.Also are the roll offs scaled to a percentage, where the total roll off is 100%. This makes possible to compare graphs of a walking measurement.

We have to note that all these data show appreciation of risk lesion in the foot by reference to the minimum risk, which can be identified on these graphs. Output equilibrium curves outside this area means that there is a risk of overloading or traumatic lesion due to lack of control or motor deficit.

Results

Our recordings provided detailed informations on the local pressures under the foot during unroll of the foot In fig. 2 is showed a screen providing the pressure information based on the automatic calculated zones under the foot. For each representation of the measured pressures, the measured forces can be displayed.. Force values (N) and pressure values (N/cm2) are represented on Y axis, and contact time is shown on X axia (ms – time of recording the pressure). According to color scale, the highest pressures are represented in red, followed by orange, yellow, green, blue, violet.

The area for each contact zone is automatically

detected and can be found in the right part of the image
(cm2).

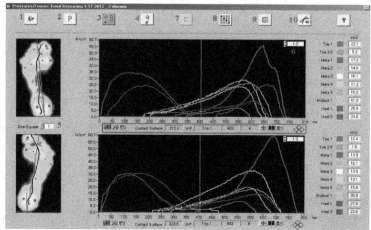

Fig. 2. A force-pressure graphic registered for a mail healthy subject, ageg 19 years. Wecan observe the presure distribution during gait reported to contact areas.

In this way is possible to look up the maximal pressure values and control the loading pattern of the different anatomical structures. It is also possible to see if a foot pronated (M1 high, red color),if there was central overloading (M2+M3 high,pink and white) or if the foot supinated (M5 high, orange).

Mean temporal characteristics of the foot roll-over during walking are given in Table 2. A normal distribution was found for all the variables studied. The values were reported to % contact time

Table 2. Recorded data of the temporal foot roll over during walking relative to total foot contact for the 8 studied sub-areas .

(N=82)	Initial contact	Final contact	Duration of contact % contact time	Time to peak pressure % contact time
	Mean	Mean	Mean	Mean
HL	0.0	40,2	39.2	3.2
HM	0.0	42.5	42.5	4.1
M5	9.2	73.9	64.1	42.0
M4	10.3	80.5	71.3	50.5
M3	12.1	98.8	79.0	52.5
M2	14.9	93.4	72.3	60.2
M1	17.5	89.5	70.4	52.3
T1	29.8	92.1	62.5	77.1

As mentioned before, the footscan software gives an overview of all the balance or gait curves.We studied the symmetry of the curves and we found assymmetries for 12 cases (fig.3 and 4).

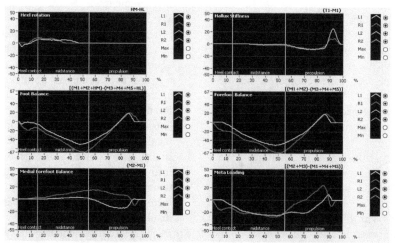

Fig. 3. Balance screen for symmetric foot patterns.

In these curves there is a very clear symmetry between left and right, which is in fact the most ideal situation, because both feet follow the same pattern.

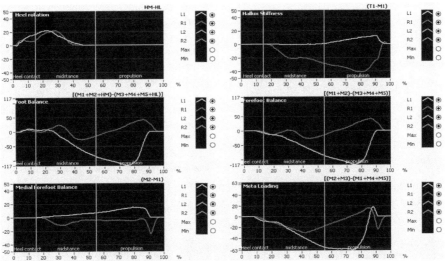

Fig. 4. Balance screen for asymmetric foot patterns.

In these curves we see a clar example of an asymmetry. There can be multiple factors causing this like> misalignment of the pelvic/spine,proprioceptive problems, leg length differences. Furher evaluation is needed. After diagnosing and the treatment, these curves an be used to evaluate the intervention..

Discussions and conclusion

The foot has a multi-functional character during the stance phase of locomotion. Balance is one of the isuues odf main importance in assesing the risk for further trauma. Here are different curves that can be analysed, like heel balance that estimates the balance between medial and lateral heel. .

If the curve is a flatline, HM and HL are in balance. If the medial side increases (because of pronation) the curve becomes positive, while a lateral increase (because of supination) causes to become negative. The white curve represents a hccl s roll off without a risk for overuse injuries, measured at a young athletic population without any injuries during a long period.

In case we look back to the biomechanics it matches perfectlly: first a pronation, caused by the internal rotation of the pelvis during the first 15%. After that a resupination caused by the external rotation of the pelvis. This means that the pronation isn t caused by muscles, but rather has to tempered by muscle. When this muscle is not working correctly a quick pronation occurs, which causes a too heavy torsion on the Achilles tendon, with little medial rupture as a result. Too eraly and extreme pronation therefore could be caused by overusage of the tibialis anterior muscle.

Forefoot balance describes the balance of the forefoot, with the formula (M1+M2)-(M3+M4+M5).

If the curve is a flatline,M1+M2 and M3+M4+M5 are in balance. If the medial side increases (because of pronation) the curve becomes positive, while a lateral increase (because of supination) causes it to become negative. The white curve represents a roll off without a risk for overuse injuries,measured at a young athletic population without any injuries during a long period.

This curve describes if the medial or lateral side of the forefoot is being used. When the graphs remains negative, you can say that M1+M2 are functionally avoided and that the lateral side is overused. This causes a disturbed roll off, because different structures have to bear the weight in a different way than it is supposed too. Too much pronation means that there is a too high loading of the medial side of the foot. In this phase the pelvis is in external rotation, causing the tibia to external rotate as well. If the foot stays unstable and doesn t supinate, torsion of the tibia is the result. This is mainly the cause for shin splints or tibia stress fractures. The next curve can help determine if there is too much force on M1, M2 or both.

Medial forefoot balance shows the balance between M1 and M2 during gait, by using the formula M2-M1. If the curve is a flat line,M1 and M2 are in balance. If M1 increases (because of pronation) the curve becomes positive, while if M2 increases (because of central overloading) causes it to become negative. The white curve represents a roll off without a risk for overuse injuries, measured at a young athelete population, without any injuries during a long period.

When in both the forefoot balance and in this curve there is a high positive value, this means there is a very high pressure under M1 alone. This is related to shin injuries and overuse injuries of the anti-pronators. This curve is only of use when M1 actually makes contact with the ground, this can be seen at patients with a too flexible first metatarsophalangeal joint. These patients can t load there first ray, so the pressure transfers to the second ray, which is more rigid.

We estimatethat our study provided a reliable and representative reference dataset for temporal characteristics of foot roll-over during walking in young healthy adults. Also this database will assist in distinguishing between normal and abnormal walking patterns

By using the results the specialists will be able to identify, classify, diagnose and propose the appropriate action or treatment, identify the risk zones, appreciate the efficiency of the treatment or rehabilitation programme.

References

1. Abboud R.J. Relevant foot biomechanics. *Current Orthopaedics* 2002; 16: 165-179

2. Hay JG. Cycle rate, length and speed of progression in human locomotion. *Journal of Applied Biomechanics* 2002; 18: 257-270

3. Blanc Y, Blamer C, Landis T, Vingerhoets F. Temporal parameters and patterns of the foot roll over during walking: normative data for healthy adults. *Gait Posture* 1999; 10: 97-108

4. Titianova EB, Mateev PS, Tarkka IM. Footprint analysis of gait using a pressure sensor system. *J. Electromyogr. Kines.* 2004; 14 (2): 275-281

5. Harrison AJ, Folland JP. Investigation of gait protocols for plantar pressure measurement of non-pathological subjects using a dynamic pedobarograph. *Gait & Posture*, 1997; 6: 50-55

6. Bryant A, Tinley P, Singer K. Normal values of plantar pressure measurements determined using the Emed-SF system. *Journal of the American Podiatric Medical Association* 2000a; 90 (6): 295-299

7. Bryant A, Tinley P, Singer K. Radiographic measurements and plantar pressure distribution in normal, hallux valgus and hallux limitus feet. *The Foot* 2000b; 10: 18-22

8. VanZant RS, McPoil TG, Cornwall MW. Symmetry of plantar pressures and vertical forces in healthy subjects during walking. *Journal of the American Podiatric Medical Association* 2001; 91 (7): 337-342

9. Giacomozzi C, Macellari V, Leardini A, Benedetti MG. Integrated pressure-force kinematics measuring system for the characterisation of plantar foot loading during locomotion. *Med. Biol. Eng. Comp.* 2000; 38: 156-163

10. Mac Williams BA, Cowley M, Nicholson DE. Foot kinematics and kinetics during adolescent gait. *Gait Posture* 2003; 17:214-224

11. Orlin MN, McPoil TG, Plantar pressure assessment. *Phys Ther.* 2000; 80: 399-409

12. Goble DJ, Marino GW, Potvin JR. The influence of horizontal velocity on interlimb symmetry innormal walking. *Hum. Movement Sci.* 2003; 22: 271-283

13. Hayafune N, Hayafune Y, Jacob H A C. Pressure and force distribution characteristics under the normal foot during the push-off phase in gait. *The foot* 1999; 9: 88-92

Attractive Ways of Practicing Physical Exercise with Medicine and Farmacy University of Craiova Students

Ciuvăţ Dragoş[1], Georgescu Luminita[2]

[1]Medicine and Farmacy University of Craiova, [2]University of Pitesti

Abstract. The systematic review of the data obtained from the study publication aimed to obtain a better information on the practicing of physical exercise by the students and the way of attracting them towards motion. The study proceeds towards the identification of the main works that have dealt with the problematics of physical education at the university level with non physical education specialization faculties and to argument theoretically its role in promoting health through motion. At the same time, the study brings into discussion for the first time in Romania, the introduction of a new concept of physical education through the use of HOPSports system.

Key words: *physical education, atractivity, HOPSports.*

Introduction

As you well know, the relationship between sports and physical and mental health represents a major concern for medicine, physiology, sports sciences and psichology. The subject belongs also to the sociologic research as public health, at statistical scale, where enquiries, questionnaires and interviews. Through such research they have outlined significantly positive connections between practicing sports and a better physical and mental health. [1]. The problem that there would be a relationship of the type dose-response between these concepts, as well as the extent to which physycal activity would be associated to important aspects such as the cognitive, physical and psicho-social one. Finally, they have proposed a multidimensional model for the examination of the mediation potential and the factor moderation in physical activity, the quality of life and the practical actions that such a model implies for the practitioners. [2]. Physical education is an obligatory discipline in UMF Craiova, to be found in the curriculum of 1st and 2nd year of study, having a frequency of 30 hours a semester. At this moment the syllabus has as major objectives the following:

a) The improvement of students' health or harmonious physical development.
b) Raising the generic motricity level and the assimilation of basic elements through practicing certain sports brances.
c) The making of a knowledge system of multilateral instruction.
d) The formation of the convictions and skills of practicing the independence of physical exercise.

Method

The systematic review of the data obtained from the study publication aimed at obtaining better information on the practicing of physical exercise by the students and the way of attracting them towards motion.

Since 2002, Ghenadi V., has stated the fact that "the positive influence of the social phenomenon –physical education and sports- must begin with the changing of general fundamental concepts about physical education and sports in a transition society. The new concepts will have to answer all requirements by social, individual and group interests. In this situation physical education and sports mst be studied as a *complex social phenomenon,* dinamic at national scale with

implications, motivations, concepts, group or individual interests, varied and always changing". [3]
E. Lupu, also believes that it would be necessary to review the concept of physical education, of tests and control procedures necessary for the evaluation of students in physical education activities as a non-specialisation subject implementing sport games less known but with a greater degree of attractiveness, with lesser effort. [4].
D. Tudor and M. Tudor, see how much a physical education course organized on sport branches succeeds to induce the growth of the biomotric potential of UMF Carol Davila students, following the evolution of fitness of students throughout the course in a semester. Thus, they appreciate the fact that introducing physical education lessons organized on sport branches, students succeed, through physical exercise, to improve both somatic profile and the biomotric potential. [5].
In "Current problems of physical education in higher non physical education specialisation " Staicovici A., advocates the diversification and harmonization of contents of physical education and sports in higher education, as a reference component of the model of professional and human training of students. [6].
Following the impact of exercise on health, Nagy A., 2011, found that there is a noticeable reduction in daily physical activity in non physical education specialisation students from Debrecen University. The author proposes a drive system based on column gymnastic exercises for a period of 14 weeks a programme based on autostreching and toning exercises, after which subjects are getting an improvement in hip muscle measurements. [7].
Rachita C., making research on modeling the characteristics of personality and development of medicine students' motivation, says that they are positively influenced by the methods and means used in physical education classes. [8].
Turcanu F., (2007)., shows the general appearance of motility levels of students in the UMF Targu Mures, noting that these students appear at the beginning of physical education courses as a heterogeneous mass with few top elements, while over 20% of them are below average for this age specific motility. [9].
As for the importance of physical education courses in the faculties non physical education specialisation Gagiu M., also reported (2003), stating that physical

education and sport education remains essentially a powerful factor of preparation for life and work, arguing that for more and more countries physical education and sports activities are activities of national interest. [10]

Belizna C., 2010, noted that, as practical, activating implications, on one hand the need of organizing the training of students in physical education classes towards promoting those structures of programmes which they join and participate with pleasure and, on the other hand the need of restructuring those rigid, obstructing and inhibitting programmes for the young people that manifest shortcomings in motiliy, as the main side of general education [11].

In 2008, I. Enache Enache C, analyzed, in the paper "Study Concerning the share of physical activities for students in the Faculty of Education Science", the lifestyle of non physical education specialisation students, noting that younger students (under 30 years) get lowest level of physical activity, not having a

regular programme of practicing it. Survey respondents (n = 190) have known mostly the positive effects that exercise has on the body, but they do not rank it among the primary physical activities of the day, citing lack of time or material conditions. [12].

Trying to make physical education and sports classes more attractive, a group of Americans have developed a HOPSports system that combined hundreds of lesson plans through video designed programmes projected on a video screen. The use of HOPSports system combines a projector, a sound system and a variety of training equipment. The lessons are conducted by athletes and celebrities or cartoons. One relatively new and novel approach to encouraging physical activity among children is the HOPSports Education Training System. According to their website, HOPSports mission is to help move a healthier generation forward by combining fitness and fun, learning and entertainment through movement (HOPSports, 2012).

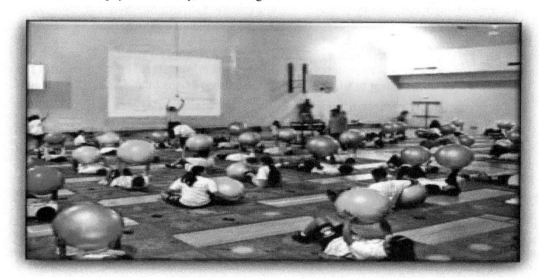

Figure 1 HOPSport System (www.hopsports.com)

This particular program involves arousal, modeling, and vicarious experience while fostering successful participation through various levels of activity, but research regarding its impact is very limited.

The founders of this system add the fact that the system does not replace the responsibilities of physical education and sports teacher but it represents an auxiliary tool, very useful for them. In the U.S., HopSports training system is currently used by over 600,000 young people a week. HopSports system is a multimedia training tool for the 21st century. The promoting of physical education is done in a fun way! HOPSports allows teachers to work with small groups or individual students while the entire group remains fully committed. Students improve their health and gain confidence to be active for life. According to a study, young people who use the HopSports system are 55% more active than those attending the traditional physical education and sports classes. [13]

From the same study, it appears that obese or overweight students using this system are 23% more

active compared to those who follow the traditional physical education and sports classes. [14]

One recent study used the HOPSports system as a means of comparing program by video and instructor supervised age-appropriate physical activities (Annesi & Vaughn, 2011). Participants were enrolled in 12 weeks of after-school care that administered the Youth Fit For Life intervention program on Mondays, Wednesdays, and Fridays, along with either after-school, instructor supervised physical activity for 45 minutes on the remaining two days per week (Youth Fit For Life plus instructor-supervised physical activity group) or HOPSports use on the remaining two weekdays (Youth Fit For Life plus HOPSports group). [15].

Conclusion

The research project "Using interactive technology in health promotion through movement" wants to improve the educational offer within the discipline of non physical education specialisation students by introducing new ways of working in order to increase their interest for an active life through movement. Thus, innovative work programs will be developed through the use of HopSports system in physical education classes. The project aims at validating these programs and the screening of the effects it has on health promotion, which will lead to a rethinking of the existing programmes in the University of Medicine and Pharmacy Craiova.

References

1. Baciu M, 2009, , *Educaţia fizică, sportul şi calitatea vieţii*, Note de curs. Universitatea Babeş-Bolyai, Cluj, p.32

2. McAuley E., 2007, State of the Art Review: Advances in Physical Activity and Mental Health: Quality of Life *American Journal of Lifestyle Medicine September/October 2007 1: 389-396,*

3. http://www.sportscience.ro/html/reviste_2002_30-2.html - accessed on 07.07.2012]

4. Lupu E., 2009, The evaluation of the motility qualities of non physical education specialisation university students, International Scientific Conference" Inovation and creation in body activities, sources of human performance", Ed Zigotto, Galati, p.62.

5. D. Tudor, Tudor M., 2009, *Scientific Competitional Annal* no.1/2009, p.71-76.

6. Staicovici A., 2009, Current Issues in physical education in higher education of non-physical education specialisation students, University of Bucharest

7. Nagy A., 2011, Improving the elasticity of hip muscle among the Population of Debrecen University Students, *Romanian Journal of Physical Therapy*, no.27/2011 vol.17, p.21

8. Rachita C., 2009, *Scientific Competitional Annal*, no.1/2009, p.71-76.

9. www.sportscience.ro/html/articole_conf-2007_-_65.html - accessed on 06/27/2012.

10. http://www.sportscience.ro/html/articole_conf_2003_-_18.html - accessed on 06/27/2012.

11. Belizna C., 2010, International Scientific Conference in Sports science, Nineteenth ed.a "Exercise and quality of life", CSSR, p.25-27.

12. whqlibdoc.who.int/hq/2003/WHO_NMH_NPH_PAH03.2pdf.

13. http://www.globalpeforumgc.org/sites/default/files/presentations/Ms._Cindy_Hensley.pdf - accessed on 07/08/2012

14. http://www.globalpeforumgc.org/sites/default/files/presentations/Ms._Cindy_Hensley.pdf - accessed on 07/08/2012

15. McNees L.K., 2012, *The impact of HOPSports on adequacy in and predilection for physical activity in children*, Northwest Missouri State University, Maryville, Missouri, p.10.

Medical Staff Opinion on the Possibility of Using Strength Development Methods Based on Combinations of Regimes of muscle contractions in Football

Ciocănescu Daniel, Stoica Doru, Barbu Dumitru, Barbu Răzvan Mihai

University of Craiova, Faculty of Physical Education and Sport

Abstract . The paper aims to provide interdisciplinary to our research, through investigation, that focused on specialists in Medical Science, in order to obtain advice from the specialists involved indirectly in preparing footballers, regarding the strength training of junior I footballers. Analyzing the answers given by the experts consulted in the sociological investigation, we have been given some conclusions about the physical training of young players, landmarks in the direction of training programs.
Key words: training, strength, investigation

Introduction

Strength development is achieved through a complex of methods, based on a solid scientific foundation, known as "muscle training" (1). Strength Junior I training must be carried out in close accordance with the recommendations of professionals in muscle preparation (2,3). A complex work on force training was designed training developed by some researchers (4,5,6,7,8). Issues connected to the theory, methodology and practice of strength training in juniors are addressed in detail, including a presentation of curricula on the development of various parts of body muscles. But there are no references to strength-training on sports branches or disciplines.

Material and Method

We used the questionnaire to obtain subjective data, some opinions from specialists involved indirectly in preparing footballers (doctors, professionals in effort physiology, biochemists etc.) on strength training junior I footballers. So I asked answers from the medical staff of Polyclinic for Sport Professionals Craiova (23.8%), the teachers from the Department of Kinethotherapy and biochemistry of the Faculty of Physical Education and Sports of the University of Craiova (23.8%), from the Department of Physical Therapy, University of Craiova FEFS and sports medicine physicians working ion the major football clubs in Dolj and the neighboring counties (38.1%).

The questionnaire was developed according to the methodology adopted, following questions to guide the subjects to express their opinions about strength training for junior I footballers, muscle training methods considered to be most effective by respondents, and possibly related to the possibility of using strength development methods based on combinations of regimes of muscle contractions.

Results

Of the 21 subjects interviewed, 23.8% of them are employed in the Polyclinic for Sport Professionals, 23.8% of them are physicians in FEFS Craiova, Department of Kinethotherapy, 38.1% work in sports clubs for football, while only 14.3% (8 subjects) are teachers at the University of Medicine and Pharmacy.

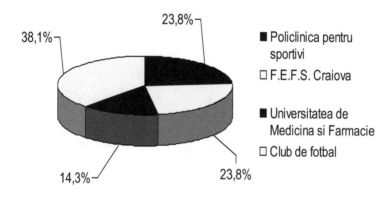

Chart no. 1 The subjects' place of work

The majority of respondents (81%) are specialized in sports medicine, 9.5% are doctors at UMF, and 9.6% have other majors (Biochemistry and Physiology).

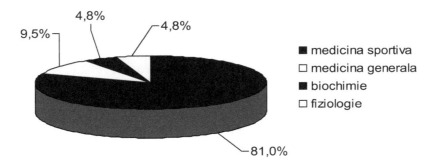

Chart no 2 The subjects' domain of activity

The physical training is of central importance in the general training of young football players for 85.7% of the respondents (18 subjects, sports medicine specialists). Only 9.5% said that physical training is minor, while one subject does not know the answer.

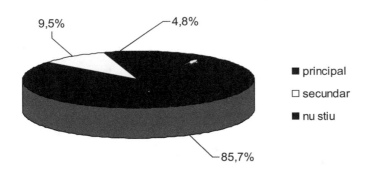

Chart no. 3 The Place occupied by physical training in the general training of young footballers

Most respondents believe that it is of central importance in physical training (85.7% - 18 subjects). This response was given by sports medicine specialists, while 14.3% (subjects with other specialties) believe that the strength training is situated on a secondary place, or do not know the answer to the question.

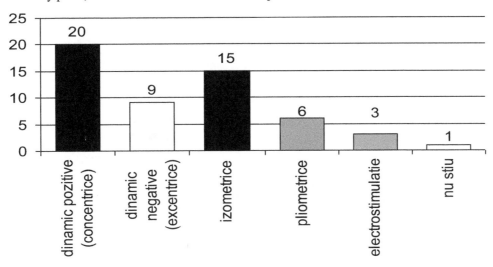

Chart no. 4. The methods of strength development recommended to football coaches

The question has multiple answers. 95.2% of the respondents recommended coaches positive (concentric) dynamic methods to football. The isometric are chosen by 71.4% of the respondents, while electro-stimulation is recommended only by 14.35% of them.

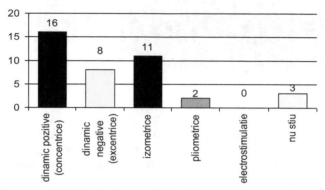

Figure no. 5 Methods of strength development recommended for competitions

For the competition periods, the answers are given only by specialists in sports medicine, 76.2% opting for the positive dynamic (concentric) ones and only 9.5% choose the plyometric. 71.4% of the respondents are unaware of strength development methods based on combination of muscle regimes. The isometric-concentric mode is selected by 5 subjects (23.8%), the concentric- plyometric being chosen by 14.3% of them, and the eccentric-concentric is chosen by a single subject.

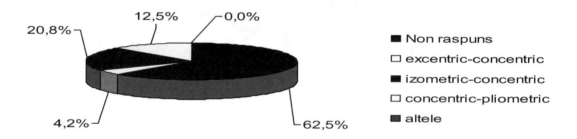

Figure no. 6 The regime of combinations known to subjects

52.4% of respondents (11 subjects) do not recommend methods to develop strength to coaches from junior I footballers. Only 6 of them (28,6%) recommend modern methods of development, based on combinations of muscle contraction regimes and 4 of them opt for the classical ones.

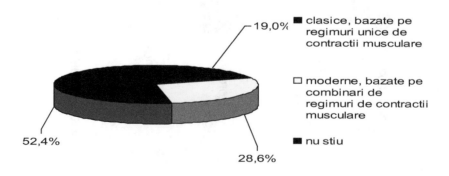

Figure no. 7 Methods of strength development recommended to football coaches of junior I groups

Medical Staff Opinion on the Possibility of Using Strength Development Methods Based on Combinations...

23

Conclusion

Analyzing the answers given by the experts consulted in the sociological investigation we have drawn some conclusions about the physical training of young footballers, landmarks in the direction of the training programs. The respondents in this field consider that physical training is particularly important in the overall process of training with junior footballers (85% of the respondents).

The same percentage (85%) of the experts consider that, in preparing the junior I footballers they have to place on the first level the strength development , as a support both for the development of specific motor qualities and for the correct execution of technical procedures specific to the football game. The respondents recommend as the main methods of strength development the concentric type (95.2%) and the isometric (71.4%) one, and less the eccentric type (42.9%) and the plyometric one (28.6%) , electro-stimulation being on the last place with only 14.3% of the vote. For the competition period, they particularly recommended those concentric (76.2%) and isometric (52.4%). Only 9 of the respondents (28.6%) say they have knowledge of methods for developing muscle strength by combination of muscle regimes, most of the (23.8% - 5 specialists) indicating the isometric-concentric type of methods.

Reference

1.Weineck, J., 2003, *Manuel d'entrainement*, Vigot Publishing House, Paris.
2.Baroga, L., (1984), *Educarea calităţilor fizice combinate*, Editura Sport-Turism, Bucureşti
3.Nicu, A.., (1993), *Antrenamentul sportiv modern,* Editura Editas, Bucureşti
4.Niculescu, M., (2001), *Ştiinţa pregătirii musculare*, Editura Universitatea din Piteşti
5. Cometti G., (1988), *Les méthodes modernes de musculation*, tome I, II, Universitaté de Bourgogne, Dijon
6.Letzelter, H., Letzelter, M., (1990), *Entraînement de la force*, Editura Vigot, Paris.
7.Weineck, J., (1995), *Biologie du sport*, trad. C.C.P.S., SDP, nr. 365-366, Bucureşti.
8.Zaţiorski, V., (2005), *The Science and Practice of strength development*, INCS, Bucharest

Effect of physical training on hemodynamic parameters in hypertensive patients

Danciulescu Daniel, Stuparu Gabriela-Lia

University of Craiova

Abstract: Objectives: The main aim of the study was to evaluate the changes of hemodynamic parameters, anthropometric and biological hypertensive patients after a rehabilitation program lasting three months. Means and methods: We conducted the study on a group of 35 patients aged 45-65 years with blood pressure values between SBP (systolic blood pressure) 150-170 mmHg and DBP (diastolic BP) 90-100 mmHg (hypertension stage I and II). Patients underwent a program of lifestyle change over a period of three months. Patients were assessed before the start of the rehabilitation program and then divided into two groups: Group A, the persons involved (20 patients) and group B, untrained persons (15 patients). At the beginning and end of the study, anthropometric parameters were monitored: weight (G), height, body mass index (BMI), hemodynamic parameters (ambulatory blood pressure monitoring): heart (FC), SBP and DBP and biological parameters: blood glucose, serum total cholesterol, LDL-cholesterol, HDL-cholesterol, triglycerides. Results: We have compared the results of anthropometric parameters, hemodynamic and biological agents before and after three months of monitoring. After 3 months we received: in group A, a significant decrease in CF (mean of 8.1 beats/minute with statistical significance $p = 0.025$), SBP (mean 8.5 mmHg, $p = 0.035$), DBP (mean 3.4 mmHg, $p = 0.041$), G (mean 2.55 kg, $p = 0.015$) and BMI (mean 0.87 units, $p = 0.037$), compared to group B where we achieved a decrease in FC on average 4.2 b / min, $p = 0.161$, SBP on average 3.6 mmHg, $p = 0.124$, average DBP by 2.3 mmHg, $p = 0.268$, and a significant decrease in G and BMI.

Keywords: *hemodynamic parameters, cardiac rehabilitation, physical training.*

Introduction

More than half of annual deaths in Europe and over two thirds of annual deaths in Romania have the main cause of cardiovascular disease (1). The incidence of cardiovascular disease is dependent on lifestyle and risk factors, whose modification undeniably demonstrated to reduce mortality and cardiovascular complications (1, 2, 3).

Research conducted over the past four decades have shown a clear link between physical activity and the occurrence of cardiovascular disease. Thus, exercise has beneficial effects in patients cardiovascular and other chronic diseases such as type II diabetes, colon cancer, osteoporosis (1, 4, 5). Alongside HTA, diabetes mellitus, obesity and smoking, lifestyle sedentary is one of major risk factors cardiovascular disease (3). Regular physical activity and exercise training are essential to improve exercise capacity, leading to increased quality of life and independence daily.

Background

Research conducted so far have shown that in patients with hypertension, exercise can contribute to therapeutic effects such as: improving functional capacity of the cardiovascular system, lowering blood pressure, improving subjective symptoms, addressing risk factors (6, 7, 8, 9). Due to the complexity of pathophysiological changes that may be present in varying proportions from a patient to another and different severity of disease from one patient to another, the possibilities of application of exercise and chances of getting therapeutic results are also very varied. In this study we followed the changes in anthropometric and hemodynamic parameters for a group of hypertensive patients with stage I and stage II hypertension, after a recovery program through exercise lasting three months.

Objectives

The aim of this study was to evaluate changes in anthropometric following parameters: weight, height, body mass index, and hemodynamic parameters: systolic blood pressure, diastolic blood pressure, and heart rate before and after the 3 months that followed patients a recovery program through exercise.

Materials and methods

Patients were specialized outpatient through general clinical examination and laboratory investigations. They watched anthropometric parameters weight, height, body mass index, hemodynamic parameters: systolic blood pressure, diastolic blood pressure, and heart rate, then conducted electrocardiogram (ECG) standard.

There have been three blood pressure measurements under standard conditions were then tested for other possible effort to detect coronary artery disease. The 35 patients selected on the basis of blood pressure between 150-170 mmHg SBP and DBP 90-100 mmHg (hypertension grade I and II) were aged 45-65 years.

All patients underwent a program of lifestyle change: smoking cessation or reduction of tobacco smoking, reducing alcohol consumption, ensuring a healthy diet based on low-salt, fats, sweets and high consumption of fruit and vegetables, dietary fiber, fish, milk and milk products (3), administered at a pace appropriate to their age, state of wakefulness and sleep, presented in a pleasant and hygienic.

After being evaluated, patients were divided into two groups - Group A (20 patients) - for persons who have been trained exercise whose intensity was determined by exercise testing previously done - Group B (15 patients) - sedentary people who did not receive exercise program. Recovery by exercise took place over a period of 3 months. Patients in group A were followed by a physical therapist. Training sessions were conducted at a heart rate between 70-80% of maximum heart rate obtained from exercise testing. The exercise was performed 5 times a week. Physical training session consisted of three parts (6): 1. heating -

with a duration of 10 minutes exercise used at this stage following muscle and cardiovascular training, 2. proper physical training, lasting 30 minutes each exercise was performed for 3 minutes with breaks of two minutes. 3. return, lasting 5 minutes.

Statistical processing

For statistical processing of initial data were used software programs Microsoft Excel and SPSS for Windows. First they built a database using Microsoft Excel, for each patient of the study group, includes values following variables:

- sex
- age
- height
- weight
- body mass index calculated according to the formula:

$$BMI = \frac{G}{H^2}$$

where: - BMI - body mass index rounded to integer
- G - weight in kg topic
- H - height in meters subject;

- heart rate;
- systolic blood pressures
- diastolic blood pressure
- if is smoker
- if consumes alcohol
- if consumes salt in excess
- if has a increased consumption of fats
- if has a increased consumption of sweets;

For variables that express weight, body mass index, heart rate, SBP, DBP, were completed two values: the first value is that at the beginning of the study and the second, that recorded three months after the change of style life. This database was then transferred to SPSS for Windows to do the math on the following statistical indicators:

- media distribution
- deviation or standard deviation (standard deviation)
- coefficient of variation
- linear correlation coefficient of Pearson (r),
- statistical significance threshold (p)

Significance Threshold (α in specialized literature, *p* or *Sig.* in statistical program SPSS) describes the chance (probability) that the maximum result is accidental, random and not derived from the research context. Under these conditions the value of materiality is a criterion for acceptance or the result obtained for the calculated parameter followed. This critical threshold has been established by the scientific community to the value $\alpha = 0.05$ ($p = 0.05$) and it corresponds to a 5% probability that the result be due to chance (the minimum probability that the result is guaranteed obtained is 95%).

Track data that shows changing parameters it been tested with test *t* (Student) of the mean difference of two dependent samples to assess the significance of the change in a parameter, the same subjects in two different situations (before and after the action of certain conditions) or in two different contexts, regardless of when their event. (Procedure *Analyze / Compare Means / Paired-Sample T Test ... of SPSS for Windows*) (10)

Results

Measurements after 3 months the two groups of the lot under study indicated the following: For group B patients (those who have not made exercise program) did not obtain significant changes in terms of weight and mass index body. In the TAS values, TAD and FC were small declines: an average of 3.6 mmHg for SBP, an average of 2.3 mmHg for DBP, 0 average of 4.2 beats / min for FC but no significant statistically (p> 0.05). For Group A patients were important changes and track parameters are described in Table I.

Table I Parameter values follow the subjects in Group A, before and after physical training

Parameter followed	Before conducting physical training physical exercise			After conducting physical training physical exercise			
	Average	Standard deviation	Coefficient of variation (%)	Average	Standard deviation	Coefficient of variation (%)	p
Weight (kg)	80,65	10,89	13,5	78,1	10,02	12,83	0,015
Body mass index	27,63	2,65	9,6	26,76	2,45	9,16	0,037
Heart rate	77,65	4,17	5,37	69,55	3,10	4,46	0,025
Systolic blood pressure (mmHg)	161,5	7,09	4,4	153,0	10,82	7,07	0,035
Diastolic blood pressure (mmHg)	95,25	4,43	4,6	91,85	6,87	7,48	0,041
Blood glucose (mg/dl)	157,3	30,9	26,3	130,0	23,6	18,15	0,032
Total cholesterol (mg/dl)	230,6	42,2	18,3	211,7	36,28	17,14	0,042
LDL-cholesterol (mg/dl)	145,1	35,0	24,1	132,2	23,6	17,85	0,038
HDL-cholesterol (mg/dl)	39,8	5,66	14,2	43,1	5,91	13,71	0,044
Triglycerides (mg/dl)	172,4	90,33	52,4	145,5	67,5	46,39	0,029

a) In respect of Group A subjects weight before and after exercise program, it is observed that subjects submitted batch kinetic recovery decreased in weight by an average of 2.55 kg. Also note that the standard deviation and coefficient of variation decreased, which indicates that group subjects became more homogeneous in terms of weight.

b) In order to correlate their height weight subjects

was calculated body mass index.

It is noted that body mass index of subjects submitted batch kinetic recovery decreased on average by 0.87 unit.

c) Another factor was clinical follow that heart rate decreased on average by 8.1 beats per minute in patients undergoing physical training.

d) Systolic blood pressure of the subjects under study batch after recovering kinetic fell on average by 8.5 mm Hg col. This decrease was not uniform, as confirmed by the increase in the standard deviation and coefficient of variation. So, the effect of exercise on blood pressure lowering for patients manifested differently from one patient to another.

e) In terms of diastolic blood pressure observed a mean decrease of 3.4 mm Hg

There is a cervical linear correlation between weight and systolic blood pressure of subjects studied group ($r = 0.61$, $p = 0.0005$) at the end the 3 months of monitoring (Fig. 1).

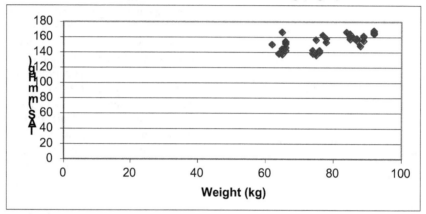

Figure 1. Correlation between G and TAS for patients undergoing trial at the end of 3 months of monitoring

There are also linear correlation between weight and diastolic blood pressure of subjects studied group ($r = 0.37$, $p = 0.029$) at the end of 3 months of monitoring (Fig. 2).

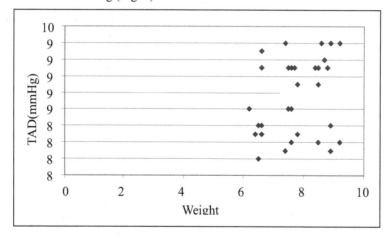

Figure 2. Correlation between G and DBP for patients undergoing trial at the end of 3 months of monitoring

Discussion

The results of this study on hemodynamic and anthropometric parameters in patients with hypertension are consistent with data found in specialized literature.

Controlled and sustained physical exercise can reduce blood pressure in both normotensive and hypertensive individuals and improves the functional capacity of the cardiovascular system. It is widely recognized role of physical activity in reducing cardiovascular risk, but many of the benefits of physical activity on cardiovascular disease prevention remains only a short time after the cessation of physical activity. Therefore, it becomes necessary daily exercise regimen.

In adults combat sedentary lifestyle may increase life expectancy and delay the onset of cardiovascular disease. Physical activity achieved even at moderate levels may have a beneficial effect on mortality but also on non-fatal coronary events.

Conclusion

- In hypertensive patients who have only program of lifestyle changes were observed insignificant changes of hemodynamic and anthropometric parameters.

Significant changes were observed in hypertensive patients, in addition to lifestyle changes have participated in a rehabilitation program with exercise. Changes are statistically based.

- There is a causal relationship (correlation) between patient weight and blood pressure levels.

- Continuing the daily exercise will lead to significant

changes and anthropometric and hemodynamic parameters followed by improving the health of patients.

References

1. Gaiță D., Avram A., Avram C., *Physical training on cardiovascular recover,* Publishing Brumaire, Timisoara 2007: 9-11.

2. Gaiță D., Avram A., Avram C., *Cardiovascular Rehabilitation - between concepts and practice,* Publishing Brumaire, Timisoara, 2007: 9-11

3. Dănciulescu D., *Health education and first aid,* Universitaria Publishing, Craiova, 2010: 11-16.

4. Paffenbarger R., Hyde R.T., Wing A.L., Lee I.M., Jung D.L., Kampret J.B. The association of changes in physical-activity level and other lifestyle characteristics with mortality amoung men, *New England Journal Medical,* 1993.

5. Thompson P.D., Crouse S.F., Goodpaster B., et. Al *The acute versus the chronic response to exercise,* Med Sci

6. Sports Exerc, 2001: 438-445.

7. Ochiană G., *The role of physical therapy in cardiac patients recover,* Publishing Pim, Iasi, 2006: 117-127.

8. Obrașcu C., *Recovering patients with cardiovascular exercise,* Medical Publishing, Bucharest, 1986, 116-119.9.

9. Poantă L., Budiu M., Albu A., Exercise and heart rate variability, *Radic III. Civilization and Sport* nr. 4(34), 2008: 34-36.

10. Vanhees L., Gaiță D., Avram A., *Cardiovascular prevention and rehabilitation,* Ed. Springer-Verlag, London, 2007, 112-113.

11. Zdrenghea D., Branea I., *Recovery of cardiovascular patients,* Publishing Clusium, Cluj-Napoca, 1995: 257-268

12. Popa M. *Statistics for psychology. Theory and applications, SPSS,* Polirom, Bucharest 2008: 298-301

Considerations about the planification and the dynamics of the training process

Dăian Gligheria[1], Shaao Mirela[1], Ilona Ilinca[1], Dăian Ioan[2]

[1]*University of Craiova*
[2]*Petrache Triscu Sports High School*

Abstract. The sport training must be well planned in order to achieve high performances. The programs are according to the physical and functional possibilities of the athletes. The high exigencies of performance sports lead to a high degree of improvement of the motor skills. Achieving performance is the result of a training process spread out over several years, during which the athlete, through an integrative system, perfects his/her motor skills, techniques, physical and volitional abilities, and consolidates his/her knowledge and health condition. The comparative estimation of the data resulted in new guidelines for the planification of the training for the next work stage in terms of the workload, the intensity of the effort and the means to be used.
Keywords: *training, adaptation, planification, results.*

Introduction

The realization of a sports activity implies making efforts of different complexities. The practical results, the effects of these activities depend primarily on the exigencies of the respective activity and on the individual's possibilities. Planification, dynamics, records and analysis of the training represent the means to ensure a scientific management of the training process.

Aim and premise of the research

The high exigencies of performance sports lead to a high degree of improvement of the motor skills. Achieving performance is the result of a training process spread out over several years, during which the athlete, through an integrative system, perfects his/her motor skills, techniques, physical and volitional abilities, and consolidates his/her knowledge and health condition.

The training itself represents the fundamental method of practice of the athlete, based on the use of the exercises in a specific sequence, repeated a specific number of times, with specific intensities, at specific time intervals.

Their fusion in various proportions leads to the global or differentiated development of the motor skills which directly condition the athlete's possibilities.

From intention to achievement there is the action, the daily sport training. Within it, the coach-athlete relationship is in a tight interdependency.

The intensity of the effort represents the fundamental element which permanently strains and leads to the improvement of sports efficiency.

This progression refers to two parameters:
• the athlete's momentary possibilities

• the demands of the proposed performance objectives. The parameters draw between them the general curve of effort and training.

In terms of the first parameter (the momentary potential), performing another training involves taking into account several aspects:

1. The effort does not reach the momentary-liminal possibilities of the athlete, thus resulting in decreasing the degree of training.
2. The effort reaches the threshold of momentary-liminal possibilities of the athlete, resulting in maintaining the degree of training.
3. The effort exceeds the liminal threshold of possibilities, resulting in the increase of the degree of training.
4. The effort greatly exceeds the athlete's threshold of possibilities, resulting in overtraining.

Materials and methods

The balance between the intensity and the volume of the stress during the training, on the one hand, and the possibilities of adaptation of the organism, on the other hand, can be expressed by the correlation between the results obtained in the Ruffier effort functional test and by the control test of 600m run, with two middle-distance runners as subjects.

Results and interpretation of data

The result of functional test is expressed by an index in the form of a figure, and the result of the 600m race in minutes, seconds and tenths allowing an immediate easy appreciation of the effort.

Results in the 600m race

	Oct.	Nov.	Dec.	Jan.	Feb.	Mar.	Apr.	May	Jun.	Jul.
Values for A	1:28.5	1:26.4	1:26.2	1:26.0	1:25.8	1:25.1	1:24.7	1:24.5	1:24.3	1:23.8
Differences		2.1	0.2	0.2	0.2	0.7	0.4	0.2	0.2	0.5
Values for B	1:30.5	1:28.1	1:27.2	1:27.0	1:26.6	1:26.5	1:26.0	1:26.1	1:26.6	1:25.3
Differences		2.4	0.9	0.2	0.4	0.1	0.5	0.1	0.5	0.3

Results in the Ruffier functional test

	Oct.	Nov.	Dec.	Jan.	Feb.	Mar.	Apr.	May	Jun.	Jul.
Values for A	3	1.6	1.4	1.4	1.2	0.6	0	-1	-1.2	-1.4
Differences		1.4	0.2	0	0.2	0.6	0.6	1	0.2	0.2
Values for B	4.2	2.4	1.6	1.4	1.4	0.6	0	0	0.4	0.4
Differences		1.8	0.8	0.2	0	0.8	0.6	0	0.4	0

Over a one-year training the Ruffier index had an increase of 4.4 units for subject A, corresponding to 4.70.00 in the 600m race, and subject B – 3.8 units corresponding to 5.20.00. It can be noticed a significant relationship between the two indices, the lowest values correspond to the best times.

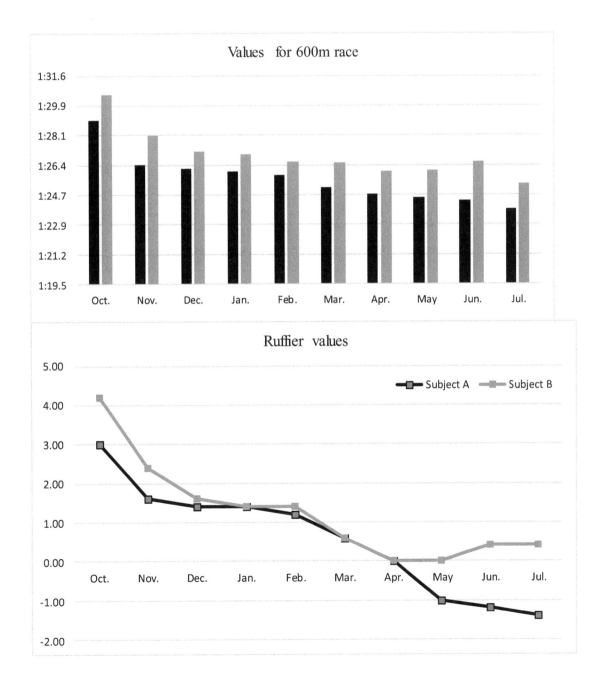

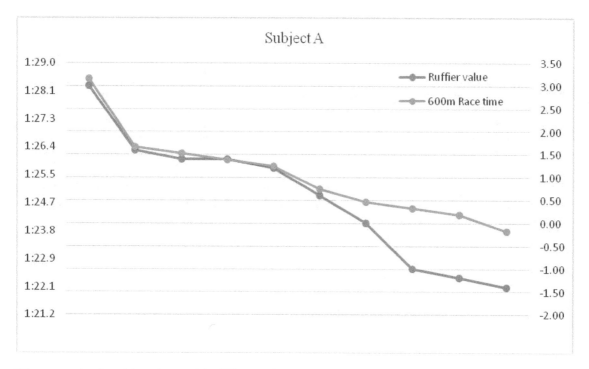

We may notice in subject A a too big difference between the progress realized in April (2" in the control test) and the qualitative leap of the values of the Ruffier index in the same period. The same finding is valid also for subject B in February, a 1" progress in the control test compared to 0.8 in the functional index.

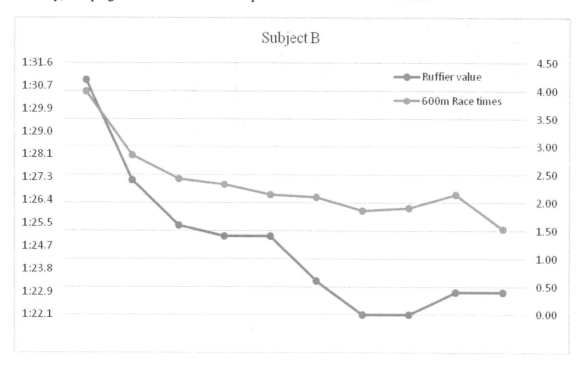

The momentary possibilities of the athletes in those periods were higher than the stress during the training.

Conclusions

The comparative estimation of the data resulted in new guidelines for the planification of the training for the next work stage in terms of the workload, the intensity of the effort and the means to be used. We went on to a reassessment of the data and to a new rescheduling of the parameters so that to eliminate the discrepancies between the values obtained during certain periods of the training year.

References

Dragnea A., Mate-Teodorescu S., 2002, *Teoria sportului*, Editura FEST, Bucureşti.

Nicu A., 1993, *Antrenamentul sportiv modern*, Editura EDITIS, Bucureşti,.

Sotiriu R., Marolicaru M., *Valenţe instructiv-formative ale structurii şi dinamicii antrenamentului*, Revista EFS nr. 10/1977.

Stănescu N., Tomescu D., 1980, *Practica medico-sportivă în fotbal*, Editura Stadion, Bucureşti,

Retrospective study on university championships of handball

Piţigoi Gabriel

UMF „Carol Davila" Bucharest

Abstract. Through its socio-cultural dimensions, the university sport gives a unique opportunity to know other students, to communicate with them, to have different roles, to gain some moral attitudes, to accept the attitudes regarding the activity, to feel some emotions that are hard to find in other spheres of life, to accept some positive elements of the life style, of adapting to the proposed objective and of becoming socially active through the performance of others. According to the FISU, handball is the first sport ever organised as a World University Championship in 1963 in the Swedish city of Lund with 90 athletes from 7 countries. As university sports, handball world showed a continuous development. In 2008 World University Championships, held in Venice - Italy, attended by a record number, 20 countries.
Keywords: *Sport University, handball, sports*

Introduction

Sports games have always aroused enormous interest among all citizens, especially among young people. This interest uncommon for practicing sports games, is largely explained by the coincidence between each individual's intrinsic desire to self-improve his personality and the beneficial effects they might have on the physical self (biological) - concerned with the body availability, the spiritual self - composed of innate or acquired mental qualities and also on the social self, concerned with the social relations and integration.

Handball is a means of physical education, which contributes positively to solve its specific tasks. Performed under competent guidance, handball will develop qualities like boldness, combativeness, courage, initiative, perseverance and moral qualities like the attitude towards teammates, the respect for the opponents, referees and the public spirit of team work and mutual assistance, a conscious discipline, etc.

As a performance sport, handball calls on athletes to make a hard work to cope with extremely heavy training loads, of which resolution claims the maximum strain of all physical, moral, capacities and the intellectual will. The requirements for the great performance and the athlete's desire to achieve it determines him to accept with conviction a regime of abuse-free life, full of restrictions and, as such, through the compliance with it, achieving his specific moral profile. Many handball players under the guidance of coaches, of sports teams were able to be successful both in sport and in society, for handball teaches the individual to be disciplined, orderly, industrious, conscious of his responsibility for the collective success, ambitious and with a continuous self-improvement will.

Students learn to train together, to relate to others through handball. All techniques involve the whole body working in a balanced and coordinated manner, resulting in a natural position.

Discussions

Through its socio-cultural dimensions, university sport offers a unique opportunity to meet other students, to communicate with them, to assume different roles, to acquire moral attitudes, to accept work-related attitudes, to experience emotions to be found less in other spheres of life, to accept positive elements of lifestyle adaptation to the set goal, that of becoming socially active through the performance of others [1].

The significance of sports competitions generally generates more intense emotional states than those generated on a daily basis. If the training and athletic training influences the student's personality formation, competitions leave deep marks on the personality of each participant, forming and transforming his qualities.

As a university sport, world handball showed a continuous development. Thus, in 2008 University World Championships, held in Venice - Italy, were attended by a record number, 20 countries (chart 1).

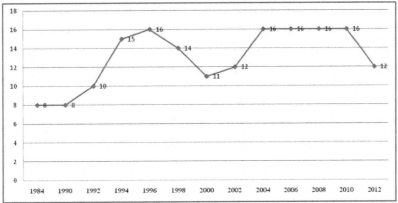

Chart no. 1 The evolution of the participating countriesto the University Handball World Championships
Table no 1 The evolution of the participating countries to the University Handball World Championships

(Source Statistics World Unniversity Championships)

Year	Country	Town	No.of countries	Ss male	Ss female	Total	Officials
1963	SWE	Lund	7	90	-	90	-
1965	ESP	Madrid	10	145	-	145	-
1968	GER	Darmstadt	15	219	-	219	45
1971	TCH	Prague	16	238	-	238	55
1973	SWE	Lund	16	228	-	228	55
1975	ROM	Bucharest	13	176	-	176	-
1977	POL	Warsaw	10	150	-	150	16
1981	FRA	-	13	189	-	189	44
1987	ROM	Bucharest	16	235	-	235	93
1990	NED	Groningen	13	186	-	186	80
1992	RUS	St Petersburg	7	98	-	98	37
1994	TUR	Izmir	13	177	-	177	60
1996	HUN	Nyiregyhaza	13	174	-	174	64
1998	YUG	Novi Sad	9	125	-	125	52
2000	POR	Covilha/Guarda	13	177	-	177	64
2002	ESP	-	12	145	-	145	56
2004	RUS	Chelyabinssk	6	81	-	81	34
2006	POL	Gdansk	15	175	96	271	34
2008	ITA	Venice	20	225	196	421	146
2010	HUN	Nyiregyhaza	12	137	97	234	69
2012	BRA	Blumenau	12	134	81	215	66

Over time the university team of Romania won 18 medals [3] as follows:

Table no 2 The evolution of the university team of Romania (Source FRF)

3d place– Sweden, 1963, masculine	3d place – Slovakia, 1994, feminine
2nd place – F.R.G., 1968, masculine	3d place – Bulgaria, 1996, feminine
3d place – Czechoslovakia, 1971, masculine	2nd place – Slovakia, 1998, feminine
1st place– Sweden, 1973, masculine	2nd place – France, 2000, feminine
1st place – Romania 1975, masculine	1st place – Spain, 2002, feminine
1st place – Poland, 1977, masculine	3d place – Italy, 2008, feminine
1st place – France, 1981, masculine	2nd place – Hungary, 2010, feminine
1st place – F.R. G., 1984, masculin	2nd place - Brazil, 2012, feminine
1st place – Romania, 1987, masculine	
2nd place – Netherlands, 1990, masculine	

Conclusion

The objective of participating in a competition is either victory or improving a previous result, which makes athletes manifest their full capacity.

The results of participating in a competition always hold a personal value for athletes - they allow establishing the form and the level reached after a sports training period.

Since 2006, men`s and women`s competitions are held in the same place. After 2012 edition, organised in Hungary, the 21st championship gathered men`s and women`s teams in Blumen. This last edition was the first in history when the World University Handball Championship took place outside Europe.

The 22nd edition of the World University Handball Championship will be held in 2014, in Portugal (Braga and Guimaraes cities).

To conclude, we can distinguish a totally varied progress, from year to year, of the number of students and participating countries during the twelve editions. Thus, the largest number of countries participating in an edition is in the 2008 edition, with 20 participating countries.

Proposals

We propose that, in addition to other departments within the Romanian Handball Federation, they establish a university department, that can assimilate and put into practice new scientific research both nationally and internationally. As can be seen above, university handball teams have had great results at university level.

References

1.Pițigoi, G., (2011). *Handbal. Basic course*, Prinrech Publishing House
2.Statistics World Unniversity Championships, FISU Magazine, 2010
3.http://www.frh.ro/

classes are: assimilating the minimum theoretical and practical knowledge about this class; transmitting and assimilating some knowledge which are necessary in case on accidents in sports games; assimilating some specific complexes of exercises and actions which can be performed in the spare time as recreational exercises.

In order to transmit and assimilate the technical, methodical and practical knowledge from the program, the following forms will be used:

• Theoretical lesson (approximately 15'-20' theoretical part)
• Practical and methodical lesson
• Contest lesson
• Individual study
• Participating as observers to different handball competitions.

2.3. Handball Class

The main string of training, the training class is the most concrete and real document of activity planning as well as the availability of the team players.

During the handball class it is ensured the conveyance of the knowledge, skills and habits, the development and improvement of technical, methodical and psychological training of the layers. Worth mentioning is the fact that during one class not all thetasks can be fulfilled. Due to this, the lessons are bound to each other and are based on each other in order to constitute a smaller or larger training period.

The structure of the handball lesson has three parts: preparation, fundamental part and closing part. These three parts are determined by the teaching and physiologic training requests and are divided in subchapters, as follows.

Preparation Part

The preparation of the body for effort starts with organizational exercises, mobilization of the functional capacity of the organism, general exercises and it ends with specific exercises, so the risk for accidents is reduced at a minimum and the level of implementing different technical actions is higher. The goal is to adapt progressively the major vital functions to effort (breathing and circulation). The analytic preparation of the locomotive apparatus means the activation and engagement of all body segments: arms, legs, body and especially the abdominal muscles.

Fundamental Part

It is the essence of the training lesson and it consists of technical and tactical exercises, specific exercises for developing the motric capacity and bilateral game with or without theme. It is the lesson itself, which is why it has the most part of the class. The content of these classes is with respect of the age of the participants, sex, training level, performance purposes and training periods.

Closing Part

Consists in all the measures necessary to gradually come-back of the body after the activity. A short assessment of the players' activity during the lesson will be done.

Conclusions

In conclusion, the teachers have the obligation to stress on the effort capacity of the students depending of individual traits and level of physical training and to give them and important volume of movements.

We consider that the importance of practicing this class is endeavor which can improve the physical and intellectual performances of the students.

Sometimes we consider the handball class useful for the students who will be engaged voluntarily in leisure sport and for improving the data base of Physical Education and Sports Class of Medicine and Pharmacy University „Carol Davila" Bucharest, but not only it.

References

1.Hector, L., Lador, I. (2005). *Physical Culture and Sports in Medicine and Pharmacy University Carol Davila, Bucharest,* UniversityPublishing House*Carol Davila*, Bucharest

2.Pitigoi, G. (2011). *Handball. Basic Class,*Printech Publishing House, Bucharest

Contribution of motion games in learning technical process in the football game at representative team

Ungureanu Aurora

University of Craiova , Faculty of Physical Education and Sports, Romania

Abstract: In the preparation of the representative football teams of technical process gymnasium methodic of teaching is very important, them having a important role, providing the basis necessary bilateral practicing of football game and for obtaining performances in competitions.The age of elementary school students is the period when development happens at all levels, including motor qualities as well as the consolidation and the learning of as many motor skills and abilities as possible.
Starting from these arguments we established the purpose of research taking the view that representative of the football teams – beginners, would be more attractive and efficient teaching of the technical process of football game through the movement games than the stantard methods.The experiment was carried out during the two semesters of school year 2011-2012, only for the period favorable to outdoor working at team representative of School with The classes I - VIII - Razvad, Dîmbovița County, which has the better material conditions. In order to prove the efficiency of the used methods there were applied testing trials. The results confirm the set goal, as follows: accurately pass (progress was 54.85% between the initial and final test), keeping the ball in the air (progress was 23.03% between the initial and final test), long pass (progress was 70% between testing the initial and final) and a technical route (progress was 14.08% between the initial and final testing).
Key words: *secondary education, teaching, the game method, control samples.*

Introduction

Middle school gymnasium is the period that it overlaps most of the time, over the period puberty, particularly important stage in ontogenetic evolution of the individual. Middle school students peculiarities of make possible the development of all of motor qualities and formation of a baggage motric adequate quantity and quality requirements for of its motion. (1)
Pubertary period is optimal, given the students' learning motor skills most specific the branches of sports. One of the the important objectives of this age is initiating in practicing some samples and sporting games by appropriating specific to them the technical and tactical elements (2). The Sporting games have their origins in emulation exercises (in general) and movement games (especially) receiving a pronounced character sporting print." (3). Football is present in the school curriculum at secondary school level, it necessitating minimal amenities materials and are greatly appreciated by pupils, especially because of the level reached performance and practicing in our country.
Through evolution, football has become a of great importance a social phenomenon thus coming back, physical education teachers and coaches of children, the task the technical preparation of the students, children and juniors, performed conscious, by an of diverse and simultaneous of basic driving skills and specific to different sports, of basic motor qualities, combined and specific, and moral qualities of character (the will, boldness, judgment, presence of mind, self-control). (6)

Material and methods

Tested subjects were the students making up the the football team representing School with the Classes I - VIII Razvad, County Dîmbovița, professor S.M.G., the experiment is carried out during the two semesters of the school year 2011-2012, only for the period favorable to outdoor work material conditions being good.
Hypothesis from whom we started was: using the movement games to teaching technical process in the appropriate methodology, and attractive (movement games in this case), with passion and well scientifically founded. Barbu D. (2008) for the activity trainers in the game plan and in workout plan, among other things recommends preoccupation for a dynamic game-oriented attack and some forms of play find attractive, rich in variety of game action in midfield. (4)
The game of movement, the physical education middle, is a variant of in which the role playing activities movement is clearly expressed. Basis is the different driving actions motivated by a theme and partly regulated by rules. Main features of the game are determined by the their nature and age those who practice them. For pupils, they constitute the main incentive psychic development, having an important role in preparing thereof for social integration.
The school's purpose is the fulfillment of the educational tasks specified in the school curriculum for each grade. To grades V-VIII the students are used movement games with dividing the collective in teams with character emulation to be dosed carefully, however, because the ability coordination of movements towards previous classes decreases due to disparity between limbs and trunk and the poor development huge muscle against bone growth. (5)
They bring the a valuable contribution to the tasks of school physical education, allowing expression football game, of the representative team of school, in secondary schools, is more efficient and also more attractive than using the standard means.
The technical process were taken from the contents of football game in physical education curriculum is selected independently of the school year but depending on the age and the level of preparation of the students on the team.
Among them we mention: kicking the ball by various variants, retrieve the ball, lead the ball, the kick on goal, marking, interception, debranding overcoming, penetration, tactics proceedings "one to two", technical-tactical actions in attack and defense. (7)
Research methods used were the classical, the researching targeting a pedagogical longitudinal type

experiment and within the statistical method we calculated the difference (D21) and the progress (D21%) recorded from initial testing of to final testing of to all control samples.

Was worked with the team representative of by the staggering annual trying to reach proposed objectives elaborated for the National School Sports Olympics football. On training lesson, she respected the classic methodology on succesion its parts, the only difference being that for the teaching specific technical procedures in football were used the movement games

and the not traditional drive systems their teaching methodology.

In each workout however was, carried out bilaterally of football playing, only in its being able to solve the concrete situations of the game and improve technical procedures specific to this sport.

Results

Under the experiment, to verify the effectiveness of the means selected, we applied the control samples, which were tested initially and the finally that we present below.

1.Accurately pass

Draw a rectangle with a width of 5m and the 10m length. On one length of the gym bench he sat reversed. The student had to send the ball in the gym bench successively adroitly foot (or both feet, your choice), with inside or across.

The assessment - registration lasted 30 seconds and counted each accurately pass, which hit the bank.

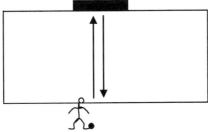

Figure no. 1. Precis care

2.Maintaining the ball in the air

Was drawn on the ground a square with of side of 10 m and the student, inside it, had to maintain the ball in the air with any part of the body besides hands.

The assessment - every contact with the ball represented one point and a sample lasted one minute.

3.Long pass

Was drawn on the ground a square with of side of 5 m, his corners being placed landmarks, to be visible from 20m from where the pupil had to execute three long passes which fall in this square

Evaluarea - pasa lungă ce a căzut în pătrat sau pe o latură a acestuia s-a considerat reuşită şi i s-a atribuit 2 puncte, rezultatul final fiind suma punctelor accumulate din cele 3 încercări.

The assessment - long pass what fell in the square or on the side of it was considered successfully and was attributed 2 points, the final result is the sum of points accumulated from the 3 trials.

4.A technical route

From a land width (handball) the pupil starts driving the ball on the 10m, executes lateral pass from movement to another student. Taking back ball before it reaches a line where starts dribbling through cones placed of 3 in 3 m and the then kicks on goal. Run back to where the center line improvised a loophole through which pass the ball situated 3 meters from it. Run the starting line where executes hitting his head on the spot, 3 times a ball discarded by the teacher. Port must have length of 50 cm and a height of 30 or may be of jumping a fence, overturned, or simply two flags, placed at a distance of 50 cm.

The assessment - stopwatch starts and stops the pupil motion after hitting the ball with his head for the third time, being recorded while he went through the entire route.

Crt. No.	Name/Class	Accurately pass		Maintaining the ball in the air		Long pass		A technical route (secunde)	
		T_i	T_f	T_i	T_f	T_i	T_f	T_i	T_f
1	C. C. / VII	11	16	67	73	2	4	20	17
2	M. N. / VII	8	15	37	50	0	4	22	19

3	O. C. / VII	10	17	40	52	6	6	23	20
4	S. S. / VII	12	17	47	61	2	4	20	17
5	I. A. / VII	13	19	76	83	4	6	22	18
6	P. S. / VI	13	20	61	72	4	6	21	19
7	P. M. / VI	12	19	58	69	2	4	22	19
8	G. E. / VI	10	14	59	71	2	4	23	20
9	I. F. / V	9	14	38	49	0	4	24	20
10	S. P. / V	10	15	42	55	2	6	23	20

Table no. 1. – Test result of control to initial and final testing

Discussions

I. Accurately pass

Statistical parameters	Iinitial test	Final test
The arithmetic average	10.08	16.6
Difference D_{21}	5.80	
Difference in percentages $D_{21}(\%)$	54.85%	

Table no. 2. Statistical parameters for sample - Accurately pass

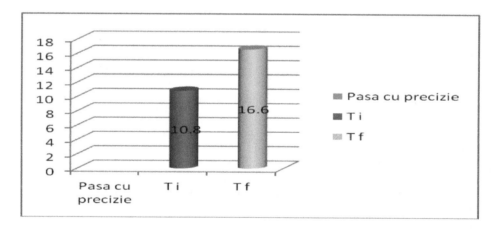

Figure nr. 2. – Graph representing the arithmetic mean initial and final testing to sample
- Accurately pass

In figure nro 2. are placed in parallel to the arithmetic mean development results to sample - Accurately pass between initial and final testing, the difference being 5.80, representing a progress to 54.85%.

II. Maintaining the ball in the air

Statistical parameters	Iinitial test	Final test
The arithmetic average	52.5	63.5
Difference D_{21}	11	
Difference in percentages $D_{21}(\%)$	23.03%	

Table no. 3. Statistical parameters for sample - Maintaining the ball in the air

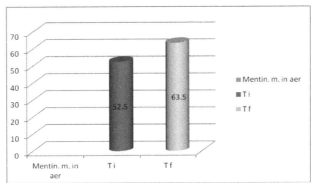

Figure no. 3. – The graph to the arithmetic average initial and final testing the sample –
Maintaining the ball in the air

The difference between the group average final and initial testing is 11, representing a progress by 23.03%.

III. Long pass

Statistical parameters	Iinitial test	Final test
The arithmetic average	**2.4**	**4.8**
Difference D_{21}	**2.40**	
Difference in percentages $D_{21}(\%)$	**70%**	

Table no. 4. Statistical parameters for sample – Long pass

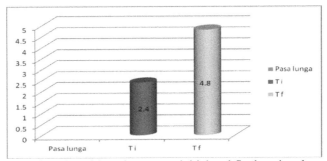

Figure no. 4. – The graph to the arithmetic average initial and final testing the sample – Long pass

Final testing of this parameter is an increase of 2.40 (70%) compared to initial testing.

IV. Tehnical route

Statistical parameters	Iinitial test	Final test
The arithmetic average	**22**	**18.9**
Difference D_{21}	**3.10**	
Difference in percentages $D_{21}(\%)$	**14.08%**	

Table nr. 5. Statistical parameters for sample – Tehnical route

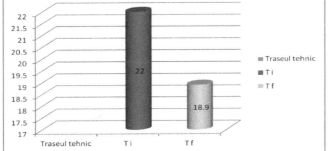

Figure no. 5. – The graph to the arithmetic average initial and final testing the sample – Tehnical route

Arithmetic mean at initial testing is 3.10 (**14.08%**) higher than the arithmetic mean final testing

Conclusions

1. Following the interpretation of the results, we conclude that the application of the experiment led to improved results of the students in the school football team at final testing, compared initial testing to all samples

2. The experiment applied by registering progress to all evidence resulted in confirmation hypothesis under which teaching of technical procedures football game by movement games is efficient and attractive also.

Proposals

Contents of the paper may be easily used in pre-secondary cycles, because the game of football is present in the curriculum of the education cycle and movement games designed may apply, requiring minimal material equipment, and is very appreciated by pupils .

References

1.Cătăneanu S. M. and Ungureanu Aurora (2011), *Physical and Sport Education in Schools – Teaching Theory and Methodology* - Universitaria Craiova, p.p 238-240.

2.Radulescu M., Cojocaru V. (2003), Guide the football coach - children and juniors - Axis Mundi Publishing House, Bucharest, pp 70, 71.

3.Colibaba-Evuleţ D. Bota, I. (1998), Sports Games-Theory and Methodology - Aldin Publishing, Bucharest, p 12.

4.Barbu D. (2008) – The technique football game - Publishing House Universitaria Craiova, page 148.

5.Ungureanu, A. (2009) ,   Methodology of Physical Education and Sport - Publishing House Universitaria Craiova, p. 132-133.

6.Ungureanu Aurora (2009), Teaching physical education lessons through movement games – Publishing House Universitaria Craiova, p. 19.

7.M.E.C.I. (2009) - Programs School V - VIII, Physical Education, Bucureşti, p. p. 9, 18, 33.

11

Coaches' personality and its role in high performance sports activity

Albina Constantin

University of Craiova
Faculty of Physical Education and Sport

Abstract: Knowing the personality of the coach is very important, first of all due to the need of forming specialists according to the needs of the upgraded model for athletes capable of performance and high performance, secondly for the fact that the coach is the educator who should form the athlete, the coach is responsible for sportive performance.

Keywords: personality, coach, model, abilities, sports performance

Introduction

Sports training is a complex process having a systematic and continuously gradual development providing the adaptation of the sportsman's body to intense physical and psychical strains, its objective being the achievement of exceptional sports performances during the competitions. Seen as a pedagogical, instructive-educational process in the past, the modern sports training tends to become more complex through its organization, content and development, offering the image of a particular interdisciplinary process.

The coach who quickly intuits the evolution orientation and the rhythm of that particular sport, who applies in practice, in a creative way, the knowledge acquired and correlates it to the discoveries of other sciences, he/she provides the premises for a real performance activity.

The reason for the coach's and sportsman's efforts is not exclusively of educational nature, the purpose being also the achievement of sports performance.

The **coach** is *that person responsible for the elaboration, planning and directing the process of training young individuals for developing their performance ability and achieving victories in competitions* [2].

His/Her status includes managerial, projective, instructive-educational, scientific research and consultancy activities.

Taking into account the research activities [9], *coach's personality* is characterized as it follows:
- the coach is the individual manifesting an obvious wish to register successful results with the sportsmen trained by him/her;
- the coach is a good organizer;
- the coach has a fair attitude towards people;
- the coach estimates to an appropriate level the cultural values;
- the coach manifests a strong self-control of feelings;
- the coach is a sincere person;
- the coach proves a leader's ability;
- the coach is altruist;
- the coach has a constant behavior.

The research **purpose** consists in investigating the coach's personality features, as well as his/her role in sports performance.

The personality analysis plays an important role in theoretical, as well as in applicative researches. Though, except for the "intelligence", any other concept of psychology is not so complex and undetermined as that of "personality". In 1931, G.W.

Allport details 50 definitions [1]. Certain authors try to express in definition the complex character of the personality structure, stressing the order and the rules of forming certain elements distinctive in kind: biological, physiological, psychological and social-cultural. Therefore, Niculescu M., defines the personality as a group of bio-physio-psychological features which allows the adjustment to the environment. Following the same idea, that of defining the personality, we should also mention:
- bio-psycho-social and cultural, individual structure, in full process of development [5];
- macrosystem of informational and operational invariants constantly expressed in conduct, defining and characterizing the subject [7] ;
- specific structure of attributes which determines a form of personal conduct in contact with the surrounding reality [4].
- relatively stable and general characteristic of an individual's way of being, his/her reactions according to different situations [10];
- series of conducts, skills, motivations, etc., whose unity and constancy represents the individuality and the singularity of each person [11];

Despite the dissimilarities between the starting points and the analysis methods, most of the modern authors point out as a common radical in defining the personality, the unity attribute, thoroughness, structurality.

Material and Method

Approaching the idea that *coach's personality* as an over-ordered dimension, having an integrative-adaptive function, is propelled by tendencies and, according to the diversity of their combinations, it involves the presence of the other dimensions: biological and physiological.

Coach's personality consists in two basic features [3]:
- stability, a way of outward expression and of inner personal undergoing which remains relatively unchanged in time;
- integration, through the creation of a psychical unity and totality.

Through observing certain *objective factors,* which determine the individual's activity, it is stated that the personality is not simple concept, but a proven reality [5,6]:
- the genetics, the genes are considered material supports of the morphological, physiological and psychological nature of an individual;
- the social factor in its entire complexity and diversity.

The society has a huge influence on the individual;
- the motivational factor, the desire to win, the determination, the aggressiveness, the leadership, the ability to respect and to consent to the coach;
- the emotional factor, the emotional stability, the self-respect, the mental rigidity, the moral sense, the social confidence, the individual's responsibility for his/her

action.

The personality, as a complex system, includes the dynamic-energetic aspect – *the temperament,* the relational-value aspect – *the moral quality*, the instrumental-value aspect – *skills* and it represents the stable feature of the individual's conduct, as well as the original, unique element [8].

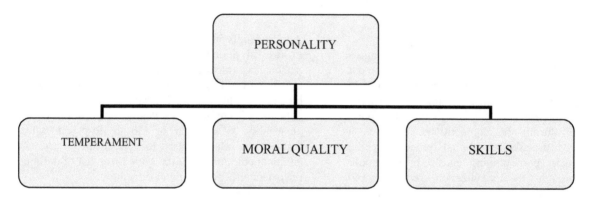

Figure 1. Personality components (7)

Coach's temperament expresses the ease or the slowness of developing psychical processes, the strain endurance, the balance of emotional processes, the dynamics of affective processes. Temperaments are classified as it follows:
- choleric;
- phlegmatic;
- sanguine;
- melancholic.
The defining elements of the temperament are:
- pure temperaments do not exist, the prevailing type of temperament being the intermediary one placed in the proximity (between the choleric and the sanguine, between the sanguine and the phlegmatic etc.);
- considering the determining factors of the personality (the genetics and the environment), the temperament is prevalent hereditary;
- the temperament do not change, it is just influenced by the social conditions or the self-control;
- the temperament expresses the attitudinal aspect of the personality, being the most accessible observation, in this sense expressing the individual's form of manifestation;
- the temperament is not reported to the human value, so it can not be appreciated as good or bad;
- the temperament analysis is necessary for the sports orientation and it is not a selection criteria.
Coach's **abilities** constitute the operational-instrumental aspect of the personality and represent the psychical and physical characteristics which are relatively stable and allow the coach to successfully perform certain forms of activity.
The *abilities* are divided into:
- simple-basic abilities (absolute eyesight and hearing);
- complex abilities, through their interaction leading to the style creation;

- general complex abilities (intelligence or sense of observation);
- specific complex abilities (didactic, artistic).
Coach's *character:* constitutes a relational-value aspect because it expresses a set of stable attitudes towards the reality, and any manifested attitude is constant, lasting in behavior acts, representing the relational quality me - the other and the value aspect generating the conduct. We may speak here about a good or bad character.
The *characteristics of the moral quality* are:
- the moral quality is considered the conscious control instance;
- the moral quality is the expression of the personality content and value;
- the moral quality is that aspect of the personality which is more acquired than inherited;
- the moral quality expresses the education and the formation availability.
Considering the ―philosophical" meaning, the personality shapes the individual gifted with a series of superior qualities and features, for which he/she contributes in a crucial way (during his/her activity as a sportsman) through special creations and results, to the development of sports, of certain sports disciplines.
From ―moral" considerations, sportsmen playing beneficial roles in the group activity (high performance sportsmen) are considered as personalities.
From a ―psychological" point of view, the personality represents the hyper-complex organized, structured, dynamic system made up of all relatively constant features and qualities psychically specific to each sports branch, according to which the sportsman adapts to the training and competition requirements.
As a *conclusion*, avoiding the polemics of different authors concerning the definition and the components

of the personality in sports, we believe that for a successful training and educational activity, the coach should admit the existence of the following components of the human being:

a) sano, the body with its physical and sensory abilities: force, speed, skill, agility, endurance;

b) the intellectual abilities characterized through the quality of moral processes, everything that the memory collects, including the capacity of using in a creator, reasoned way the theoretical-tactical material;

c) the emotionality and the temperament: totality of emotions, factor which depends on the inherited temperament of the sportsman, correlated to, intensified and enhanced by the competition experience;

d) the motivation: total amount of interests, needs;

e) the moral quality: moral component of personality.

Knowing the personality of the coach is very important, first of all due to the need of forming specialists according to the needs of the upgraded model for athletes capable of performance and high performance, secondly for the fact that the coach is the educator who should form the athlete, the coach is responsible for sportive performance.

The sports activity should become very efficient, the coach's concerns should be focused on the harmonious development of all structures of his/her personality and of that of the sportsmen trained by him/her, by means of the sports training and competition.

Reference

1. Allport G.W., 1981,Structura şi dezvoltarea personalităţii.Bucharest: Didactică şi Pedagogică Publisher, 580 p.

2. Dragnea C. A., Mate-Teodorescu S. 2002, Teoria sportului. Bucharest: FEST Publisher, p.187.

3. Epuran, M., Holdevici, I., Toniţa, F. 2001, Psihologia sportului de performanţă: teorie şi practică. Bucharest: FEST Publisher, p.77.

4. Holban I. 1972Realizarea personalităţii – Hazard sau ştiinţă? Bucharest: Orizonturi Publisher, , p.21.

5. Mărgineanu N. , 1973 Condiţia umană. Bucharest: Ştiinţifică Publisher, p.31

6. Niculescu M. 1999, Elemente de psihologia sportului de performanţă şi mare performanţă. Bucharest: Didactică şi Pedagogică Publisher, p.54.

7. Popescu-Neveanu P. 1978, Dicţionar de psihologie. Bucharest: Albatros Publisher, p.553.

8. Popescu C. 1979, Antrenorul – profilul, personalitatea şi munca sa. Bucharest: Sport-Turism Publisher, p.24.

9. Weinberg R. S., Gould D., 1997,Psychologie du sport et de l'activité physique. Toronto: Edisem Vigot Publisher, , p.234-237.

10. Grand dictionare de la psychologie. 1991, Paris: Larousse Publisher , 862p.

11. Le petit Larousse – Dictionaire Encyclopedique., 1995, Paris: Larousse Publisher, 1784 p.

12

Impact of physical exercise on the cognitive impairment in the elderly

Fita Ioana Gabriela[1], Mihaela Macovei-Moraru[2], Luminita Diana Marinescu[2], Gabriel Ioan Prada[1]

[1]*"Carol Davila" University of Medicine and Pharmacy Bucharest, National Institute of Geriatrics and Gerontology "Ana Aslan" Bucharest,* [2] *University of Medicine and Pharmacy of Craiova, Romania*

Abstract: The cognitive disorder is a common disease, specific to the elderly, with a significant social and economic impact. The current treatment of this disease is mainly symptomatic; that is why prevention is essentially important in the development of this disease. One of the most affordable methods of prevention is physical activity. This article is based on the case study of a72 years old patient suffering from a mild cognitive impairment, who has been included in a program of light physical activity.

Key words: *physical activity, elderly, cognitive impairment*

Introduction

In the general context of a world-wide aging population, cognitive impairment is a frequent condition which is often underdiagnosed or incorrectly diagnosed. It is a fact that the polipathology and associated polypharmacy are the most common features of hospitalized elderly patients. Another characteristic is the significant delay in asking for specialised medical help based on a general but inadequate impression that certain symptoms are normal in the intricate context of ageing.

The following case study highlights these issues. We consider it representative for both the elderly population admitted to INGG "Ana Aslan" and those patients included in the clinical trial called "Impact of physical exercise on the clinical debut and development of the cognitive impairment in the elderly".

Clinical case presentation

This case-study concerns PT-a 72 years old patient, who was admitted into our clinic for the following symptoms grouped as it follows:

1) Impairment of recent memory - a symptom that both patients and caregivers noticed to have appeared about a year ago; it slowly and progressively worsened;
2) Initiation insomnia, mood swings, tearfulnes, ideas of hopelessness, depressed mood- symptoms observed during the last six months;
3) Postural dizziness and occipital headache - the patient could not specify a time of onset;
4) Epigastric chronic pain progressively worsened during the last two months;
5) Progressive bilateral, chronic knee joint pain, but worsening during last month;
6) Mixed urinary incontinence, dysuria, polakiuria, nocturia occurred a month ago.

History of significant pathological events:

1) Depressive disorder -1996- for which the patient was hospitalized in a psychiatry clinic; the patient has been on antidepressant treatment with Sertraline 100 mg/day and Bromazepam (3 mg/day) for 2 years.
2) Essential hypertension diagnosed in 2005 (TA max. 190/100 mmHg),
3) Vertebral basilar circulatory insufficiency diagnosed in 2009
4) Essential tremor in 2009.

The patient is a physician retired for old age, doesn't smoke and occasionally consuming ethanol. PT lives alone and is daily visited by a caregiver.

The patient is currently being treated for depression with chronic Tianeptin 1 HP 12.5 mg/day, for insomnia with Zolpidem 10 mg 1 cp/day, for hypertension with Nebivolol 5mg 1 cp/day, for vertebral basilar circulatory insufficiency with Gingko biloba 40 mg 3 hp/day and for severe joint pain with Ketoprofen SR 200mg 1 cp/day.

On physical examination were found varicose veins, Heberdeen and Bouchard lumps, increased thoracic kyphosis and lumbar lordosis, bilateral crackles on knee joint mobilization, mild epigastrium tenderness to palpation .

The patient has a good personal and space orientation sense. A bilateral hand tremor could be noticed.

All laboratory tests performed were within normal limits, except for total serum cholesterol 250 mg/dl, triglycerides 175 mg/dL, and the urine culture – that highlighted the presence of Escherichia coli.

The patient's standard geriatric assessment included:

1. **Mini Mental State Evaluation (MMSE, Folstein)**,a test developed by Folstein et al. in 1975 [1]. The patient MMSE score of 27 points was considered normal.

2. **Clock drawing test**. This test is a simple method that can be used to assess neuropsychiatric functions [2]. The patient TDC score recorded 8/10 points, significant for possible mild cognitive impairment on Sunderland scale [3].

3. **Geriatric Depression Scale**. This scale was developed as a depression screening measure for the elderly [4]. The patient showed 7/15 points, a significant score for depression.

4. **Evaluation of Static and Dynamic Balance while walking (Tinetti test)**. Fall risk assessment was done using the Tinetti test [5]; the patient's results were: the static balance score was 14/16 points and the dynamic balance during walking score was 11/12.

5. **Evaluation of Daily Basic Activities and Complex Daily Activities**. The patient was evaluated in terms of ability to perform both various common tasks and/or complex activities using the two scales mentioned above (ADL and IADL) [6, 7]. At daily basic activities (ADL) the patient had a score of 5/6; the complex activities (IADL) score showed that our patient received 5/8 points.

6. **Nutritional Geriatrics Assessment**. The nutritional assessment of the patient showed a body mass index (BMI) of 27 kg/m2.

Psychological examination was performed. It showed mild difficulties regarding concentration, attention, a slightly impaired evocative efficiency of the immediate events, slight mental rigidity, irritability, low tolerance to frustration, strong compulsive attitude-**conclusion**-mild depression associated to a mild cognitive impairment.

The carotid Doppler exam - showed plaques with no significant hemodynamic effect situated on both internal carotid arteries and bilateral carotid bulb levels.

Front and profile knee X-ray exam - showed specific gonarthrosis changes.

Abdominal Barium X-ray exam - small transhiatal gastric hernia.

Brain CT scan- showed cortical atrophy, located mainly at the right temporal lobe level , cerebral leukoaraiosis, multiple lacunar strokes. (Fig. 1)

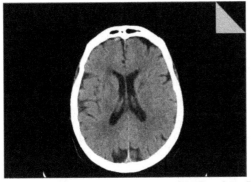

Figure no.1   CT PT patient, 72 years

EEG examination revealed: a general α wave pattern with a low voltage structure highlighted in some sectors; we could also notice isolated, unorganised subalfa elements, (that make the transition from normal to pathological patterns) ; irregular θ deficiency type elements sporadically present > 10% - are characteristic for mild cognitive impairment. The presence of fast track β type structure elements > 10% was characteristic for mixed depressive disorder. (Fig. 2, Fig. 3)

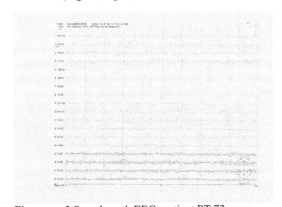

Figure no.2 Sample path EEG, patient PT 72 years

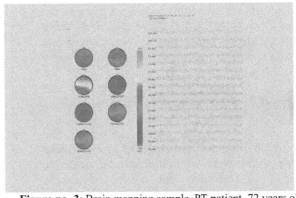

Figure no. 3: Brain mapping sample, PT patient, 72 years old

Intermediate diagnosis
1. Mild cognitive impairment (Petersen criteria [8])
2. Depressive disorder
3. Hypertension
4. Mixed dyslipidaemia,
5. Vertebral basilar circulatory failure,
6. Transhiatal gastric hernia,
7. Low tract urinary infection with E. coli,
8. Osteoarthritis,
9. Varicose legs.

Treatment
Medication: 10 mg atorvastatinum 1 cp / day, 12.5 mg tianeptin 1 cp / day, 10 mg zolpidem necessary, nebivolol 1 cp / day Ginkgo biloba 40 mg 1 HP x 3 / day, Gerovital 1 ampoule i.m. / day 10 days, Tylenol for joint pain, Detralex 2 cp 500 mg / day

Physical therapy and kinetotherapy.
P.T. is included in a clinical trial that investigates the implications of exercise on the emergence and development of elderly cognitive impairment. Daily physical activity consists of a 2 km walk three times a week. This program was originally initiated under medical supervision.

The patient and his caregiver returned to our clinic for the 6 months evaluation. According to his late medical personal history, the patient has respected both the medical treatment and exercise program.

Identical tests were used in order to assess the patients' evolution; the results are as follows:
1. MMSE test score is 27/30 points
2. TDC test revealed 9/10 points
3. At GDS patient received 6 points.

There is a slight improvement in score TDC and GDS score. Carergiver confirms the positive evolution of the patient's condition, especially in terms of improving his depressive mood and insomnia. The caregiver cannot however confirm an improvement of memory disorders. Blood pressure, cholesterol and triglycerides are normal. Medical advice for PT is to continue medical treatment and physical activity.

1 year clinical evaluation- the patient returns for a reassessment feeling much improved.

Identical tests were carried out again:

1. MMSE test -score of 28/30 points
2. TDC test - 9/10 points
3. GDS test- 5 points.

The carergiver confirms a slight improvement in patients symptoms related to memory disorder and depression. He also noted that the patient has reassumed his social activities and the fact that he has initiatives regarding domestic and leisure activities. Patients blood levels in cholesterol and triglycerides were normal. The complex daily activities score improved from 5/8 points to 7/8 points which indicates a decrease in the dependence level.

Disscution:

Noticeable to this case is the polipatologia and associated polypharmaceutical treatment. Another characteristic feature is the delay in asking for specialised medical advice, because both patients and carers felt that they could consider patient' s symptoms as being normal according to ageing popular standards. It is also interesting to mention the positive progressive evolution of the patient's mild cognitive disorder and depression, during a year of consistent medical and physical therapy and surveillance. Patient is included in a clinical trial that investigates the implications of exercise on the emergence and development of cognitive impairment in the elderly. Daily physical activity is represented by walking a distance of 2 km three times a week. The antidepressant treatment associated to gingko biloba treatment could positively influence the cognitive disorder and the depression. This does not rule out the hypothesis that physical activity carried out consistently could also have a positive influence on cognitive function and depression. We cannot be sure of physical effort influence on total cholesterol, triglycerides and blood pressure, because the patient was under antihypertensive and statin treatment.

Medical literature shows undoubtable evidence of positive influence of physical activity represented by walking towards the cognitive status [9, 10] and the patient's functional level measured by specific daily activity scales (ADL and IADL) [11].

There is also data showing an improvement of depressive disorder after physical activity performed consistently [12-15].

Conclusions:

This patient is representative for the type of patients

admitted to INGG "Ana Aslan". He is also representative for the target population of the Nostrum clinical trial. Our observations confirm the literature data. They also support the hypothesis that sustained physical activity has a positive influence on cognitive status and over the general well-being of non-institutionalized elderly.

There is no doubt that in order to confirm the statistical significance of the information we provided, it is required for statistical processing of data from all patients enrolled in the clinical trial, data that will be published later.

References:

1. FOLSTEIN MF, FOLSTEIN SE, McHUGH PR ""Mini-mental state". A practical method for grading the cognitive state of patients for the clinician". Journal of psychiatric research 1975 12 (3): 189–98.

2. SHULMAN KI. *Clock-drawing: îs it the ideal cognitive screening test?* Int J Geriatr Psychiatry 2000;15:548-561.

3. SUNDERLAND T, HILL JL, MELLOW AM, LAWLOR BA, GUNDERSHEIMER J, NEWHOUSE PA, GRAFMAN JH: *Clock drawing în Alzheimer's disease, a novel measure of dementia severity.* J Am Geriatr Şoc 1989; 37: 725–729.

4.http://www.chcr.brown.edu/gds_short_form.pdf

6. TINETTI ME, WILLIAMS TF, MAYEWSKI R: Fall risk index for elderly paţient based on number of chronic disabilities. Am J med 1986, 80:429-434.

[6] KATZ S. Assessing self-maintenance: activities of daily living, mobility, and instrumental activities of daily living. J Am Geriatr Şoc. 1983 Dec;31(12):721-7

7. LAWTON MP, BRODY EM. Assessment of older people: self-maintaining and instrumental activities of daily living. Gerontologist. 1969 Autumn;9(3):179-86.

8. PETERSEN R.C., SMITH G.E., WARING S.C., IVNIK R.J., TANGALOS E.G., KOKMEN E. *Mild cognitive impairment: clinical characterisation and outcome.* Archives of Neurology 56, 303-308, 1999.

9. PROHASKA TR, EISENSTEIN AR, SATARIANO WA, HUNTER R, BAYLES CM, KURTOVICH E, KEALEY M, IVEY ŞL. *Walking and the preservation of cognitive function în older populations.* Gerontologist. 2009 Jun;49 Suppl 1:S86-93.

10. PATERSON DH, WARBURTON DE Physical activity and funcţional limitations în older adults: a systematic review related to Canada's Physical Activity Guidelines. Int J Behav Nutr Phys Act. 2010 May 11;7:38.

11. STRAWBRIDGE WJ, DELEGER S, ROBERTS RE, KAPLAN GA *Physical activity reduces the risk of subsequent depression for older adults.* American Journal of Epidemiology 2002, 156(4):328-34

12. MARTINSEN, E. W., *Physical activity and depression: clinical experience.* Acta Psychiatrica Scandinavica, (1994) 89: 23–27. doi: 10.1111/j.1600-0447.1994.tb05797.x;

13. DR KENNETH R FOX *The influence of physical activity on mental well-being* Public Health Nutrition:1999 2(3a), 411–418 411 Accepted: 7 May 1999 Published online: 02 January 2007;

14. SAMUEL B. HARVEY, MRCPsych and MATTHEW HOTOPF, PhD *Physical activity and common mental disorders,* The British Journal of Psychiatry (2010) 197: 357-364. doi:10.1192/bjp.bp.109.075176

13

Comparative study concerning training methodical line to junior I athletes of 400m flat running

Albină Alina Elena

University of Craiova, Faculty of Physical Education and Sport

Abstract: Training planning and scheduling to athletes performing the 400m flat running trial should consider the training factors, and the physical training should solve in an individualized and, at the same time, balanced way, the development of basic motor skills. The athletes on 400m flat sprint need skills, such as: speed, specific endurance, force, joint mobility and muscle flexibility.
Key words: *methodical line, training sessions, sportsmen, results.*

Introduction

The performance sport is correlated to intense physical effort which is materialized through the achievement of sports results in training and, mainly, in competitions.

Sports performance determines the validation or the cancellation of applied methods and means during the training sessions, having the opportunity to discover the optimum aspects or the gaps in sports training, which involves the completion or the optimization of the applied training methodology. Without a diligent work from the sportsmen and a rigorous elaboration and control of training schedules, the sports performance can not be achieved. Only through a combination of the biomotor, bioenergetic and biomechanical parameters as part of a well-planned training sessions, we may achieve remarkable performances in sprint trials. In order to underlie the scientific-methodical aspects of the research, it is mentioned in the studied field literature that the athletes, practicing the 400m flat running, register the following essential characteristics: time reaction to the start, which is the time collapsed from the start command and the runner's first movement (value of the start time reaction), ability for burst of speed assessed as the necessary distance for reaching the maximum running speed (ability for launching from the start point), maximum running speed and ability to maintain it as long as possible and ability to prove high efficient actions in order to cross over the finish line. These characteristics differ from one athlete to another, considering certain individual features, the running distance and the sportsmen's level of training [5,8,11].

Research Purpose

The research purpose consists in pointing out the training particularities (methods and means used during the training) applied for sprinters on 400m flat included in our research, as well as how these particularities comply with the methodical line enforced by the Romanian Athletics Federation for this specific trial according to the level of age.

Research Hypothesis

The research aims at finding new solutions of improving the training process, through the elaboration of new methods and means concerning the education of high motor skills able to provide a continuous increase of sports performances.

Research means: the training planning elaborated by us for 12 runners on 400m flat, attending ―ParacheTrişcu‖ Sports Program High School of Craiova and the planning proposed by the Romanian Athletics Federation, according to the training methodical line for junior I category.

Research theoretical substantiation

The multilateral training and development are important aspects in the athlete's practice, and there is a correlation between these aspects [1,4]. The general physical training is in direct ratio to the technical aspect of the trial, to the time interval between the training stages and the peak competitions (indoor and outdoor competitions), and in inverse ratio to the level of sports skills reached by the sportsman [7].

The physical training *"provides the energetic background of the performance through stimulating the evolution of functional and morphologic indices (joint, ligament strengthening, muscle development) and, consequently, of motor skills, the enhancement of the strain general ability of the body which allows the acquirement of technical-tactical knowledge necessary for the practiced trial"*[2].

The use on a large scale of different training drills specific to other sports and their application in practice may provide the evaluation of dissociated and integrative effects on the body, as well as the selection of highly efficient exercises according to the sportsman's age, sex and level of training.

According to I. Şiclovan [9], the physical training implies:

• the improvement of motor and coordination skills;

• the formation, consolidation and improvement of basic and specific motor skills and abilities;

• the development of morpho-functional and psychical indices.

Considering an organized training program (Table 1), the physical training has the following structure [3]:

• *general physical training (GPT);*

• *specific physical training (SPT);*

• *improvement of specific biomotor skills.*

The first two stages are included in the pre-training period, when a strong basis is needed, the third phase is specific to the competition period, when the objective is to maintain and to improve the level of training achieved following the pre-training period.

Table 1. Sequential approach of the physical training evolution according to the annual planning of training [3, p.49]

Training stages	Pre-training stage		Competition stage
Development stage	1	2	3
Objective	General physical training	Specific physical training	Improvement of specific biomotor skills

The main objective of the general physical training is to improve the strain ability necessary for the sports performance practice. For the young promising sportsmen, the GPT is very important as it generates subsequent performances. For the high performance sportsmen, the GPT is correlated to the trial demands and to the sportsmen's individual features. The general physical training implies exercises used during the specific training, namely, exercises for developing endurance, force, take-off and speed. The young sportsmen practicing the 400m flat gradually pass to the specific training. The specific physical training is built up on the basis of the GPT. The main objective of this training is to provide the sportsman's physical development according to the physiological and methodical features of the sports trial. The GPT needs a high volume of training which becomes possible only through a decrease in intensity.

The improvement of specific biomotor skills begins when the pre-training period ends, and the objective of this phase is to develop the specific biomotor skills and to adjust the sportsmen's potential in order to satisfy the specific demands of the practiced trial.

The 400m flat trial represents a speed trial as considering its particularities specific to the strain which can be of physiological and biochemical nature [6]:
- an increased deficiency of oxygen following the physical strain – 92%;
- the deficiency of oxygen generates an important debt of lactates -84%, as compared to that of alactates – 16%;
- the highest concentration of lactic acid in the blood (277mg%).

Considering the 400m flat running trial, good results may be achieved by the sportsmen having special abilities, through different methods of training.

Training staging considering the sportsmen's age:
- the basic training structures the functional support for the training focused on the systematic development of future maximum performances, therefore, the biological and pedagogical standards for children development, as well as the main exigences of the discipline will be considered;
- the training generates specific suppositions related to the potential (trial technique, limited coordinate conditioning ability, knowledge and conduct) of the background in a group of athletic trials and, later, in a single trial; sports performances should be still the prevailing result of the multilateral training;
- the connection training develops exigences specific to the practice of a certain trial; the practice derives from a particular planning; the athlete heads from a high level to competitions meant to allow him/her the inclusion in the national team. The determining factor for reaching the adequate level of potential and involvement necessary for the junior category is the process of ―refinement" for the trial during the juvenile training period. This process is reflected by the correlation between the general and the specific training.

Taking into account the fact that the sports training focused on the efficiency always represents a refinement stage, this process should be divided as in the following outline (Table 2) [10]:

Table 2. Training staging according to the sportsmen's age [10]

Age	Juvenile training stages	Level of refinement	Training for competitions	Indices for the training task
10 - 14 years	Basic training	All the athletic trials asjusted to the age category; mainly combined trials.	Completely useless	Multilateral task, but focused on all sportsmen's demands
15 - 18 years	Development training	Refinement in a group of trials. refinement in a certain trial.	General introduction in the competition training. Introduction in the competition training for a certain trial.	Partially multilateral functional level of a group of trials. Functional level specific to a certain trial.
19 - 20 years	Link-up training	Complete refinement in a trial (competition and training).	Specific training for a trial.	Specific functional refinement; functional level for high performances of a trial.

―alent" hunting in sports, in default of a well-developed system of juvenile training, represents an error which highly afflicts and quickly eliminates

young gifted individuals interested in athletics. Given the rivalry existing between different sports branches, the system does not afford to reject young individuals willing to practice high performance sport.

Sprint trials training constitutes a delicate and complex issue, because there is a high risk of being wrong about the strain dosage considering the practice volume and intensity. In sprinters' training, the running technique occupies the first place and it should reveal a perfect accuracy as gesture, a very good neuromuscular coordination, amplitude and a high level of relaxation.

The sprinter should have a very well trained —sense of speeding up" which involves a developed —speed ability", both aspects contributing to the maximum improvement of the individual's speed potential.

The second aspect of great importance is the sprinter's force training which contributes to the individual's speed potential improvement; as well, an inappropriate force training may —strangle" this potential.

The force training is also focused on the appropriate development of the muscles at the level of the abdomen and on the hip lifting, and concurrently, it provides the coxofemoral joint flexibility.

A third important aspect is the development of the endurance against a speed background, which should provide the maintenance of the maximum speed or of the performance speed (for long distance running), as long as possible.

Following-up the research, we have tried to compare the level of general indices to that of specific ones complying with the training methodical line enforced by the Romanian Athletics Federation and that applied by us including the sprinters on 400m flat running selected for the experiment group (Table 3).

Table 3. Pattern of the main training indices to junior I runners on 400m flat

Code		Indices	F.R Athletics methodical line		Personal training
			15-17 years	17-19 years	**16-19 years**
1	General	Period of training (no of days)	272	290	**277**
2		Training sessions (no of sessions)	250	280	**277**
3		Training hours (no of hours)	556	670	**518**
4		Starts (no)	14	21	**30**
5	Specific	a. start from stnding for 60m 95-100% (km.\)	20	25	**25.8**
6		a. start from stnding - 80m $\geq$95% (km.)	20	32	**39**
7		a. start from stnding - 100m $\geq$ 95% (km)	20	35	**57.1**
8		a. start from stnding – over 100m 80-90% (km)	210	250	**248.1**
9		a. start from stnding – over 100m $\geq$ 75% (km)	26	125	**79.8**
10		a. long distance trial, a.Fartlek type (km)	100	160	**708**
11		Force (exercises with weights) (tones)	120	180	**150**
12		Take-off (detachment from the ground) (no)	6000	8000	**8450**

Analyzing the values indicated in Table 3, one may observe that the training program conceived by us for the sportsmen group, all runners on 400m flat, presents numerous similarities with the methodical line required by the Romanian Athletics Federation for the junior I category. Our training program includes the same values as those registered by the sportsmen aged between 17 and 19 years and pretty significant differences as compared to the group including sportsmen aged between 15 and 17 years. Therefore, we will consider the group made up individuals with ages varying between 17 and 19 years – the methodical line required by the Romanian Athletics Federation and the values achieved by our sportsmen group.

Almost even values are indicated for the number of training sessions (280-277), for the standing start for 60m 95-100% (25-25.8 km), for the standing start for over 100 m 80-90% (250-248.1 km), for the take-off

(ground detachment) (8000-8450 no of repetitions).

On the other side, we register differences for the following trials, such as: the long distance trial, Fartlek type (160-708km) and the standing start for over 100m ≥75% (125-79.8km) and the number of training hours (670-518).

The general indices of training are somehow similar for both training categories due to the planning structure applied for junior I training when dealing with the 400m flat running trial.

For the specific indices, there are significant differences due to the fact that the training planning conceived by us is focused on the running speed on distances of 100m and 80m with short active rest periods. As well, the training sessions oriented on the development of the specific endurance, we register significant increases for the type Fartlek running with changes of rhythm and on various distances. The trials consisting in sprints on 500m and 600m, register reduced values due to the fact that they have been performed mainly during the pre-training winter stage and less during the pre-training spring period.

Conclusions

The parameters volume-intensity considered for the young individuals' training, play an important role according to the effects they generate. The intensity parameter produces long-term effects as a main characteristic, and as a secondary one, immediate effects, while the intensity parameter registers opposite features, meaning, immediate effects and as collateral features long-term effects. The two parameters are distinctively combined according to the young individual's level of training, and, as the athlete evolves, they tend to reduce the importance of the long-range training, while the training focused on immediate objectives gains value.

For the training planning to junior I category, we should consider the following requirements: the physical training optimization through the increase of the motor skill indices specific to the trial; the optimization of the selective development of motor skills applying the most efficient means and methods; the improvement of the performed trial technique following two main ways: through global physical exercises with variable intensity and using special double-oriented exercises (technique and motor skills); the optimization of the competition tactics; the improvement of the level of field theoretical and methodical formation.

During this training stage, various standards and norms specific to the high performance sports training are enforced, though, we should consider that high performances to the junior level should result from a multilateral training focused on performance and an early specialization of the training leave irreparable traces for the next stage oriented on higher performances.

References

1. Alexa N., 1986, Rolul şi importanţa pregătirii fizice a sportivilor. In: Physical Education and Sport, no 1, Bucharest, p. 5-7.
2. Alexa N. 1993, Antrenamentul sportiv modern. Bucharest: Editis, 255p.
3. Bompa T.O., 2001, Teoria şi metodologia-periodizarea antrenamentului sportiv. In: CNFPA. Bucharestp. 49-50.
4. Dragnea A. 1993, Antrenamentul sportiv, teorie şi metodologie, Bucharest: ANEFS,286 p.
5. Dragomir M., Albină A.E., 2009, Atletismul în şcoală. Craiova : Universitaria,. p. 88 – 117.
6. Dumitrescu V.,1968, Alergări pe 100m, 200m, 400m. Bucharest : CNEFS, 210 p.
7. Pradet M., 2000, Pregătire fizică tome I. Bucharest : CCSP, 252 p
8. Stoica M. 1999, Optimizarea pregătirii la sprint a juniorilor de nivel I în raport cu modelul ritmic al alergării în proba de 100m.p.PhD Thesis, Bucureşti,. p. 20.
9. Şiclovan I., 1984, Teoria şi metodica antrenamentului sportiv. Bucharest : INEFS, 1984. p. 359.
10. Tshiene P. 1995, Aspectele adaptive ale competiţiei. Bucharest: In Competition Theory, MTS, CCPS no 362, 363, 364, , p.45-59.
11. Winckler G., 1991, O privire asupra anduranţei de viteză, (View on Speed Endurance) New Studies in Athletics, Londra,. In : Traducere FRA şi MTS, CCPS. Bucharest, 1993, p. 24-25.

14

Rhythm Development Through Means Specific to Rhythmic Gymnastics on Female Students Attending Physical Education and Sport Faculty

Cosma Germina[1], Orţănescu Dorina[1], Paunescu Mihaela[2]

[1]Department of Theory and Methodology of Motricity Activities, University of Craiova, Romania
[2]National University of Physical Education and Sport, Bucharest, Romania

Abstract. This paper shows the impact of the working programs of the rhythmic gymnastics shape the body expression of female students in the first year (aged 20±), as well as the level of appropriation of the movement general basis. Therefore, 30 female students have been selected and they have been intensely involved for 14 weeks, performing 2 hours of rhythmic gymnastics per week. We observe a better ability of reproducing the rhythm and the tempo and a better correlation between the music and movement after 14 weeks of practicing.
Key words: *rhythmic gymnastic, music, rhythm.*

Introduction

Rhythmic gymnastics is a sports discipline included in the school curriculum of female students in the first year of school within the Faculty of Physical Education and Sport of Craiova. This type of movement is necessarily performed all of a piece with the musical backup.

Music plays an important role for sports events such as rhythmic gymnastics, synchronized swimming, skating and so forth. From a musical perspective, it is found that the lack of congruence between music and movement is observed through videos such as the Olympics and the Commonwealth Games. Interviews were conducted with coaches and the study reveals the limitations faced by coaches including the musical background of gymnasts and the editing of music for a routine (1). Music is the soul of Rhythmic Gymnastics, if there was no music this sports would become uninteresting. This article, through the analysis of Rhythmic Gymnastics music theme, gives a brief explanation of how to select the music of rhythmic gymnastics individual performance and the important issues in making music selection (2).

The favorable influence of music on the movement depends on providing an harmonic discipline between the strength and resources of the musical expression and those of the movement. The complete harmony between movement and music contributes to a faster learning of motor skills, to the development of the motor ability, to the improvement of the cultural and spiritual life of trainees.

Music plays an important role in calisthenics gymnastics and music rhythm is one of the most important elements in music expression. Rhythm is the marrow of music and the (emotional) basis of movement intensity. In calisthenics gymnastics, the speeds of all the movements such as running, jumping and circling are based on the rhythm of music melody (3). The musical backup represents an acoustic-aesthetic component associated to the specific motor behavior focused on the conduct, the adjustment, the organization and the arrangement of movement structures (4). This approach is necessary for every rhythmic gymnastics class, but it should be suitable for every stage, motor structure and level of training.

Method

Through the tests applied, the research aims at observing the way in which the working programs of the rhythmic gymnastics shape the body expression of female students in the first year (aged 20±), as well as the level of appropriation of the movement general basis. Therefore, 30 female students have been selected and they have been intensely involved for 14 weeks, performing 2 hours of rhythmic gymnastics per week. In order to analyze how the selected means may influence the rhythm and the tempo education, and their perception by the subjects, rhythmic series expressed through clapping the hands have been elaborated, the female students being asked to reproduce them immediately.

The trial included two sub-tests, the subjects having to reproduce with accuracy two rhythmic series at a time. As well, motor structures have been achieved, keeping the 2/4 time signature meant to conserve the correlation between music and movement. The subjects were tested at the beginning of the class and, subsequently, at the end of the class after 14 weeks, registering, thus, the number of mistakes made by the female students.

Rhythmic series applied during the class:

ST1 – reproduction: four quarter notes tied together;
- reproduction: one quarter note, two eighth-notes, one quarter note, two eighth-notes;
- reproduction: two eighth-notes, one quarter note, two eighth-notes, one quarter note;

ST2 – reproduction: one half note, two quarter notes;
- reproduction: one half note, two quarter notes;
- reproduction: one half note, two eighth-notes, one quarter note.

The motor structure (2/4 music time signature):

PI – standing on the toes, hands on the hips
M I and II T1-4   Four paces
MIII and IV T5-8   Left turn with successive paces
M I and II T1-4   Four paces
MIII and IV T5-8   Right turn with successive paces
M I and II T1-4   Four curved paces
MIII and IV T5-8   Left turn with curved paces
M I and II T1-4   Four curved paces
MIII and IV T5-8   Right turn with curved paces

Results

Considering the test application, we have registered the following results:

Table I Results of the rhythmic series

| | SUB-TEST I | | SUB-TEST II | |
	T1	T2	T1	T2
Number of mistakes	13	5	10	4
Percentage mistakes	43%	17%	33%	13%

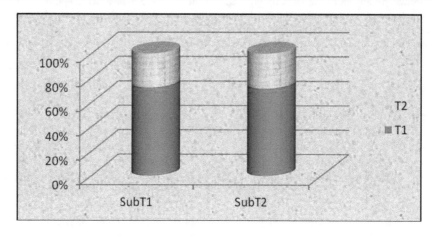

Chart no 1 Results of the rhythmic series

Following the test focused on the ability of reproducing the rhythm and the tempo, we have noticed, considering the two rhythmic series initially and finally tested, that the sportswomen achieve 43% for the first sub-test, meaning a total number of 13 mistakes and, subsequently, to the second testing their results are better: among the 30 sportswomen only 5 have registered mistakes, 17%, therefore, half of those who have initially a wrong performance, have improved their activity. To the second sub-test, at first there was a number of 10 mistakes, meaning 33% of the female trainees, while to the final testing we have registered 4 mistakes (13%). (chart 1)

Table II Results of the music-movement
Music-movement Test

	T1	T2
No of wrong executions	8	3
Percentage	27%	10%

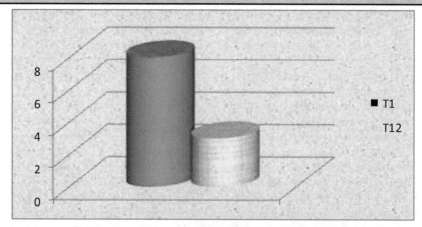

Chart no 2. Results of the music-movement Test

Following the test focused on the correlation between the music and movement, we register a reduced number of mistakes than compared to keeping the rhythm through percussion which provides accessibility to movements leading to an accurate conservation of rhythm. We may notice an improvement of the tested parameters to the final testing, the difference between T1 and T2 being of 17% (table 2)

Conclusions

Through an optimum excitability of the nervous system, through a high level of sensibility of the auditory analyzer for perception, through the stimulation of the main functions of the body (breathing and blood flow), music constitutes an important educational method for the achievement and the improvement of a motricity based on neuromuscular coordination providing a right and fast development of motor skills.

The space and time orientation and the sense for rhythm and tempo are abilities with a positive influence on the achievement of superior performances. The means applied for the expression training have contributed to the creation of a movement form involving expressiveness and honesty, as well as to the improvement of the execution indices through the enhancement of the reproduction ability of the rhythm through percussion and movement.

The correlation between movement and music should not be simply considered as a musical measure, rhythm, tempo, but, as well, through its emotional content, it should correspond to the physical exercises it accompanies.

Reference

1.Loo Fung Chiat Loo Fung Ying, (2012), Importance of Music Learning and Musicality in Rhythmic Gymnastics, *Procedia – ocial and Behavioral Sciences,* Volume 46, *2012,* Pages 3202–3208

2.Jiang Yu, (2002), A Study on Rhythmic Gymnastics Individual Performance's Music Selection, *Journal of Hubei Sport Science,* 2002-04 (http://en.cnki.com.cn/Article_en/CJFDTOTAL-HYKJ200204035.htm)

3.Deng Wei, (2004), Cultivation of calisthenics gymnastics athletes' sense of music rhythm, *Journal of Wuhan Institute of Physical Education,* 2004-04, (http://en.cnki.com.cn/Article_en/CJFDTOTAL-WTXB200404032.htm)

4.Macovei S., (2007), *Manual de gimnastica ritmica,* Editura BREN, Bucuresti

15

Some key points in neuromuscular diseases (nmds) rehabilitation therapy

Zavaleanu Mihaela[1], Rosulescu Eugenia[1, 2], Ilinca Ilona[1], Danoiu Mircea[1]

[1.] *Faculty of Physical Education and Sports, University of Craiova, Romania*
[2.] *Children Residential Rehabilitation Center DGASPC Craiova*

Abstract. Neuromuscular diseases (NMDs) represent a heterogeneous group of disorders, including motoneuron diseases, disorders of motor nerve roots or peripheral nerves, neuromuscular transmission disorders, and muscle diseases. The results of those are always muscle dysfunctions. Rehabilitation management is important in order to maintain function and functionality of body or some body parts and systems, for as long and better as possible, and to reduce all the principal risks due to the disease and also reducing the secondary risks due to the time of being ill.

This paper presents some key points that we consider important for the rehabilitation therapists, physiatrists, occupational therapists or any other member of the rehabilitation teams.

Key Words: *neuromuscular disease, rehabilitation, disability.*

Introduction

Neuromuscular disease (NMD) is a term that encompasses broad diseases and ailments that either directly or indirectly impair the function of the body's muscle system, via the nerves. [1] Neuromuscular disorders can affect many people; the diseases are not age dependent, sex, race, geographic area etc. Most of rare neuromuscular disorders (NMD) forms have genetic aetiology. Neuromuscular diseases represent a heterogeneous group of disorders, including motoneuron diseases, disorders of motor nerve roots or peripheral nerves, neuromuscular transmission disorders, and muscle diseases [2], and there are approximately 600 different NMDs with great variety in referral to physical therapy (PT) [3]. The progression of the diseases varies considerably. The deficits can range from muscle weakness, sensory loss, pain, fatigue, and autonomic dysfunction in varying combinations. These deficits combine to lead to impairments of musculoskeletal and sensory functions, limitations in activities, and restrictions in participation. [2] Some key points in NMD management rehabilitation therapy are important because the signs and symptoms, that are the peripheral effects of the disease, must be manage to maintain function or the patient life even we don't have yet a therapeutic intervention to definitively cure. Simply, all therapists must know the fact that NMDs stand for a group of maladies that affect any part of the nerve or muscle, which can involve motor neurons from the brain, spinal cord, or periphery, and like major symptom that lead to weakening the muscle. If we talk about Charcot-Marie-Tooth disease (CMT), or different peripheral neuropathies, myasthenia gravis (MG), Pompe disease or the lack of other metabolic enzyme, Duchenne muscular dystrophy, Becker dystrophy, all affect the muscular and nervous tissue, NMDs may directly affect all forms of muscle, particularly skeletal, respiratory and cardiac muscle. The physiatrist may be called on to manage these conditions and at times may be required to diagnose in patients presenting with new complaints of weakness, cramps or functional difficulties. [4]. The risk due to the diseases per se and also the secondary risks and complication resulting from the function changes due to the long period when all the complication determines other functional modifications. The complete the signs and syndromes from the start of diseases can be totally different from those that are present after 1, 2 or even three years and must be manage by the therapy.

Symptoms, clinical signs and the NMDs

The NMDs worldwide prevalence estimate, together, is 1:3500 individuals [5]. In childhood, the most frequent NMD is Duchenne muscular dystrophy (DMD), a recessive X-linked inherited disorder with worldwide incidence around 1 in 4.000 newborn boys [6]. The onset of the disease frequently occurs before the age of five years. The first symptoms are walking problems due to symmetrical weakness of the lower limbs muscles, often associated to calf pseudo hypertrophy. There is a slowly weakness progression over time with involvement of the upper limbs and respiratory muscles [7]. It is well known that the most common symptomatology in NMDs is the weak or progressive decreasing of muscular strenght. Treatment is goal-oriented, using numerous modalities that are validated over the years and after many studies. Impairment and disability after a NMD should be methodically assessed based on the World Health Organization criteria as applied to neuromuscular diseases (Table 1). *Impairment* is evaluated by measurements of strength, range of motion, spine deformity, cardiac and pulmonary function, and intellectual capacity *Disability* is evaluated by measuring of mobility and upper extremity function, cardiopulmonary adaptations, cardiac and pulmonary complications, and psychosocial adjustment. Diniz citing Mutarelli underlined that one of the most significant findings in the DMD patient's neurological exam is the muscle weakness [6, 9]. Regardless of the dystrophic types, functional deficits common to this population include joint contracture, limited mobility, poor respiratory function, as well as impaired activities of daily living. [10,11]. Taking in account the facts that concern the guides that are available on internet, regarding the management of care for Duchenne patient in special and other studies and guidelines, we present here just some key points, in a shorter version that can be apply for the care management in all NMD. An aggressive approach to the patient with disease of motor unit is essential [4].

After de Lisa [4], the rehabilitation treatment may be *anticipatory, symptomatic or restorative.*

Table 1. Disability in neuromuscular diseases [8].

Organ	Impairment (usually progressive)	Disability	Disadvantage (handicap)
Skeletal muscle	Strength and endurance	Motor performance Mobility	Quality of life Educational opportunities
		Upper extremity function	Employment opportunities
		Fatigue	Dependency and disadvantage
Bone and joint	Joint Contractures Spine Deformity	Function Pain and deformity	
Lungs	Pulmonary function	Restrictive Lung Disease (RLD) Fatigue	
Heart	Cardiomyopathy Conduction defects	Cardiopulmonary adaptations Fatigue	
CNS	Intellectual capacity	Learning ability Psychosocial adjustment	

In the case of NMD patient *anticipatory care* mean the prevention of contracture and functional decline, is the first stage of rehabilitation treatment of disease. Contractures are problematic because they limit motion, alter the centre of gravity, and accentuate weakness by limiting the potential tension a residual muscle can produce [12].

Symptomatic care or maintaining functionality addresses the problems that already exist, due to the disease or existing before the symptomatic manifestation of NMD [4].

Restorative care represents the optimal result of rehabilitation that mean the return of the patient to his higher level of function or to reverse the complication of simultaneous acute or chronic illness that can affect the patient with a NMD or any adverse effects of treatment [4].

Rehabilitation management of neuromuscular disease

The rehabilitation is planned to treat the clinical expression of those diseases, to maintain patient function and functionality, participation of the child or adult, to try to fulfil the patient life [4]. The best way to apply therapy in case of NMDs for healthcare providers from the rehabilitation domain is to treat various symptoms of the neuromuscular disorder and adapt to an array of functional changes. Best therapeutic management is carried out by an interdisciplinary team consisting of specialists in different area of expertise (rehabilitation, orthopedics, neurology, genetics, etc.), physical therapist, occupational therapy and speech therapists, social workers, vocational counsellors, and psychologists etc. And with every new symptom the team is enlarge.

Like we said before, the muscles are the affected by NMD, this determine clinical problems and also associated problems. A number of well-controlled studies have documented the effect of exercise as a means for NMD patients to gain strength, although much remains to be learned in this area [13].

Treatment plans may be designed principally in few steps meant to deal with some key points like:

- Educate the patient and parents/families/carers regarding the diseases and the changes that will occurred in the future of pathology, use of assistive devices, adaptation of the house etc.
- Recommend the prevention and supportive treatment, orthoses, assistive equipment,
- Prevent complications;
- Determine which diagnostic tests are necessary to clarify the diagnosis;
- Help to maintain maximum function and desired quality of life.

De Lisa proposes some management principles for the neuromuscular diseases, which can encompass many NMD (See Table 2).

Table 2. Management principles after DeLisa for the neuromuscular diseases [4].

Ambulatory stage	Establish the diagnosis and provide genetic counselling
	Provide early and informed counselling and psychological support to prevent counterproductive family psychodynamics. encourage goal-oriented activities and prepare the patient and family for current and future therapeutic intervention. the advantages of early intervention during each stage should be stressed.
	Manage and prevent musculotendinous contracture and decreased pulmonary compliance.
	Use appropriate supportive physical and occupational therapy, including splinting and therapeutic exercises.
	Prolong ambulation by the above, plus surgery (musculotendinous release or transfer, spinal stabilization) plus lower extremity bracing as indicated
	Monitor for, and prevent, cardiac complication
	Manage dysphagia and nutritional concerns
Wheelchair – dependent stage	Enhance ADL independence with assistive devices
	Prevent or correct spine deformity
	Monitor for and manage cardiac insufficiency
	Maintain pulmonary compliance and alveolar ventilation
	Manage dysphagia and nutritional concerns as appropriate
The stage of prolonged survival	Educate the patient and encourage taking responsibility for management decisions and directing caregivers
	Facilitate ADL independence with assistive devices
	Introduce noninvasive respiratory muscle aids to assist alveolar ventilation and clear airway secretions

| Manage dysphagia and nutritional concerns as appropriate

Education for patient and parents/caregivers

After the diagnosis is established, the patient and family should be well organized by the case manager and must be well educated about the expectation and real results achieved by therapy and warned regarding also the different problems encountered and regarding the prognosis of disease.

Many studies sustain that the rehabilitation program can maintain the patient's quality of life, as well as maximize the patient's physical and psychosocial functions, an effective rehabilitation program hope minimize secondary comorbidity, prevent or limit physical deformity, and ease the patient participation in ADL. [14]

The physician should then assess the goals of patient and family and orchestrate a palliative and rehabilitative program that matches those goals. [14]

All the NMD can benefit from the different rehabilitation treatment techniques. The team must be always ready to face the acute symptomatology in the case that other new problems occur, or while different stages of the disease are reached.

Exercise hypotheses to improve strength

Outcome measures had to be at the level of body functions, activities, or participation according to the definitions of the *International Classification of Functioning, Disability and Health* (ICF) [8].

Individuals with neuromuscular diseases (NMDs) are characterized by a progressive weakening and loss of functional skeletal muscles [15]. Reduced functional muscle mass is common to all neuromuscular diseases and results from both atrophy of disuse secondary to a sedentary lifestyle and muscle degeneration secondary to the disease itself [16]. Fatigue is a significant

limiting factor in physical performance in patients with NMDs and it is likely to be multifactorial, related to deconditioning and impaired muscular activation [17]. Thus, the primary clinical goal is to maintain strength, function, independence, and quality of life [15]. Submaximal, low-impact aerobic exercise (walking, swimming, stationary bicycling) improves symptoms of fatigue by enhancing cardiovascular performance and increasing utilization of oxygen and substrate by muscle [17]. In addition to general health benefits and disease prevention, improved physical activity may provide a number of disease-specific benefits to people with cardiac, pulmonary, and musculoskeletal impairments, improved physical activity is likely to contribute directly to improved community locomotion and community integration and to improved ability to participate in a variety of recreational activities [16].

Cup and all, in a review article from 2007 summarize and critically appraise the available evidence on exercise therapy and other types of physical therapies for patients with NMDs (*Table 2*), and present the best evidence synthesis based on the information presented for each subgroup of NMD and each type of intervention [18], evidence synthesis based on a classification of the Dutch Institute for Healthcare Improvement [19].

Effective stretching of the musculotendinous unit requires a combination of interventions, including active stretching, active-assisted stretching, passive stretching, and prolonged elongation using positioning, splinting, orthoses, and standing devices. [20,21,22–25] For the Duchenne patient, K. Bushby and her team consider that as standing and walking become more difficult, standing programmes are recommended [26].

Table 3. Summarized and critically appraise the available evidence on exercise therapy and other types of physical therapies for patients with neuromuscular diseases [18].

Motoneuron Disorders	Muscle strengthening exercises Aerobic exercises. A combination of muscle strengthening and aerobic exercises. Lifestyle modification with or without muscle strengthening exercises.
Motor Nerve Root Disorders and Peripheral Nerve Disorders	Muscle strengthening exercises. A combination of muscle strengthening and aerobic exercises
Neuromuscular Transmission Disorders	Breathing exercises.
Muscle Disorders	Muscle strengthening exercises. Aerobic exercises. A combination of muscle strengthening and aerobic exercises. A combination of muscle strengthening and breathing exercises and mud/massage/bath. Breathing exercises.
Heterogeneous Group of Patients with NMD	Muscle strengthening exercises. Aerobic exercises. Muscle strengthening and aerobic exercises.

Stretching, bracing, and surgery for contractures and scoliosis

Joint contractures and scoliosis are also some major clinical problems in NMDs, particularly in patients with DMD and spinal muscular atrophy (SMA) type II [27]. In ambulatory patients, upper-extremity contractures may occur and can be complicated by joint subluxation, particularly in the shoulder girdle;

contractures appear to be related to maintaining a prolonged positioning, shortly after the patient becomes wheelchair-dependent [27]. Stretching and positional splinting may slow the progression of contractures, although the actual effectiveness of this has not been well studied or documented in the literature; surgical release of contractures in the lower extremities may allow a patient to be functionally braced. This may prolong ambulation, although a number of studies have shown that weakness, not contracture, is the factor that makes the greatest contribution to the loss of functional ambulation [27].

With regard to scoliosis, there does not appear to be an etiologic relation with loss of ambulation. Although both scoliosis and wheelchair dependence are age-related, several studies have found there to be no relation between the 2 phenomena. A large study by Lord et al reported an almost 4-year difference between wheelchair dependence and the onset of significant scoliosis in patients with DMD [28]. Patients with DMD typically develop scoliosis around the time of the adolescent growth spurt [29]. In DMD and SMA, studies have shown that thoracolumbar curves are much more common than lumbar curves; patients, especially those with DMD, should be monitored closely with serial radiographs because the curve may suddenly progress [14]. Unfortunately, correction of the scoliosis with fusion does not appear to improve pulmonary function [35]. But can bring some ease in posture and transfers.

Knee–ankle–foot orthoses (KAFOs; eg, long leg braces or callipers) for prevention of contracture and deformity can be of value in the late ambulatory and early non-ambulatory stages to allow standing and limited ambulation for therapeutic purposes but might not be well tolerated at night. Patient and caregivers must be aware of apparition of pressure sore that can diminish the use of othoses and replaced with other aid supports. Any patient with weakness due to an NMD may benefit from bracing, depending on the distribution of weakness, gait problems, and joint instability. The decision to brace should include the risk of the brace's added weight and the willingness of the patient to use the brace. [14]

National Institute of Neurological Disorders and Stroke Muscular Dystrophy [38] on their web page make also the next recommendations to help maintain the functional motion:

- *Support aids such as wheelchairs, splints and braces, other orthopedic appliances, and overhead bed bars (trapezes) can help maintain mobility.*
- *Braces are used to help stretch muscles and provide support while keeping the patient ambulatory.*
- *Night splints, when used in conjunction with passive stretching, can delay contractures.*
- *Orthotic devices such as standing frames and swivel walkers help patients remain standing or walking for as long as possible, which promotes better circulation and improves calcium retention in bones.*

Discussions and conclusions

NMDs are a lagre group of diseases that are presented in the rehabilitation clinics. The diagnosis of a neuromuscular disorder inevitably means the beginning of a new journey for the patient and his family they did not expect to be making. Rehabilitation management of this complex group of disorders is an arduous task under the best of circumstances. For this reason, a multidisciplinary comprehensive approach, as some key points we mentioned above, is more effective for

everybody. Many patients with severe NMD may now live through child-bearing years, possibly bearing children, and expecting to enjoy a high quality of life [39]. Patients, families and specialists believe that, even where before was not hope, the new technology era will bring more satisfaction and prologue life for many persons, not only increasing life expectancy but also improved quality of life.

Even the number of patients is not large in our Romanian district area, we notice that the terapeutic and care treatments are a majore component of those patients life after the diagnosis. The functionality and the normality in daily lifes of those patients are important from the patient and his family, and this is the major challenge for the rehabilitation therapist. To function on a day-to-day basis, is the single most important change of life and has greatly improved the social and functionality quality of life, doing things really makes life worth living for the NMD patient.

After we worked to this article we discovered some more need for us like therapists and for the patients also. Some of those are the facts that for all persons involved in the NMD care in Romania we need to improve quality standards for treatment and care, vocalization and do more promotional work of the NMD educational materials for physicians and patients, also do further research about the cost of care for patients with NMD, promote the knowledge. All of that can be done by implementing research multidisciplinary clinics and centers that include rehabilitation specialists, genetics counselors, cardiologists, pulmonologists etc. with the purpose to epidemiological, therapies follow-up etc. in order to improve efficiency of medical care.

References

1.Nanette Joyce, Craig McDonald (2012) Neuromuscular Disease Management and Rehabilitation, *Part II: Specialty Care and Therapeutics, an Issue of Physical Medicine and Rehabilitation Clinics*, Saunders,
2.Dombovy ML. (2005) Rehabilitation management of neuropathies. In: Dyck PJ, Thomas PK, editors. *Peripheral neuropathy. 4th ed. Philadelphia: Elsevier Saunders*; p 2621-36.
3.Cup EH, Pieterse AJ, Knuijt S, et al. (2007) Referral of patients with neuromuscular disease to occupational therapy, physical therapy and speech therapy: usual practice versus multidisciplinary advice. *Disabil Rehabil*;29:717-26.
4. DeLisa, Joel A.; Gans, Bruce M.; et all (1998) *Physical Medicine & Rehabilitation: Principles and Practice*, 3th Edition, Lippincott-Raven Publishers, chapter 61, Rehabilitation of the patient with diseases of the motor unit, p 1545:1573
5.Strehle EM. (2009) Long-term management of children with neuromuscular disorders. *J Pediatr*;85:379-384.
6.Diniz GPC et al. (2012) Motor assessment in patients with Duchenne muscular dystrophy *Arq Neuropsiquiatr*;70(6):416-421
7.Grange RW, Call JA. (2007) Recommendations to define exercise prescription for Duchenne muscular dystrophy. *Exercise Sports Sci Rev*;35:12-17.
8.World Health Organization. (2001) *International classification of functioning, disability and health*. ICF full version. Geneva: WHO,

9.Mutarelli EG. (2000) *Propedêutica Neurológica: do sintoma ao diagnóstico*. São Paulo: Editora Sarvier; 23-58.

10. Brooke MH. (1986) *A clinician's view of neuromuscular diseases,* second edition. Williams & Wilkins.

11. FowlerWMJr, Abresch RT, Aitkens S et al (1995) Profiles of neuromuscular diseases. Design of the protocol. *Am J Phys Med Rehabi*l; 74: S62-69.

12. Sutherland DH, Olsen R, Cooper L, et al. (1981) The pathomechanics of gait in Duchenne's muscular dystrophy. *Dev Med Child Neurol*; 23:3-22

13. Jansen M, de Groot IJ, van Alfen N, Geurts ACh. (2010) Physical training in boys with Duchenne Muscular Dystrophy: the protocol of the No Use is Disuse study. *BMC Pediatr*. Aug 6;10:55.

14. Gregory T Carter, Consuelo T Lorenzo, Teresa L Massagli, Richard Salcido, Francisco Talavera, *Rehabilitation Management of Neuromuscular Dise*ase, (2012) http://emedicine.medscape.com/article/321397-overview

15. Abresch R. Ted, Jay J. Han, Gregory T. Carter (2009) Rehabilitation Management of Neuromuscular Disease: The Role of Exercise Training, *Neuromuscular Disease* Volume 11, Number 1 September

16. McDonald CM. (2002) Physical activity, health impairments, and disability in neuromuscular disease. *Am J Phys Med Rehabil*; 81(Suppl):S108 –S120.

17. Sharma KR, Kent-Braun JA, Majumdar S, et al. (1995) Physiology of fatigue in amyotrophic lateral sclerosis. *Neurology*. Apr; 45(4):733-40.

18. Cup Edith H., Allan J. Pieterse, Jessica M. ten Broek-Pastoor, Marten Munneke, et al. (2007) Exercise Therapy and Other Types of Physical Therapy for Patients With Neuromuscular Diseases: A Systematic *Review Arch Phys Med Rehabil* Vol 88, Issue 11 November, p 1452: 1464

19. Kwaliteitsinstituut voor de Gezondheidszorg CBO. (2005) *Evidencebased Richtlijnontwikkeling. Handleiding voor werkgroepleden*. Utrecht: Kwaliteitsinstituut voor de Gezondheidszorg CBO;. Appendix A-1. Levels of Evidence.

20. McDonald CM, Abresch RT, Carter GT, et al. (1995) Profiles of neuromuscular diseases. Duchenne muscular dystrophy. *Am J Phys Med Rehabil*; 74 (suppl): S70–92.

21. Dubowitz V. (1964) Progressive muscular dystrophy: prevention of deformities. Clin Pediatr (Phila); 12: 323–28.

22. Hyde SA, Fløytrup I, Glent S, et al. (2000) A randomized comparative study of two methods for controlling Tendon Achilles contracture in Duchenne muscular dystrophy. *Neuromuscul Disord*; 10: 257–63.

23. Scott OM, Hyde SA, Goddard C, Dubowitz V. (1981) Prevention of deformity in Duchenne muscular dystrophy. A prospective study of passive stretching and splintage. *Physiotherapy*; 67: 177–80.

24. McDonald CM. (1998) Limb contractures in progressive neuromuscular disease and the role of stretching, orthotics, and surgery. *Phys Med Rehabil Clin N Am*; 9: 187–211.

25. Johnson EW, Kennedy JH. (1971) Comprehensive management of Duchenne muscular dystrophy. *Arch Phys Med Rehabil;* 52: 110–14.

26. Bushby K, Finkel R, Birnkrant DJ, et al. (2010) Diagnosis and management of Duchenne muscular dystrophy, part 2: implementation of multidisciplinary care. *Lancet Neurol*; 9: 177–89 www.thelancet.com/neurology

27. Gregory T. Carter, *(*1997) Rehabilitation Management in Neuromuscular Disease, *J Neuro Rehab*; 11:69-80, http://usuarios.discapnet.es/adm_peru/carter.htm

28. Lord J, Behrman B, Varzos N, et al. (1990) Scoliosis associated with Duchenne muscular dystrophy. *Arch Phys Med Rehabil*. Jan;71(1):13-7

29. Cambridge W, Drennan JC. (1987) Scoliosis associated with Duchenne muscular dystrophy. *J Pediatr Orthop*. Jul-Aug; 7(4):436-40.

30. Sussman M. (2002) Duchenne muscular dystrophy. J Am *Acad Orthop Surg*; 10: 138–51.

31. Shapiro F, Sethna N, Colan S, Wohl ME, Specht L. (1992) Spinal fusion in Duchenne muscular dystrophy: a multidisciplinary approach. *Muscle Nerve*; 15: 604–14.

32. Heller KD, Wirtz DC, Siebert CH, Forst R. (2001) Spinal stabilization in Duchenne muscular dystrophy: principles of treatment and record of 31 operative treated cases. *J Pediatr Orthop*; 10: 18–24.

33. Alman BA, Kim HKW. (1999) Pelvic obliquity after fusion of the spine in Duchenne muscular dystrophy. *J Bone Joint Surg Br*; 81: 821–24.

34. Sengupta DK, Mehdian SH, McConnell JR, Eisenstein SM, Webb JK. (2002) Pelvic or lumbar fixation for the surgical management of scoliosis in Duchenne muscular dystrophy. *Spine*; 27: 2072–79.

35. Miller RG, Chalmers AC, Dao H, et al. (1991) The effect of spine fusion on respiratory function in Duchenne muscular dystrophy. *Neurology*. Jan;41(1):38-40

36. Bakker JP, de Groot IJ, Beckerman H, de Jong BA, Lankhorst GJ. (2000) The effects of knee-ankle-foot orthoses in the treatment of Duchenne muscular dystrophy: review of the literature. *Clin Rehabil*; 14: 343–59.

37. Archibald KC, Vignos PJ Jr. (1959) A study of contractures in muscular dystrophy. *Arch Phys Med Rehabil*; 40: 150–57.

38. National Institute of Neurological Disorders and Stroke Muscular Dystrophy: Hope Through Research http://www.ninds.nih.gov/disorders/md/detail_md.htm, accesed on line 10.03.2013

39. Carter GT, Bonekat HW, Milio L. (1994) Successful pregnancies in the presence of spinal muscular atrophy: two case reports. *Arch phys Med Rehabil*: 75(2):229-31

16

Simple and effective means of treating the achillean tendinopathies caused by overuse, in athletes

Mârza-Dănilă Doina, Mârza-Dănilă Dănuț Nicu

"Vasile Alecsandri" University of Bacau, Faculty of Movement, Sports, and Health Sciences, Department of Physical Therapy and Occupational Therapy, Bacău, Romania

Abstract. Tendinopathies are frequent injuries, caused generally by an overuse of the tendon. The overuse hurts and disorganizes the tendon fibers, taking them weeks to fully recover. A coherent treatment should be based on the analysis of the biological and mechanical factors that caused the tendinopathy, and on the use of techniques that have proven to be useful for rehabilitation (evidence-based physiotherapy). For treating the achillean tendinopathies in athletes, caused by overuse, one can use a combination of sports massage and deep tissue massage; both methods imply a movement of the injured muscle fibers (replacing the effect of normal movement, which would constitute a risk), the appearance of hyperemia, maintaining it long enough to allow the treated anatomical part to respond to the following exercises, and ensure a durability of the effects, a fact that allows the athletes to perform better after the treatment. By treating properly and gradually not just the tendon, but also the attached muscle, and the proximal areas, one can ease the pain, extend the range of motion, and facilitate the healing process. The combination of these two methods of massage gives us a simple and effective means of treating the overuse-caused achillean tendinopathies in athletes.

Key words: *achillean tendinopathy, sports massage, deep tissue massage*

Introduction

Tendinopathies are frequent sports injuries, caused generally by an overuse of the tendon. The overuse hurts and disorganizes the tendon fibers, taking them weeks to fully recover. A coherent treatment should be based on the analysis of the biological and mechanical factors that caused the tendinopathy, and on the use of techniques that have proven to be useful for rehabilitation (evidence-based physiotherapy).

Current studies show that "the most effective treatments for tendinopathies seem to be, beside rest, cryotherapy, for pain management, stretching, for gaining more articular mobility, and progressively put the tendon under tension, performing especially eccentric exercises. In case of failure, radial shock waves can be tried. Any treatment of tendinopathies must comprise at least these elements" (1).

Among the factors considered to favor and/or cause the tendinopathies, there is (2):

• *Intense physical exercise.* Tendons allow the transmission of forces from the muscles, or from the environment, to the body. Physical exercise can be associated with both types of forces, intensely using the tendon. This can lead to the inflammation of the tendon - tendinitis. Tendinitis can appear after a too intense physical effort, if no time for recovery is given. Overuse of the tendon can be due also to an unbalance between the tendon and the muscle. If the muscle becomes too strong, the attached tendons will be overused. Intense physical exercise provokes an increase in the tissue acidity (acid energy), and the acid favors the production of uric acid, hence the apparition of tendinitis.

• *Decreased muscle elasticity.* When the muscle is not used to perform stretching exercises, its elasticity is reduced. A less flexible muscle is often a less relaxed muscle. The more contracted is the muscle, the more the sum of the tensions using the tendon increases. Muscle contractures during, or after prolonged efforts cause a poorly trained tendon to have its fibers in a permanent state of tension, which can lead to overuse.

• *Stress-generated muscle hypertonia* that uses the tendon is susceptible to cause tendon injuries. If the tendon can stand a passing hypertonia, normal when performing movements that can be taken to extreme in sports, a long-term hypertonia can make the tendon more fragile, and more vulnerable, as a result of bad gestures that exert forces on it inadequately.

Referring to sports massage, Meagher, J. and Boughton, P. (1984) wrote the following: "Repeated, deep compressions performed through muscle fiber stretching techniques in sports massage, produce not only a drainage of the tissues, but also hyperemia. The method causes the hyperemia to extend in all muscles, in depth, and over a long surface, persisting due to histamines and acetylcholine released through repeated deep compressions. Muscle fibers are worked in this manner, through separated stimulation, repeated multiple times, for improving their elasticity, contractility, and functional potential. By improving the muscle elasticity, we increase the freedom of movement for a longer period of time, because a supple muscle responds quicker to the demands of contraction and relaxation. Hyperemia leads to an improvement in the oxygen flow, and to a more effective elimination of wastes, thus delaying the anoxia, and the accumulation of toxins that provokes glycolysis."

Deep tissue massage is used mostly in treating posttraumatic muscle-tendon and joint capsule-ligament pains. In parallel with its painkilling effect, it can also lead to a functional re-harmonization by cleaning the proprioceptive afferents that were initially perturbed by nociceptive messages.

The mechanisms on which the effects of deep tissue massage are based on are (4):

• "The friction increases the temperature in the area where it is applied (a hyperemia appearing right in the area of the injury), which has a painkilling effect.

• The mobilization is realized on two levels:

- an entire mobilization of the tendon in the proximity areas, or a mobilization of the sheath on the previously stretched tendon; in the latter case, the transversal

massage eases the sliding of the tendon back in its sheath, smoothening out the rough surfaces;
- a mobilization of the treated anatomical part fibers, one after the other."

Material and methods

This study comprised 10 athletes with pains in the achillean tendon (above the heel), after a period during which they had a sensation of blocked tendon. The athletes comprised in this group practice various sports (volleyball, handball - within the Stiinta Bacau University Sports Club, and track and field - within the Bacau Municipal Sports Club). Their problems were identified during clinical and functional tests conducted in September 2012, and, right after that, were included in individualized treatment and training programs. Each athlete benefited, over the course of 7 weeks, of 15 treatment sessions (3 sessions in the first week, and 2 in each of the other weeks), consisting of sports massage and deep tissue massage. Each treatment session lasted approximately 15 minutes.

For the functional assessment of the athletes the following were used:
- examination by palpation, to identify the points of maximum pain intensity (signaling the stress of the tendon);
- test exercises, to identify passive and/or active signs that can suggest the injury of a certain anatomical element;
- a combined numbers and adjectives scale (5), to assess the pain felt during palpation and during normal,

tiptoe, and heel walking (in which 0 represents the absence of pain, and 5 represents a maximum intensity, unbearable pain);
- range of motion assessment for the ankle joint.

The tests were conducted at the beginning and at the end of the treatment period.

It has been identified in all of the assessed athletes, during the palpation examination, a thickening on the lateral-external side of the tendon (and an increased sensitivity in this area), and 2 points that were sensitive to pressure, one on the external side of the heel, and the other at approximately 7.5 cm above the ankle, also on the lateral-external side of the calf.

The testing of the lower side of the calf has identified the presence of pain during isometric contraction in inversion-adduction of the leg, and during passive dorsal flexion, and passive forced eversion of the leg.

The pain felt during palpation, in the stress points, recording values of 4 and 5, the one felt during normal walking recording values of 3 and 4, and the one felt during tiptoe and heel walking recording maximum values, associated with reflex pain contractures, had generated also a decrease in the ankle joint range of motion.

The intervention program was oriented toward dealing, through sports massage, with the 3 sensitive points identified during the palpation examination, and through deep tissue massage, with the lower side of the calf

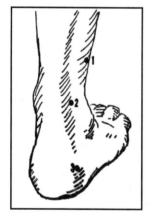

The treatment scheme used for applying the sports massage was as follows: $1P_{15}" \rightarrow R \rightarrow 1P_{+15}" \rightarrow R \rightarrow 1P_{++15}" \rightarrow R \rightarrow 1FL_{10}" \rightarrow R \rightarrow 1FL_{+15}" \rightarrow R \rightarrow 1FL_{++20}" \rightarrow R + 2P_{15}" \rightarrow R \rightarrow 2P_{+20}" \rightarrow R \rightarrow 2C_{15}" \rightarrow R \rightarrow (2C_{+15}" \rightarrow R) \times 2 + 3FL_{15}" \rightarrow R \rightarrow 3FL_{+15}" \rightarrow R \rightarrow 3FC_{15}" \rightarrow R \rightarrow 3FC_{20}' \rightarrow R$

Legend:
  P = direct pressure;
  R = relaxation;
  FL = linear friction;
  FC = circular friction;
  + = increase in pressure;

Figure 1. The points of maximum pain intensity (that showed the stress of the tendon) on which the sports massage intervention was applied

The lower side of the calf was approached while the patient was in supine position, his leg in abduction and slight plantar flexion, and his hip in a slight external rotation, applying transversal frictions, with low amplitude, and slowly moving the fingers to cover the whole area.

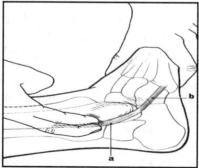

Figure 2. Deep tissue massage applied to the lower region of the tibialis posterior

Results

The removal of residual muscle tensions, the increase of blood flow in the treated areas, and the disappearance of reflex pain contractures, as a result of the diminished and/or disappeared pain, have led to the rehabilitation of the functional potential of the achillean tendon, and, implicitly, of the ankle joint. The range of motion has been considerably improved, or even completely rehabilitated at the end of the sports massage and deep tissue massage intervention program (Charts 4 and 5), while the pain felt during palpation and during walking was gone, or has been considerably diminished (Charts 1, 2, and 3). Only 4 of the athletes comprised in the treatment program, at the end of the 15 sessions, have recorded sensations of slight discomfort during palpation, and during tiptoe and heel walking. Also, the range of motion in these athletes was not completely rehabilitated. This situation called for an extension of their treatment by another 5 sessions (one per week), until the set goals were reached.

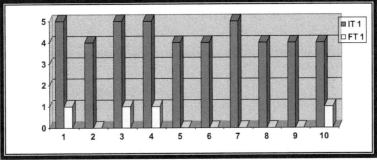

Chart 1. Development of pain felt during the touching examination

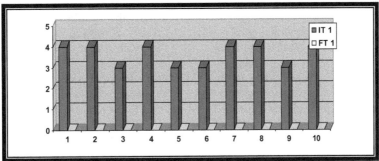

Chart 2. Development of pain felt during normal walk

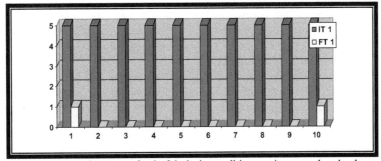

Chart 3. Development of pain felt during walking on tiptoes and on heels

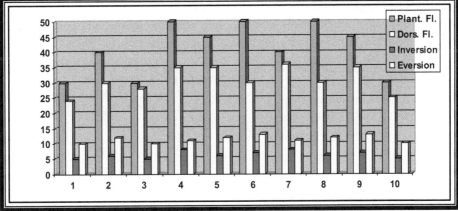

Chart 4. Development of the ankle joint range of motion during the initial testing

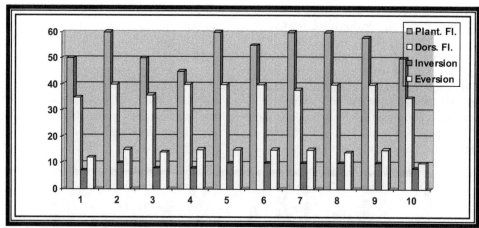

Chart 5. Development of the ankle joint range of motion during the final testing

Discussions and Conclusions

When a muscle is contracted (more or less), this does not affect only that particular group of muscles, but also the neighboring muscle groups, the result being a rapid and simultaneous drop in the muscle's ability to contract and in movement coordination. Also, the muscle that is in a permanent state of tension will overuse its attached tendon.

Any resistance opposing the normal functioning of the muscle (e.g. accumulated residual muscle tensions) makes the contraction process more difficult to perform, a surplus of energy and oxygen per working unit now being necessary. Residual spasms and muscle contractures amplify even more the resistance opposed to the contraction, and lead to a faster degradation of these areas, transmitting the fatigue faster to the proximal areas of the body.

Sports massage discovers these muscle spasms and removes them, keeping the body of the athlete in an optimal state of functioning, making it apt to perform its activity to maximum capacity. Either it is applied to the entire body, or on just one spot that is responsible for that particular discomfort, before performing the athletic effort, the principle of muscle fiber relaxation is the same: preparing the muscle to function at its full mechanical effectiveness, and to be able to perform the movement with full range of motion.

As the use of deep tissue massage is concerned, the following observations were made: at the beginning of the session, for 2-3 minutes, the pain in the injured area increased, then it gradually decreased, until it totally disappeared; after the decrease or disappearance of the pain due to applications during the session, the local pain reappeared, but at a lower intensity than at the beginning of the treatment; the gradual drop in the pain intensity (from one session to another) has confirmed the good development of the treatment (the pain disappearing completely after approximately 7-9

weeks); after the massage session, the tension of the tendon became less painful (at the beginning of the treatment), or even not painful at all (toward the end of the treatment).

Therefore, at the end of this study, the following conclusions can be drawn:

Sports massage, by acting on sensitive points that signal the achillean tendon stress, can be used effectively to fight the residual muscle contractures, to fight pain, and to functionally rehabilitate the structures on which it acts.

Deep tissue massage, acting directly on the injured tendon, can be used to fight the pain localized in that spot, to prevent and/or fight the posttraumatic or post-inflammatory adherences, and to rehabilitate the functional properties of the tendon.

The combined use of sports massage and deep tissue massage in treating achillean tendinopathies caused by overuse, in athletes, contributes effectively to the functional rehabilitation of the tendon, by cleaning the proprioceptive afferents that were initially perturbed by nociceptive messages.

References

1.Gard, S. (2007), *Tendinopathies : quels sont les traitements efficaces en physiotherapie?*, Revue Médicale Suisse, Nr. 120, accessed 15.07.2010, www.medhyg.ch
2.Hess, G.P., Cappiello, W.L., Poole, R.M., Hunter, S.C. (1989), *Prevention and treatment of overuse tendon injuries*, Sports Med. 8 (6), accessed 10.01.2013, http://www.voloden.com
3.Meagher, J., Boughton, P., (1984), Sportmassage - un programme complet pour améliorer la performance et l'andurance dans 15 sports populaires, Québec, Canada, L'Etincelle
4.Cyriax, J.H. (1971), *Textbook of orthopaedic medicine*, vol. II, Paris
5.Raveica, G. (2008), *Terapia durerii – abordare kinetoterapeutică*, Bacău, Editura Alma Mater

17

Sociological study on an active lifestyle among students at the non-specialized faculties

Popescu Sorin, Cosma Germina
University of Craiova

Abstract. In order to achieve a standard harmonious physical development envisioned by the university curriculum, we considered necessary to develop together with the female students an awareness activity in which everyone to realize the importance of the physical activity organized for persons of their age and the multiple influences the physical exercise has on the body. The enquiry was made on 58 female subjects, students at the Faculty of Letters within the University of Craiova, office automation section, at the beginning and at the end of the academic year, period in which there were executed programs of aerobic gymnastics within the physical education courses. At the end of the experiment more than 85% of the subjects go to gym at least once a week.
Key words: exercise, health, motivation

Introduction

The American Association of Healthcare, Physical Education and Recreation (1970) consider that ―physical education is an integral part of the total education which contributes to the development of each individual by means of human exercise" (1). Everybody, regardless of ender, age, occupation, needs *exercise* in order to maintain all vegetative functions to a higher level (respiration, circulation, metabolism, thermoregulation) in order to fight the new physiologic attitude because of vicious body postures (from the labour process, incorrect sitting at the desk, and so on), in order to strengthen the muscles and nervous system. We especially advocate for the ―sport for all" concept, where the benefit is particularly high, considering the low exercise rate for most members of the society. The individual benefits which an active person has are both physical – *a better lung capacity and cardiovascular functionality, stronger muscles, the person rests and sleeps better, lifts, pushes and pulls easier, is more resistant to effort, has surplus energy, is full of life, energetic, has a correct body posture, has a low risk of illness, both* psychological and social – *is able to withstand stress, is good-humoured, cheerful, quits smoking easier, has more time for herself, is sociable and makes new friends, upkeeps pleasant conversations (2).* In the past three decades, the demands of ordinary life increased, and along with them the lack of exercise, both young and adults. The phenomenon has been globally noticed, which lead to efforts of the organizations interested in human health to recommend and *stimulate making exercises* ―atall ages, for the entire life―.Among the indicators of quality of life we also find health, stimulated and maintained by exercise, but not by any kind of exercise, but by rational, systematic exercise, which became a habit (3).

To form a controlled, figurable body posture, – however modifying the tonus and aiming an elevated body tonicity leads to emotional changes of the structure of personality, improving self-image, self-confidence, creating the joy of looking and being fine.

Material and Method

In order to show the extent to which the female students are interested in physical exercise we have made a survey by means of the quiz, which helped to discover the reasons for which the inquired persons wish to make physical activity and the expected effects thereof. In order to get acquainted with the reasons for which the subjects included in research wish to make physical activity and the expected effects thereof, we have elaborated a multiple-choice quiz made up of 8 questions, which aims to evaluate the following elements: the concept of active living, exercise and health; making physical exercises, aerobic gymnastics. The quiz has been answered by 58 female respondents, female students at the Faculty of Letters of the University of Craiova, Office support section, at the beginning and the end of the academic year, during which aerobic gymnastics programs have been conducted within the physical education classes.

Results

Processing and interpretation of the investigation results consisted of the denudation and analysis operations of the obtained results. During the denudation we have checked the completeness and accuracy of the answers given by the inquired respondents. The analysis of the obtained results has been made in terms of the objectives and hypotheses of the investigation. The answers have been classified and analyzed in detail. The McNemar test has been used for the dichotomous items (applicable for nominal variables, for two independent samples) indicating the number of subjects who have changed or not their opinion after getting through the aerobic gymnastics lessons proposed for the experiment. For the other items, with multiple-choice answers, the frequencies and percentages of total subjects have been calculated.

Table 1. *The important activities for respondents in an active life*

What activities do you consider more important in an active life?	T_i		T_f	
	Nr.	%	Nr.	%
Sporting activities	14	24,14	34	58,62
Complementary professional activities	4	6,90	2	3,45
Friends meetings	21	36,21	15	25,86
Disco, entertainment	15	25,86	5	8,62
Housework	1	1,72	0	0,00
Others	3	5,17	2	3,45
Total	58	100,00	58	100,00

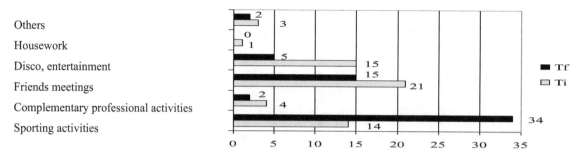

Figure 1 *The important activities for respondents in an active life*

At the initial testing, the sporting activities are the most important in an active life for 24.14 % of the subjects, while at the final testing this percentage increases to 58.62%. The friends meetings also occupy an important place – 36.21% at the initial testing, and 25.86% at the final testing. For 25.86% of the female students, participating in entertainment is an important element in active life, this percentage decreasing to 8.62% at the end of the research.

Table 2 *Exercise is for my health*

Exercise for my health is:	T_i		T_f	
	No.	%	Nr.	%
Very important	21	36,21	29	50
Important	18	31,03	24	41,38
Little important	12	20,69	5	8,62
Not important	7	12,07	0	0
Total	58	100,00	58	100,00

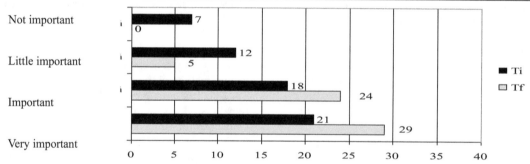

Figure 2 *Exercise is for my health*

For more than 60% of the enquired subjects, the exercise is important and very important in order to have a good health condition. This percent rises to over 90% at the end of the research.

Table 3 *Exercise and health*

Exercise and health:	T_i		T_f	
	No.	%	Nr.	%
I exercise enough to maintain my health	26	44,83	34	58,62
I don't exercise enough to maintain my health	14	24,14	24	41,38
I don't know	18	31,03	0	0
Total	58	100,00	58	100,00

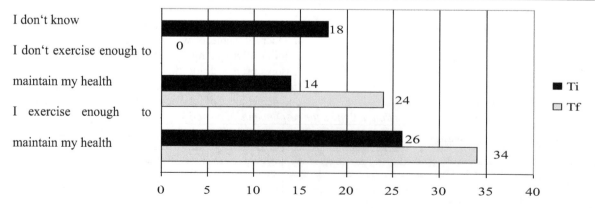

Figure 3 *Exercise and health*

Only 44.83% of the female students say they exercise enough to maintain their health, the percentage increasing to 58.62% at the end.

Table 4 *I do physical exercises in my free time*

I do physical exercises in my free time:	T_i		T_f	
	No.	%	Nr.	%
Never	17	29,31	0	0,00
Once a week	20	34,48	16	27,59
Several times a week	16	27,59	34	58,62
Every day	5	8,62	8	13,79
TOTAL	58	100,00	58	100,00

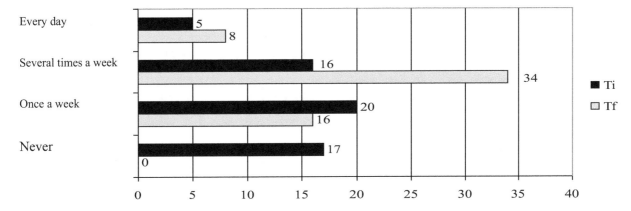

Figure 4 *I do physical exercises in my free time*

Physical exercises are practiced several times a week by 27.59% of the subjects at the beginning of the academic year. After the performance of the aerobic gymnastics program, the percent increases to 58.62%, the other female students making physical exercises once or several times a week.

If at the beginning of the experiment 36.21% of the female students considered they mainly make the physical exercises to maintain their health, at the end the percent was of 50%. At the end, a percent of 18.97% considers that by making physical exercises you get a great muscle shape.

Table 5 *Reasons for practicing aerobic gymnastics*

	T_i		T_f	
	No.	%	Nr.	%
Harmonious physical development	14	24,14	37	63,79
Weight loss	19	32,76	16	27,59
Socialization	4	6,90	3	5,17
Mental balance	3	5,17	2	3,45
Others	1	1,72	0	0,00
I don't practice	17	29,31	0	0,00
Total	58	100,00	58	100,00

32.76% of respondents practice aerobic gymnastics for weight loss, and 24.14% for a harmonious physical development. The socialization is chosen only by 6.9% of the female students.

At the end of the experiment 63.79% of the subjects consider that they practice aerobic gymnastics for a harmonious physical development, while 27.59% say that it contributes to their weight loss.

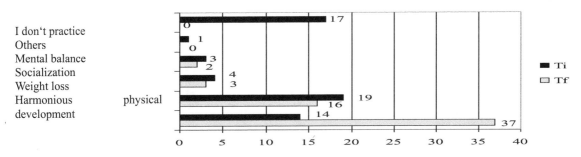

Figure 5 *Reasons for practicing aerobic gymnastics*

Table 6 Period of practicing aerobic gymnastics

I've been practicing aerobic gymnastics:	T$_i$	
	No.	%
For several months	3	5,17
for a year	4	6,90
For more than a year	9	15,52
Occasionally	25	43,10
I don't practice	17	29,31
Total	58	100,00

More than 70% of the subjects practice aerobic gymnastics, the frequency of the training variable, 43.1% of them practicing it occasionally. At the end of the experiment, 29.31% of the female students, who initially didn't practice aerobic gymnastics, go to gyms. The question was asked only in the initial phase of the project. In the final phase it had no sense as the subjects have constantly attended the aerobic gymnastics classes during the experiment.

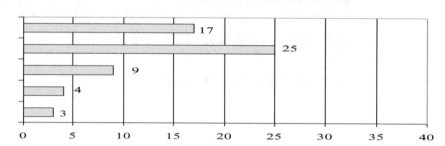

Figure 6 Period of practicing aerobic gymnastics

Table 7 *Attendance at aerobic gymnastics*

I attend the aerobic gymnastics gym:	T$_i$		T$_f$	
	No.	%	Nr.	%
One session a week	17	29,31	31	53,45
Two sessions a week	16	27,59	19	32,76
Three sessions a week	6	10,34	6	10,34
More	2	3,45	2	3,45
Never	17	29,31	0	0,00
Total	58	100,00	58	100,00

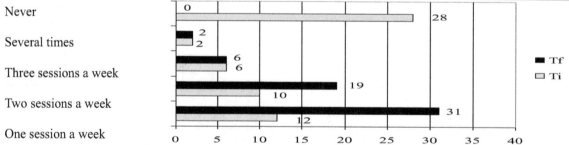

Figure 7 *Attendance at aerobic gymnastics*

Regarding the training attendance in a week, more than half of the female students attend a session or two, while only 3.5% attend the gym several times. At the end of the experiment more than 85% of the female students go to gym at least one session a week.

When using the McNemar test, it has been noticed that the number of female students whose choice changed after practicing the sessions of aerobic gymnastics is 21, while 37 subjects haven't changed their choice from the initial test. (Table 9)

Table 9 McNemar test

Final	Initial	
	Yes	No
Yes	26	0
No	21	11

The significance level being less than 0.01, it results that it existed a significant change in the number of subjects who changed their answer to the question after getting through the session of aerobic gymnastics. (Table 10)

Table 10 McNemar test

	Final and initial	
N	58	
Exact Sig. (2-tailed)	.000	

Conclusion

The interest showed by the female students during the experiment, to have an active, efficient, conscious participation, has given the best results regarding the performed activity.

The increased efficiency has been achieved as a result of the rigorous organization of the gymnastics lessons, particularly consisting of attractive exercises, individualization through personal conversations, counselling, and implementation of the desire to exercise. The attractive physical education lessons have a variety of aspects on the training process itself. Implementing the theories of modern didactics, integrating them in the lesson systems, we have created a systemic model and a broader training and educational system of the female students. The female students of the investigated group have acquired practical experience, beliefs to support this leisure activity and certainly strong motivations which contributed to the systemic participation and not to sporadic participation in the aerobic gymnastics program. They have understood that only by practicing constant exercise throughout life one can get all the other benefits of exercise – health, a special body posture, good humour, "well-being", an optimal weight.

References
1. Dragnea A., (2002), T*eoria educaţiei fizice şi sportului*, Editia a II-a, Editura F.E.S.T., Bucharest, p. 27
2. Popescu S., (2009), *Căi şi mijloace atractive pentru promovarea in rândul studentelor a principiului vieţii active*, PhD Thesis, UNEFS, Bucharest, *p.29*
3. M. Epuran, (2006), *Caracterul autoplastic al unor activitati corporale*, UNEFS, Bucharest

18

Sociological study on the use of psychomotility skills during the junior fencers' training

Forțan Cătălin[1], Popescu Cătălin[1], Mangra Gabrie[1], Popa Gabriel Marian[1],Podeanu Radu[2]

[1] University of Craiova,L.P.S. Petrache Triscu[2]

Abstract. This paper analyses coaches' opinions regarding the use of psychomotor skills in training fencers, mandatory approach which provides precise data on the current action methodologies in fencing. The questions referring to the use of the psychomotility components in the fencers' training, the sample used 40 coaches representing several sports clubs and schools in the country. The respondents consider very important the psycho-motor training, although not all work in this direction, most using less specific and nonspecific means to develop the psychomotility components.
Key words: *fencing, junior, skills*

Introduction

The role of psychomotor training of the fencers is extremely useful in the use of the strategies to be winners. The book is a manual for coaches and athletes who need psychological skills development. (1)
Learning and development of motor skills and techniques in fencing and other sports with open motor habits are based on perceptual processes involving the senses of vision, touch, and hearing. In fencing, the same stimuli can yield defensive or offensive actions, which are strictly related to the tactics and strategy. (2). The psychomotor education process that has as orientation the accumulation of certain behavior, which is gradually building basic components, belonging more or less instinctively, which contribute to a more accurate representation of body movements. The authors present also action means for the education and rehabilitation psychomotility through games. (3).

Material and method

In order to research the role of psychomotility in fencing we considered necessary the analysis of coaches' opinions on the use of psychomotor skills in training fencers, mandatory approach which provides precise data on the current action methodologies in fencing. We appealed to the sincerity of the respondents; the questions referring to the use of the psychomotility components in the fencers' training, the sample used 40 coaches representing several sports clubs and schools in the country. Of the 40 coaches, 12 have been employed in teaching up to 5 years (30%), 10 between 5-10 years experience in teaching (25%) and 18 more than 10 years (45%) having trained lots of children aged between 10-12 years. According to our research, the components of the psychomotility on which the experiment focused - coordination (static and dynamic), the rapidity of the movements can be positively influenced between the ages of 6-11 years.

Results

The survey achieved through a questionnaire highlights the opinions of coaches from Romania who with 10-12 year-old fencers training. After centralizing the data from the questionnaire, it is shown that 12.5% believe that the primary selection in fencing should start less than 10 years old. Most coaches believe that the best age selection is between 10-12 years old (75%) and a percentage of 12.5% of coaches considers that the selection should be delayed until after 12 years old.

Optimal age selection in fencing	Number of answers	Percent
Under 10 years old	5	12,5%
Between 10-12 years old	30	75%
Over 12 years old	5	12,5%
Do not know	0	0%

Table 1. The age of the selection

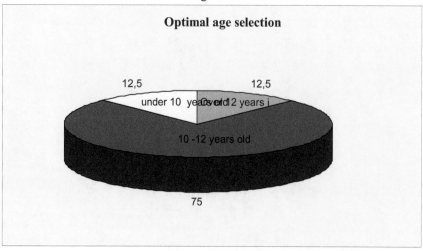

Chart 1. Optimal age selection according to the fencing coaches

Regarding the parameters taken into account in the selection process, the majority (85%) believe that the assessment for the junior fencers' selection must include, in addition to the somato-functional and motor criteria, the evaluation of the psychomotor parameters.

Decisive parameters of selection	Number of answers	Percent
Somato-functional	2	5%
Somato functional and motor	3	7,5%
Somato functional, motor and psychomotor	34	85%
Do not know	1	2,5%

Table 2. Selection indices

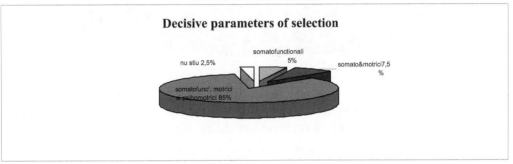

Chart 2. Selection parameters in fencing

On the third question of our survey, most of the respondents (65%) believe that action must be taken during the training on skills coordination and speed of movement of the junior fencers, which means we should actually act on the psychomotility.

Dominant psychomotility components in fencing	Number of answers	Percent
Static and dynamic coordination	6	15%
Speed of movement	8	20%
Both	16	65%
Do not know	0	0%

Table 3 Dominant psychomotility components in fencing

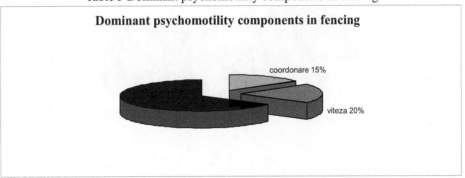

Chart 3. Psychomotility components in fencing

With regard to the means used to develop the psychomotility components, those were only examples of specific ways, some coaches (37.5%) acting on both components (speed-coordination), 22.5% consider most important the coordination and 35% acting with specific means for the speed development.

Means used to develop psychomotility	Number of answers	Percent
Means for coordination	9	22,5%
Means for speed	14	35%
Means for coordination and speed	15	37,5%
Do not know	2	5%

Table 4 Means used to develop psychomotility

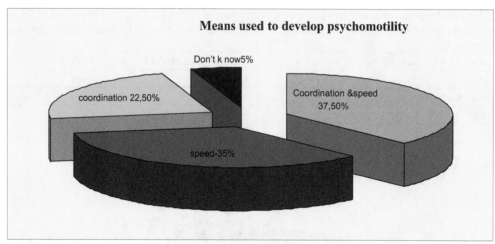

Chart 4. Means used

The last item of this questionnaire raised the issue of finding a new methodological guidelines, the majority of coaches (80%) believing that it is necessary to find new ways to develop the psychomotility components.

Development of a new methodology	Number of answers	Percent
Yes	32	80%
No	7	17,5%
Do not know	1	2,5%

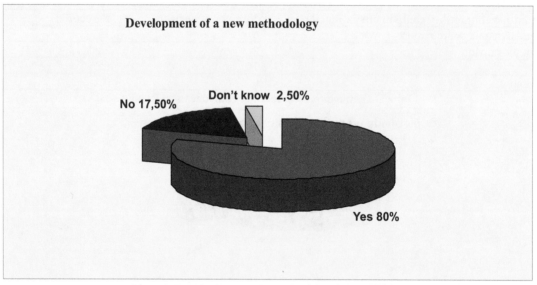

Chart.5. Developing a new methodological guidelines

Conclusion
After analyzing the questionnaire presented we conclude:
The inquiry performed by the questionnaire reflected the opinions of the coaches who are responsible for training junior fencers in Romania. The respondents consider very important the psycho-motor training, although not all work in this direction, most using less specific and nonspecific means to develop the psychomotility components. However, almost all (80%) consider a re-orientation of the working methodology that acts on training the junior fencers based on the development of the psychomotor index taking into account the fact that the maximum operating level on them is between the ages of 6 - 11

years. We also consider it necessary to elaborate work programs in order to develop the fencing psychomotility in view of the fact that there is little information currently in this respect in Romania.

References
1.www.fencing.net/training-tips/mental-training-for-fencing/psychological-skills-manual.html - accesat in data de 14.02.13
2. Borysiuk, Zbigniew1 / Waskiewicz, Zbigniew, (2008), Information Processes, Stimulation and Perceptual Training in Fencing, Journal of Human Kinetics. Volume 19, Issue -1, Pages 63–82
3. Albu C., Albu,A., Vlad T., Iacob I., (2006), *Psihomotricitatea – Metodologia educarii si reeducarii psihomotrice,* Bucuresti

19

Role of Mass-media for Promoting a Physically Active Lifestyle

Păsărin Daniel[1], Orţănescu Dorina[2]

[1]*National University of Physical Education and Sport, Bucharest, Romania*
[2]*University of Craiova, Faculty of Physical Education and Sport, Romania*

Abstract. This paper is counting the impact of the radio programs focused on the potential benefits of sports on the grown-ups' action determination. Thus, we have applied the inquiry method. For this reason, we have elaborated a questionnaire including 10 items and we have used it for a group of 60 persons made up of 30 men and 30 women aged between 20 and 40; these subjects being selected among those who listened at least once Radio Craiova Oltenia broadcast airing information concerning an active lifestyle through physical exercise, promoted under the slogan –Sports means life, enjoy sports." The inquiry indicates us the fact that grown-ups are aware of the role of the physical exercise for an optimum health condition, one of the reasons for which they are practicing sports activities during their spare time. We may conclude that the way in which the spare time is spent, highly depends on the individual's education and on the information the individual receives from exterior sources. The results deriving from the data interpretation, during the questionnaire, indicate us that most of the subjects positively appreciate the broadcasts on this topics and consider that the promotion of an active lifestyle through mass media means may considerably improve the quality of their life.
Key words: radio, active, lifestyle.

Introduction

Nowadays, in highly developed countries, sports activity, in its broad meaning – sports for everyone, sports for health, represents a state policy, a performance and a viability criteria of the social system, and on the European level, the area concerns, efforts and achievements are much more numerous and substantial. Concerning the effects of the sports practice, as physical exercise, on the psyche, it is stated that the aerobic and fitness activities, but also, the competitive sports, such as tennis, volleyball and football, *reduce* the short-term*anxiety*, as well as the *depression* (longer-term depression)(1). The persons in charge of promoting an active and healthy lifestyle have always confirmed the educational potential of sports and exploit it by integrating it into educational policies and actions meant to improve people's life quality, particularly, their health.(2).

Method

In order to point out the impact of the radio programs focused on the potential benefits of sports on the grown-ups' action determination, we have applied the inquiry method. For this reason, we have elaborated a questionnaire including 10 items and we have used it for a group of 60 persons made up of 30 men and 30 women aged between 20 and 40; these subjects being selected among those who listened at least once Radio Craiova Oltenia broadcast airing information concerning an active lifestyle through physical exercise, promoted under the slogan —Sorts means life, enjoy sports." The questions addressed had as an objective the identification of the impact of mass media on the current lifestyle of adults, of the obstacles encountered in sports activity practice, of their choices for certain sports disciplines and their direct involvement in the performance of certain motor structures according to a radio or TV show recommendation.

Results

Following the questionnaire, we have observed that:
From the 60 selected subjects , 30 of them are women and 30 men.
Among the 60 responders, 35 are aged between 20 and 35 years, 14 register ages varying from 35 to 50 years, 10 have ages between 50 and 65 years and 1 subjects exceeds the age of 65.
Most of the responders (72%) are highly educated, 25% have finished the high school and 3% are post-graduated.
To the question concerning the spare time, 75%, meaning, 45 subjects assert the fact that they spend their spare time through physical activities, while 15 subjects admit that they do not practice physical activities during their spare time. (chart 1)

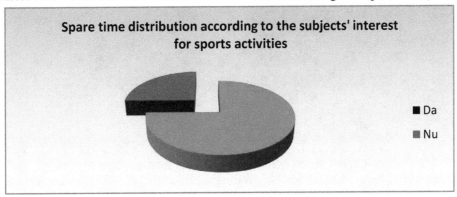

Chart 1. Spare time distribution according to the subjects' interest for sports activities

Among the 60 responders, 10 practice physical exercises several times per week (1-3 times), 35 of them on a weekly basis, while 15 on a monthly basis.

Most of the interviewed subjects (70%) consider that as a first obstacle in practicing sports activities is the lack of time, being, thus, unable to allocate time to such activities. 17% of the subjects do not afford to attend a sports club or a gym and 13% of them invoke other reasons which restrain them from practicing sports. (chart 2).

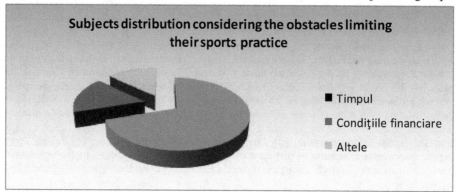

Chart 2. Subjects distribution considering the obstacles limiting their sports practice

To the question referring to the primary components necessary for the improvement of the life quality, 34% consider that the nutrition is the most important, 25% opt for the frequent practice of physical exercises, 20% hope for stress factors elimination, 13% consider that, through relaxation, the quality of life is improved, while 8% vote in favor of the entertainment as a basic component of an improved quality of life. (chart 3)

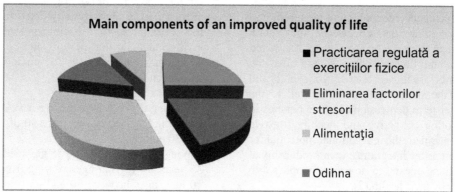

Chart 3. Main components of an improved quality of life

Considering the preferred sports disciplines the subjects are currently practicing or wish to practice, we have achieved the following data:

• 11 of the male subjects (37%) consider football as a primary sports discipline, 4 of them (13%) wish to practice tennis, 9 (30%) attend or wish to attend fitness programs and 6 of them (20%) enjoy jogging. (Figure no 4)

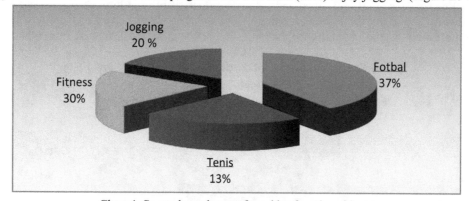

Chart 4. Sports branches preferred by female subjects

15 female responders (50%) have practiced aerobic gymnastics, 10 of them (33.3%) attend or wish to attend dance classes, 5 (17%) are interested in swimming disciplines. None of the female responders practice sports games. (Figure no 5)

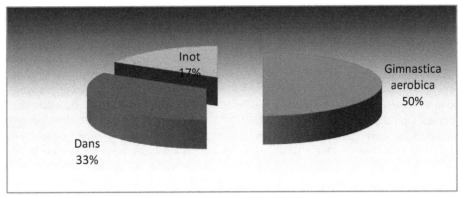

Chart 5. Sports branches preferred by female subjects

• Analyzing the opinions of the 60 subjects, most of them (62%) prefer to perform independently sports activities, for example, football with the friends, jogging, while 38% of the subjects, mostly women, practice organized physical exercises (sports clubs, gyms).

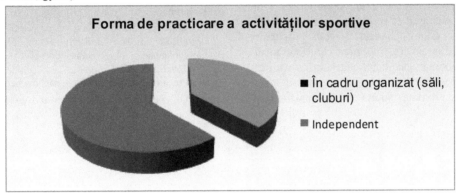

Chart 6. Forms of sports activity practice

Even though, lately, numerous gyms are open in Craiova city, most of the subjects (78%) are not satisfied with them. They consider that there are not enough spaces equipped for sports practice, being exposed to numerous risks and the parks are very crowded. The individuals who are not satisfied with sports courts are those who afford to attend a private sports club.

Being selected among the auditors of Radio Oltenia Craiova station broadcast, 58 of them frequently catch radio programs providing sports information.

A large number of the interviewed individuals (75%) appreciate the positive effects generated by certain shows promoting an active and healthy lifestyle through sports, being highly convinced that the message they transmit may lead to an improved quality of life.

Asked whether the project —Sports means life, enjoy sports." may contribute to a reconsideration of their lifestyle, 33% consider that it has a positive impact on the quality of their life, 35% answer that it may be possible, 17% are not so sure and 15% believe that the project does not influence their lifestyle.

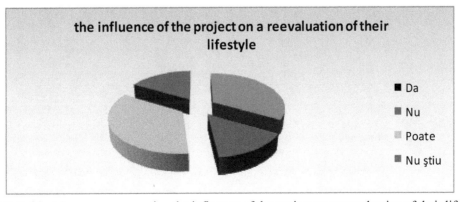

Chart 7. Subjects' answers concerning the influence of the project on a reevaluation of their lifestyle

Conclusions

The inquiry indicates us the fact that grown-ups are aware of the role of the physical exercise for an optimum health condition, one of the reasons for which they are practicing sports activities during their spare time.

We may conclude that the way in which the spare time is spent, highly depends on the individual's education and on the information the individual receives from exterior sources.

The results deriving from the data interpretation, during the questionnaire, indicate us that most of the subjects positively appreciate the broadcasts on this topics and consider that the promotion of an active lifestyle through mass media means may considerably improve the quality of their life.

The mass media means have an essential role in pointing out the potential of sports as a form of social integration and equal chances. Sports thematic broadcasts should stress the important contribution of sports to the economic and social cohesion, as well as to the creation of well-integrated societies.

O society which promotes sports and understands its value, provides a strong component of the population health, of wellness and social optimism. Released from the necessity empire included in the working time extent, the subject is free to —consume" his/her spare time by interacting with those shows through direct involvement, his/her being reacting like a tuned-up instrument, the merger between the activity and the individual proving to be almost complete. Included in school curricula, highly frequent in mass media and assiduously practice by certain individuals, the sports activity is a modern phenomenon impossible to neglect. More and more people are aware that the practice of physical exercises provides a high quality of their lives, being really a formula (a healthy one) of fashion, all media channels turning to celebrities' support for transmitting this massage.

Reference

1. Iluţ, P., 2010, *Efectele practicării mişcării fizice organizate asupra calităţii vieţii, Teză de doctorat,* Universitatea —Babeş-Bolyai" Cluj-Napoca, http://web.ubbcluj.ro/ro/pr-acad/rezumate/2010/sociologie/sabau_gheorghe_ro.pdf, p.8

2. Official Journal of the European Union, (2012), C 9/75

20

Sport completes human condition

Chirițescu Ileana Mihaela

Department of Foreign Languages, University of Craiova, Romania

Abstract. „Sport completes human condition" –Bernard Guillemain says – thus mentioning the many benefits it brings in the personal development of each of us. In this paper, we want to show that game and sports offer every person the chance to assert his true personality. Practicing a sport is both a pleasure and a need. People choose to do sport because this way they manage to break free from everyday worries, to forget the shortcomings and build more self-confidence. The release of everyday stress - this is purpose of practicing sports for maintaining vigour of mind and spirit. Sport releases mind, spirit, it gives us freedom that we cannot otherwise gain. Therefore, people who practice sport for pleasure are always open to new ideas, creation, to perform the tasks that most of the population denies from the start. Sport doesn't only have the quality to liberate the mind and spirit, it has the great ability to shape the character and of course, the body. And this modelling of character and body is the more efficient as it does not represent a harmful process to human beings, quite the contrary. People shape their body through physical exercise. Sport organizes, calms heated spirits and burdened consciences.

Key words: *game, sport, passion, courage, development·*

Introduction

„Sport completes human condition" –Bernard Guillemain says – thus mentioning the many benefits it brings in the personal development of each of us. Starting from childhood, the child perceives sport as an activity devoid of responsibility. But the game is not without its share of „seriousness" because by playing, the child develops his/her imagination, creativity, team spirit, ambition, courage, devotion to team partners and respect for his /her opponents. We can tell a lot about the „game". The term was analyzed in specialized works, being given many definitions. „The game is a voluntary activity that can be done in certain limits fixed by time and place, following a rule freely consented and fully defined, followed by an end in itself, accompanied by a feeling of tension and joy and security that you manifest completely different than in everyday life".(1)

„Passion for the game can be compared to the emotion of hope that maintains all our actions, but equally, is crushed by everyday activities. Through sport, man escapes from everyday activities, thus managing to revive a totally new hope and stop fear which he overcomes. Therefore, this passion is somehow noble, it provides pleasure because it requires a „deliberate work" and does not know the disappointments of everyday life. That is why this passion is felt by ferocious souls".(2)

We can say that children play and adults practice certain sports. After all, sport is based on accurate rule-based games, in well defined conditions. Both, the game and the sport, develop techniques and tactics. „Games and sports train for life, improve physical, intellectual and moral characteristics, develop reflexes, muscle, attention, self-control, angry resistance".(3)

Game, sport and society

1. People feel the need to compete. Both on the playground and in social life.

Game and sports offer every person the chance to assert his true personality. The society we live in limits the chances for people to be themselves.

„Through sport, man finds what he lacks: freedom, invention, poetry, harmony, understanding from a group or a community. Game and sports are born from a necessity and fulfil a need. «People feel fulfilled only when playing» - Schiller said".(4)

Practicing a sport is both a pleasure and a need. People choose to do sport because this way they manage to break free from everyday worries, to forget the shortcomings and build more self-confidence. The release of everyday stress - this is purpose of practicing sports for maintaining vigour of mind and spirit.

Sports and game are not binding practices in human existence. You cannot compel someone to practice sport, at most, you can guide him/her to this activity. For example, a child plays because through game he feels the pleasure of discovering new things. The child creates a new world through play, a fantasy world filled with beauty and tests that he must overcome to feel a hero. The child is not required to play; he does so willingly, with pleasure and joy of discovery. Initially, adults, parents choose the toys they deem appropriate for their children. But not always, the toy the adult considers most suitable is, in reality, the child's favourite.

By convention, the toys are chosen according to the sex of the baby. Like outfits. But it is not mandatory that all girls should love pink and boys, blue. Equally, is not imperative that all boys should love toy carts, horses, and all the little girls should love dolls.

It is exactly the same when we choose the path in life. It is not mandatory that all girls should want to become teachers or doctors, and all boys, aviators or astronauts. It is true that the balance tilts towards the highest percentage. But the „majority" is not the decisive factor in making personal decisions. But individuality. And one of the best represented areas in terms of individuality and strength of character is sports. Moreover, a clear conscience is based on assumed individuality. The child becomes an adult when he assumes individuality. Child strengthens his self-confidence when he falls, bruises, stands up and moves forward. He does not only go on, but is even more ambitious and eager to accumulate more. Ambition requires courage, courage involves ferocious desire. And where else can we see these qualities more pronounced than when we practice sports? Any sport. At any time. But not arbitrary. Sport does not mean chaos, at all. On the contrary. Sport organizes, calms heated spirits and burdened consciences.

Sport releases mind, spirit, it gives us freedom that we cannot otherwise gain. Therefore, people who practice sport for pleasure are always open to new ideas, creation, to perform the tasks that most of the population denies from the start.

„Liberated through game, the individual gradually detaches from reality which he transforms, creating a new world, a world of amusing ideas and game. Excitement or fear is quite wanted in sports. They arise from real or perceived danger. Where would the fun of game be if we did not feel fear or adrenaline? Through human nature itself, people search for things that are afraid of, driven by their own will."(5)

Since childhood, life is a game or an excuse for constant playing. The child is delighted that he can play imposing the rules himself. Later, in adulthood, the adult loses this freedom of imposing his own game. Adults long all their life for freedom of being their own masters, long not to „play" by the rules imposed by society or tradition. Here is another reason why adults choose to practice sports. Practicing sports one become his own master, one feels stronger, or why not, a hero?

By playing, both the child and the adult want to assert their superiority to others. Nobody starts to play a game wanting to lose. In fact, such an attitude would not be normal. Permanently, people feel the need to compete. Both on the playground and in social life. People grow through comparison with others. They look up to models they consider successful and, driven by the desire to attain the performance of the hero or model, they compete with other people who have the same ideals. The whole life is a competition. People play to win something: respect, self-confidence, appreciation of others, medals, awards, diplomas, money.

Society we live in determines us to want extra, more and more. This is called competition. We are in constant competition. Even with ourselves. And perhaps this is the real task we must successfully accomplish.

From this test we must emerge truly winners. Competition with oneself is the most difficult of all. If one feels victorious within then one can certainly say he had a matching competitor. Himself. There can never be more dreadful opponent than oneself. If you have the courage at least to try and overcome yourself, then you have the courage to compete with anyone else.

The whole life is a test. As it is in sports competition so is in everyday life, man must overcome tests, standards, burdens. Full success comes when the game is fair play.

Real athletes and real people cannot feel truly fulfilled when they know that they have won the competition with someone's help or by means other than those required by the rules of the game. Any type of game: sport, social, personal.

As the game is self-affirmation and fulfilment of their desires, completion of life. If the game is not played by clearly defined „rules" and if „standards" are not attained, the human being cannot possibly feel

completely fulfilled. Because of the limits of human nature, you cannot feel the sun from anyone else's soul. But surely you can feel the one in your soul. To really play and truly gain, this is the only victory that can be recognized by everyone and cannot be challenged by anyone.

2. Sport sculpts both the character and the body

Sport doesn't only have the quality to liberate the mind and spirit, it has the great ability to shape the character and of course, the body. And this modelling of character and body is the more efficient as it does not represent a harmful process to human beings, quite the contrary. People shape their body through physical exercise.

Even if they come from different social backgrounds, although they have careers in distinct fields, people like to look good, to be admired, to maintain a long-term beauty, to be considered true models in terms of physical appearance, for their peers. Conservation of beautiful appearance, youth longevity represents things that can be considered true medicine for body and soul.

Some people understand since childhood that the only possible way to maintain the balance of life is in the nets of the idea of motion exercise. Marin Sorescu said that „aging starts with a sigh", and certainly premature aging occurs in people who do not move, and do not release themselves from the accumulated stress, through sport.

There are delicate tricks that people use to „escape" from the practice of sport, for example, they excuse by saying that exercise causes some discomfort or use as an excuse the long hours of work, or a requesting family life. In fact, all these ways to avoid physical movement are at their personal expense. The beauty of sports practice consists precisely in the release of all these shortcomings.

When we talk about sports, we do not mean professional sports, but the exercise so necessary at any age. There is no other activity that people do, that can be compared with the practice of movement. A slim and healthy figure cannot be maintained through starvation, or by avoiding certain foods, or by diets. Likewise, no sound mind can be maintained only by choosing strictly cultural programs or training. A balanced conscience needs a slender body and a free mind. And behold, whatever spin the discussion might take, whether we like it or not, we conclude in sports practice.

There is also some weirdness in people's way of thinking. When they are in the position to be parents of young children, adults guide their children to play; they buy them multiple toys, and even play with them. Parents prefer walking outdoors with their children. When children grow up and go to school, most often parents change their behaviour by limiting hours of outdoor play for their children. There are also parents who encourage their children to practice sport, giving them the chance for a harmonious development.

If parents stop the progress or limit physical activity of children, this kind of behaviour entails the desire of children not to attend sports classes in school. If in elementary school, children do not attend sports classes they are prone to exclude, when they reach maturity, exercise from their favourite activities. People only need determination to practice exercise outdoors. For walking, for ball games so dear to children, people need a dose of will and responsibility for themselves or for their children.

People have an obligation to themselves to find the objective pleasure to practice movement because the contemporary society does no longer offer the individuals the opportunity to find oneself through natural means. If science has advanced so much, in terms of power of chemical combinations, that people knowingly and voluntarily provide so often and so easily to their bodies, it is because of the lack of information that people have begun to trust the artificial rather than the natural.

The artificial, whatever the form and shiny packaging might take, can never be more effective than the natural. On the contrary. Therefore, the phrase „healthy mind in a healthy body" should be told by each of us at least once a day, and thought of, constantly.

At an early age, teenagers, because of the lack of credible information, prefer to swallow slimming pills, without being prescribed by physicians, rather than exercise.

Whether we like it or not, whether we admit it or not, lack of exercise leads to disease whose causes are sought in ways that have nothing to do with reality. It is very difficult to convince sedentary people that movement is vital. It is difficult but not impossible. It's strange to want to convince a sedentary person that joint pain are based on lack of exercise, that physical numbness that is the first step towards mental numbness and that this is the starting point of „disasters" regarding human beings.

Conclusions

To be confident, to feel the master of the world, to have the courage to face life - these are the elements that can only develop from a healthy mind and body. To have the courage to climb the ups of life like climbing a mountain - this is an attitude one encounters in active people.

A difficulty represents a question, the endeavour one gives to answer it, is the saving solution. It is true that it may seem easier to take things for granted, but it is certainly healthier to do it for you, in your own terms and personal benefit.

To practice sport can seem difficult when you have the alternative of swallowing some pills you were told they are the miracle of life. This is homework for all of us, regardless of age, social status, the hierarchical level of professional membership. Learning life practices for personal gain and benefit without feeling this as a chore - it is the way that people could choose thus daring to strive for the supreme.

References:
1. Huizinga, Johan, (1938), *Homo ludens, Essai sur la function sociale du jeu*, translated in French in 1951, Gallimard éd., apud Colette Becker, *Jeux et Sports*, Classiques Hachette, 79, Boulevard Saint-Germain, Paris, 1973, p. 4; Thèmes et parcours littéraires sous la direction de Jean Pierrot.
2. La Pléiade, Gallimard éd., *Les Arts et les Dieux*, «Définitions», apud Colette Becker, *Jeux et Sports*, Classiques Hachette, 79, Boulevard Saint-Germain, Paris, 1973, p. 5; Thèmes et parcours littéraires sous la direction de Jean Pierrot.
3. Becker, Colette, (1973), *Jeux et Sports*, Classiques Hachette, 79, Boulevard Saint-Germain, Paris, p. 9;
4. Becker, Colette, (1973), *Jeux et Sports*, Classiques Hachette, 79, Boulevard Saint-Germain, Paris, p. 9;
5. Becker, Colette, (1973), *Jeux et Sports*, Classiques Hachette, 79, Boulevard Saint-Germain, Paris, p. 10;

21

Sociological Study on Students' Favourit Sports

Chivu Daniel[1], Nanu Marian Costin[2], Cosma Germina[2]

[1] National University of Physical Education and Sport, Bucharest, Romania, [2]Department of Theory and Methodology of Motricity Activities, University of Craiova, Romania

Abstract. This study aimed to identify the preferences of high school students on the possibility of diversifying the syllabus of physical education discipline within the curriculum on school's decision. This survey involved 50 students who responded to a set of nine questions. Among the subjects mostly opted by the respondents, we have found Basketball, Dance, Volleyball, Tae-Bo and Pilates.
Key words: *physical education, preferance, students*

Introduction

Students' concern for new, exciting activities requires a reconsideration of physical education and sports media for their structuring in order to lead both to the domain's objectives achievement physical, harmonious development, health, etc..) and to the increase of interest of those interested (the students) in practicing exercise initially in an organized form and then independently, according to the opportunities of leisure, to the objectives and the satisfaction provided. (1)

Social practice has shown that the young generation has a greater appetite for relatively new sports (fitness, aerobics, tae bo, pilates, skateboarding, dancing, etc..) so that we should deduce the importance of the aspect that school must meet the requirements of students, offering, thus, new study contents in an organized framework. The need to display a certain physical condition daily , both aesthetically and in terms of health, is an important issue for the young generation. "Traditional" physical education is not a point of attraction anymore, the young changing directions towards new physical activities in accordance with the present day's requirements (2). The intention is not to give up what is currently used in schools in physical education and sport but to include, in addition to existing procedures, already checked in time, a number of alternative subjects in the school curriculum. The alternative disciplines that we propose based on the preferences of the subjects falling within the area of interest of teenagers, fact revealed both by the Romanian society trends and by what is going on in Europe and worldwide in physical education and sport. Approaching these subjects in the school curriculum

will contribute to the achievement of physical education and sport objectives, both in attractiveness and efficiency, and, doing it also, through the impact they have on the younger generation they are addressing. We believe that such subjects will improve the bio-motional potential of students by involving them affective-volitionally.

Material and method

The purpose of this study is to identify the preferences of high school students on the possibility of diversifying the syllabus of physical education discipline within the curriculum on school's decision (CDS). The sociological survey conducted by us can provide important information on sports subjects preferred by students, subjects that are not in the current curriculum, for a future reassessment of the CDS. This survey involved 50 students who responded to a set of nine questions.

Results

The term curriculum is widespread today, being the bearer of a new conception about selecting and organizing content and, more broadly, about designing and organizing learning in a particular class for a number of disciplines or a specific module.Maybe this is why all respondents answered affirmatively to the first question (Are you familiar with the concept and content of the school curriculum?).

To the question assessing physical education and sports activities within the curriculum on school's decision, 46% of students appreciate the physical education and sports activities in the school curriculum as important. Interestingly, none of the respondents consider these activities as

worthless,which is a good thing.

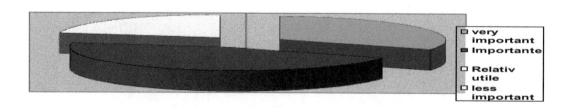

Fig. 1. The assessment of physical education and sports activities, within the curriculum on school's decision, by students (very important, important, relatively useful, less important)

To the question assessing physical education and sports activities within the curriculum on school's decision, those organized in the school, 60% of the students responded that they participated in such events.

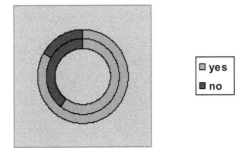

Fig. 2. The participation of students and respectively of teachers to (organization) the physical education and sports activities within the curriculum on school's decision

On the top sports disciplines necessary to be introduced in the curriculum on school's decision we have obtained interesting results.

Students have opted in large numbers for Basketball , followed by dancing and volleyball disciplines. Immediately below the top we gather among students' options two new disciplines, namely Tae-bo and Pilates, but this can not be considered surprising, as long as out of the 50 students -respondents, a number of 37 were girls.

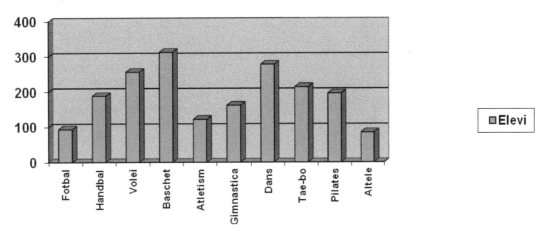

Fig. 3. The ranking of sports disciplines necessary to be introduced in the curriculum of on school's decision (students)

Analyzing students' interest in the physical education and sports activities within the curriculum on school's decision, we observed that 66% of the respondents state a great interest for the physical education and sports activities within the curriculum on school's decision.

Another question was related to organizing the sessions in the curriculum on school's decision. Half of the students surveyed believe the first version (organizing particular sessions for each class) as being the most useful. The next option has been organizing the session on classrooms at school level (24%).

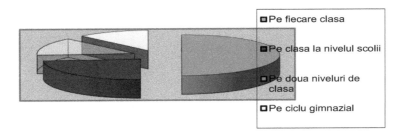

Figure 4. Organising the sessions within the curriculum on school's decision

As expected, the question on the number of hours in the curriculum on school's decision, brought expected results, a rather high percentage of 84% for the variant of 2 hours / week, which states almost everything about students' options in this regard.

Another question that got large percentages and expected results was that on students' participation in activities related to physical education and sport within the curriculum on school's decision. A percentage of 64% of the respondents consider the participation to such activities as obligatory. Other 30 percent were directed to the optional participation in these activities, and only 6% of students consider that their participation should be voluntary.

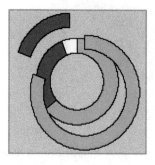

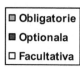
□ Obligatorie
■ Optionala
□ Facultativa

Figure 5. Student participation to the physical education and sports activities within the curriculum on school's decision (OBLIGATORY/OPTIONAL/FACULTATIVE)

The questionnaire ended with a question that will come as a conclusion to all the other questions and that will confirm to some extent the purpose of this investigation. Thus, when asked: Would you consider necessary a syllabus for physical education classes and sports in the curriculum on school's decision?, 88% said yes.

Conclusions

1. Physical education and sport are considered indispensable for the development of the individual personality, being an integral part of the overall education program for each student.

2. Following the survey by questionnaire we observed students' interest towards the physical education and sports activities in the CDS.

3. Among the subjects mostly opted by the respondents, we have found Basketball, Dance, Volleyball, Tae-Bo and Pilates.

Reference

1. Colibaba, E., D, (2007), Praxiology and curricular design in physical education and sports, Universitaria Publishing House, Craiova

2. http://www.edu.ro/Programe scolare accessed on 20.02.2013

22

Sports Activities and Leisure Budget of Students from the University of Targu-Jiu

Neferu Florin[1], Stăncescu Camelia[2]

[1]*University of Tg.Jiu, Romania*
[2]*University of Craiova, Faculty of Law "Nicolae Titulescu", Romania*

Abstract. The paper proposes a budget leisure radiographs of students from the University of Targu Jiu, in order to determine the place that occupy sporting activities occupy in their life. After applying a call and questionnaire-based surveys has shown a lack of a sporting activity among students, some of them motivated by the lack of materials needed to perform it.
Keywords: sports, leisure, questionnaire

Introduction

According to opinions issued by Duck, G., 2007, our age, leisure has become a social, educational and cultural problem, which relates to the same extent, society and the individual. Interested society as its going forward and progress of mankind depends on health, intelligence and creative power of its members.(1) In physical education can be developed a modern approach to non-formal physical education activities in university environment, in line with the interests and motivations of young people in a rapidly evolving social context and in light of their becoming later, the full development of their personality. (2) Sufficient physical activity 50 minutes walking, 30 minutes running at moderate tempo per day for 5 days per week, or 20 minutes running at a sustained tempo 3 times per week, subtract the number infarcts and heart

adapt more easily to changes in the intensity of effort in time, shrinks better and becomes less sensitive to stressors. (3)

Material and Method

In this study aimed to interest young people to exercise and an overview of the lifestyle of students (age 20 ± 1.5). Present research has as subject the study of students concern for sport at the moment, especially as practiced sport and recreation and maintenance, regardless of physical education classes. Method of leisure is thus a relevant dimension, referring to the activities it conducts subject directly, unconditionally. In order to understand the concerns of leisure youth through sports, we have initiated a sociological research based on questionnaire that included 10 items that were applied to a total of 50 subjects, 35 female and 15 male.

Results

Following centralization of responses, we found the distribution of hours in a typical day:

Activity	Average no. hours
Organized activity of school training	5
Reading	1
Hours of sleep	7
Fun activities	4
Sports activities	1
Watching TV and Computer	6

Table no.1 Activities during the day

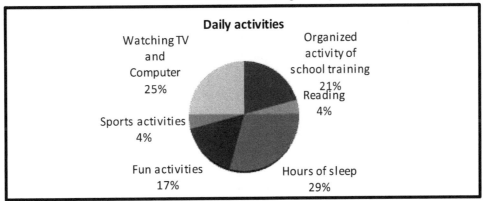

Chart no.1 Student's activities

It is important for budget tracking to observe the importance they attach to certain activities young menus daily during the week. We can see from the above table (table no.1) the fact that young people today manage their budget for the following:
- First fall sleep 7 hours, followed a short time spent in front of the TV or computer.

- Third ranks in the life of college students finds that activity by an average of 5 hours
    - Unfortunately, the last places are sports and reading.
Regarding the number of hours spent practicing sports at the weekend, the situation is as follows:

ANSWER OPTION	NUMBER OF RESPONSES	PERCENT
Between 5-6 hours	3	6%
Between 1-2 hours	28	56%
I do not practice this activity	19	38%

Table no. 2 Number of hours for sporting activities during weekends

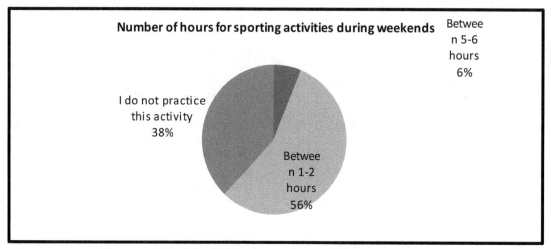

Chart no. 2 Number of hours for sporting activities during weekends

We observe that young people's interest in sports increase in weekend, phenomenon favored by the existence of a greater range of leisure, escape from everyday life. This is particularly important considering the social environment and lack of bases and places for practicing sports activities, of clubs to organize some sports events that do not require large financial efforts.

Despite these obstacles a rate of 6% of respondents practice on weekends between 5-6 hours of sports, 56% practice between 1-2 hours while 38% are not interested in such activities.

Obstacles in practicing physical exercise	Number of respondents	PERCENT
Time	15	30%
The lack of sports bases	13	32%
Financial reasons	22	44%

Table no. 3 Impediments practice sports exercise in leisure time

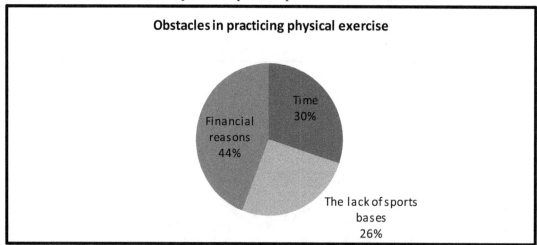

Chart no. 3 Impediments practice sports exercise in leisure time

Sport activities suffers not only from lack of time students (30%) but a lack of sports and favorable conditions of practicing sport, there has been a condition for those who have the financial resources necessary to cover the costs of within private sports clubs.

Regarding how sporting or recreational activities practiced at present the situation is as follows:

TYPE OF ACTIVITY	NUMBER OF PRACTITIONERS	PERCENT
Jogging	5	10%
Fitness	8	16%
Aerobics	15	30%
Sports Games	10	20%
Other (cycling, roller)	12	24%

Table no.4 Sports activities performed by subjects

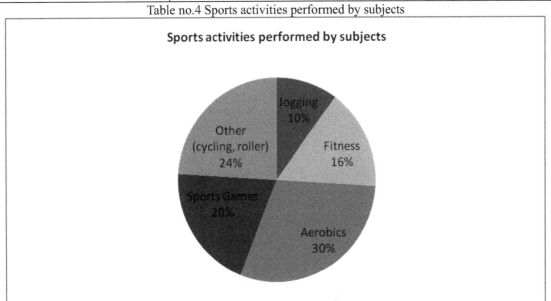

Chart no.4 Sports activities performed by subjects

Notice in Table 4 that 30% of respondents like the idea of practicing aerobic gymnastics, actually justified by the presence of upper female respondents, 24% prefer cycling or rollerblading, 20% are followers of sports-dominated subjects here male, 10% tend to run, while 16% attend fitness facilities.

Conclusion

In the study undertaken, we found that sports activities are underrepresented among students during the week, becoming for some of them, one of the favorite activities for youth as a means of leisure over the weekend. Unfortunately, there is a fairly large percentage 38% of respondents who do not practice any sports activity on weekends. Leisure arrangements depend largely on socio-economic context, the material conditions existing on the specific local traditions and not least the degree of culture of individuals. Practice of physical exercise in leisure is active rest, one of the most effective forms of rehabilitation and recreation of the body. Society and authorities empowered to be more involved in creating optimal conditions to practice physical exercises.

Reference

1. Duck G., 2007, *Free time management strategies*, Course for master, Ed.PIM, Iasi
2. Nichitov Florentina, 2012, *Non-formal activities and physical education. values, motivations and strategies formative*, Summary Thesis, University of Bucharest, p.25
3. Brîndescu, S., 2010, Benefits of practicing leisure activities, *Marathon, vol.II, nr.2,* http://www.marathon.ase.ro/4/brinescu.pdf

23

Sociological inquiry concerning the physical training to tennis beginners

Lică Marcelina Eliana, Dragomir Marian

University of Craiova, Faculty of Physical Education and Sport

Abstract. The paper aims at identifying the parameters of the physical training in the practice of table tennis players for discovering the weaknesses on which we should react and to point out the type of the performer in this sports area. For analyzing the role of the physical training in the practice of table tennis players, we have considered the need for achieving a sociological investigation applying the questionnaire method which has provided us the trainers' opinions concerning the use of working methods, a compulsory approach which reveals accurate data on the activity methods applied for this sports branch. According to the answers received from the interviewed trainers, the physical training plays an important role in the sportsmen's activity. Though the physical training is considered as being highly important, most of the trainers allot it only 30% of the training activity within the annual planning.

Key words: *table tennis, inquiry, beginners*

Introduction

The physical training includes a whole system of measurements which provides a high functional potential of the body through an intense development of basic and specific motor skills, optimum values of morphofunctional indices, full mastery of the physical drills applied and a perfect health condition. (1). For the physical activity the evolution of the general motricity is given by the level of physical training, which, in reality, represents the sportsman's ability of performing motor acts given different speed, force, flexibility, endurance systems etc., in order to develop individual and group actions which belong to the sports technique (2). Lately, the tennis game became very powerful, seen as a sport of speed performance, it transformed into a force sport, namely, the force for ball hitting.

Material and Method

The paper aims at identifying the parameters of the physical training in the practice of table tennis players for discovering the weaknesses on which we should

react and to point out the type of the performer in this sports area. For analyzing the role of the physical training in the practice of table tennis players, we have considered the need for achieving a sociological investigation applying the questionnaire method which has provided us the trainers' opinions concerning the use of working methods, a compulsory approach which reveals accurate data on the activity methods applied for this sports branch.

The questionnaire addresses to a number of 40 trainers and includes 10 questions, each one having only one possible answer and an accurate goal, namely, the achievement of certain real data on the way in which the physical training to the level of the table tennis beginners is performed.

Results

The inquiry undertaken by means of the questionnaire points out the Romanian trainers' and teachers' opinions involved in the training of table tennis players, aged between 8 and 11 years.

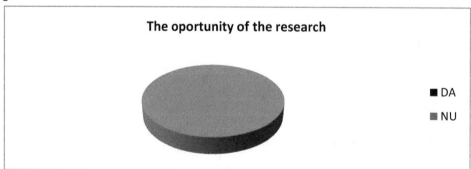

Chart 1. The trainers' opinion referring to the research opportunity of physical training to the level of table tennis beginners

The opportunity of a research concerning the improvement and the evaluation of physical training in table tennis to the level of beginners is clearly expressed by all the trainers submitted to the investigation. The unanimous answer shared by the trainers, confirms their interest for the physical training of the sports practice in table tennis.

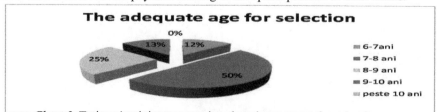

Chart 2. Trainers' opinion concerning the adequate age for selection

Considering the answers, 45% of the trainers agree on the fact that selection should include individuals aged between 7 and 8 years. A reduced percentage, namely, 11% places the selection process to the age level of 6 or 7, which is unexpected because this age interval is considered as being appropriate according to the criteria elaborated by the Romanian Table Tennis Federation (RTTF). Their arguments being the risk of losing them and, therefore, they would be forced to undertake a new selection after one or two years.

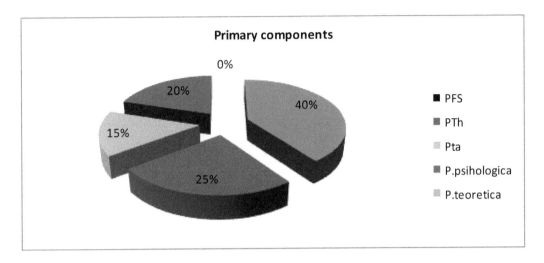

Chart 3. Trainers' opinion concerning the **primary components**

In order to establish the primary components of the table tennis training, most of the interviewed persons consider that specific physical training prevails (40%), followed by the technical training (25%), the psychological training (20%) and, eventually, the tactical training (15%). The fact that most of them have appreciated the specific physical training as being a primary component, determines us to allot it a special role in achieving high sports performances.

To the question concerning the importance of physical training in table tennis, all the responders (100%) have attributed it an important role.

Table 1. Trainers' ratings related to the current level of PT registered by their players

Current level of PT	No of answers	Percentages
- very good	6	15%
- good	14	35%
- average	18	45%
- low	2	5%
Total	40	100%

45% of the trainers consider that their trainees register an average level of physical training, 35% indicate a good level, only 15% confirm a very good level and 5% place their players to a low level.

Table 2. Trainers' considerations regarding the PT and the ThT ratio

PT and ThT ratio (technical training)	No of answers	Percentages
PT > ThT	16	40%
PT< ThT	10	25%
PT = ThT	14	35%
Total	40	100%

One may notice that 40% of the trainers attribute greater importance to the physical training as compared to the technical one, 25% consider it less important while 35% agree that they are equally important.

Table 3. Trainers' opinion related to the importance of PT for the annual planning

Importance of PT for annual planning	No of answers	Percentages
30%	20	50%
40%	12	30%

50%	3	7%
60%	3	8%
Other	2	5%
Total	40	100%

For most of them (50%), the physical training occupies 30 percentages of the total interval of annual planing, 30% attribute it 40% of the total volume of training, while 7% deal with physical training half of the interval.

Table 4. Trainers' opinion concerning the importance of GPT and SPT for the annual planning

Importance of GPT and SPT for annual planning	No of answers	Percentages
20% GPT – 80% SPT	12	30%
30% GPT – 70% SPT	10	25%
40% GPT – 60% SPT	5	12%
50% GPT – 50% SPT	8	20%
60% GPT – 40% SPT	5	13%
Total	40	100%

The interviewed trainers have different opinions concerning the importance of the general and the specific physical training in the activity programs of tennis beginners. Therefore, most of them consider that at this level of age, the focus should be on the specific physical training. 33% of the responders equally treat the general physical training or even more, within the annual activity program.

Table 5. Use of non-specific means in physical training

Use of non-specific means	No of answers	Percentages
- YES	24	60%
- NO	16	40%
Total	40	100%

From the total number of responders, 60% prefer to use during the physical training means which are not specific to the table tennis game and 40% occasionally recur to these means.

Table 5 Introduction of force training to beginners

Introduction of force training to beginners	No of answers	Percentages
- YES	30	75%
- NO	10	25%
Total	40	100%

For the physical training, 75% agree on the force training to the level of beginners, while 25% consider its introduction as being to early.

Results

The investigation based on the questionnaire has provided important data on the current working methodology applied by table tennis trainers within their groups of beginners. According to the answers received from the interviewed trainers, the physical training plays an important role in the sportsmen's activity. Though the physical training is considered as being highly important, most of the trainers allot it only 30% of the training activity within the annual planning. For educational reasons, we have treated separately the two training factors (physical and technical training) as they correspond in features and functions and interact with each other, as they do with the other factors of the training process, and, at the same time, these two factors adequately correlate according to the training period and stage.

Reference

1. Dragnea A, (1996), *Antrenamentul sportiv*, Didactică și Pedagogică Publisher, Bucharest, p. 163
2. Simion, Ghe., Mihăilă I., Stănculescu G., (2011), *Antrenament sportiv. Concept sistemic*, University Press Publisher, Constanța, p. 118

24

Role of gymnastic and acrobatic elements in volleyball players' physical training

Cosma Alexandru[1], Pascu Dănuț[2], Lică Eliana[3]

[1] National Colleges "Nicolae Titulescu" Craiova, Romania
[2] University of Craiova, Faculty of Physical Education and Sport, Romania

Abstract. The purpose of the study was to determinate whether gymnastic and acrobatic elements would increase the vertical jump performance to 12 volleyball players (age 16±1). They have followed a physical training program for a period of 3 months, 2 training sessions of 45 minutes each per week, focused on means specific to the gymnastics, namely, acrobatic elements. The scores achieved were compared to those registered by the control group, made up of 12 volleyball players having the same level of training, following similar tasks and a classic program of physical training. Applying the Student test, one may notice that for the vertical jump with take-off, touching a fixed point with one hand or both hands, the difference between the two groups is significant, certifying the value p – 0.023, which reveals an increased significance threshold.
Key words: volleyball, training, gymnastic

Introduction

The current standards enforced by the superior forums charged with the evaluation of trainers'/ physical education and sport teachers' activity, through which the fast achievement of sports performances points out the schoolteachers' merit, have automatically led to a short-term prognosis of performances through the early background of the volleyball player; the training adaptability being inappropriately figured in sportsmen's concrete and real training. Therefore, there are sportsmen whose results are acceptable just for a certain level of training, their way towards high performance and senior level being suddenly closed because they do not manage to handle top performance requirements; the physical training through non-specific means tends to be neglected in modern volleyball. (1).

Physical training includes an entire assessment system which provides a high functional capacity of the body through the high level of developing basic and specific motor skills, through optimum values of morphofunctional indices, an absolute mastery of all the exercises applied and a perfect health condition. (2) The great advantage of the practice of acrobatic drills combined with basic gymnastic ones consists in the mattress, a carpet or a mat, they can be well performed. The development of critical motor skills registered by a sportsman becomes insufficient when there are consequences which lead to a limited training, inefficient whenever various strategies and tactics are approached. Given certain game situations, when sportsmen are neutralized and defeated on their strong points, it is obvious that they do not dispose of suitable physical resources for changing the challenge range. A general conditioning and hypertrophy training along with specific volleyball conditioning is necessary in preseason for the development of the lower-body strength, agility and speed performance in volleyball players.(3)

Method

The present study aims at checking the working means and determining certain issues revealed by the recommended pattern. The subjects submitted to the experimental activities formed the experiment group, including 12 volleyball players (age 16±1) performing for the team of —Niolae Titulescu" National College of Craiova. They have followed a physical training program for a period of 3 months, 2 training sessions of 45 minutes each per week, focused on means specific to the gymnastics, namely, acrobatic elements. The scores achieved were compared to those registered by the control group, made up of 12 volleyball players having the same level of training, performing for the team CNMB School Ramnicu Valcea, following similar tasks and a classic program of physical training. In order to validate the working programs, we have chosen the following tests recommended by the Romanian Volleyball Federation:

1. *Vertical jump with take-off, touching a fixed point with one hand (cm)*
Objective: evaluation of the explosive force at the level of lower limbs.
Applied means: special scaled device allowing the accurate assessment of the jumping height; flat surface.
Trial performance:
The total height with the skillful arm extended is measured.
The vertical jump (the device placed above) is performed, with take-off from attack, lower limbs flexion and arm-swing, followed by feet detachment from the ground and touching the device with the hand. Two jumps are performed, the best score being registered.

2. *Vertical jump with take-off, touching a fixed point with both hands (cm)*
Similar to the previous test, except for touching the maximum height with both hands.

Results

Following the application of working programs, several parameters have been registered:

Tabel 1. Data registered by the control group when performing the vertical jump with take-off, touching a fixed point with one or both hands on experimental group

No	Subjects	Vertical jump with take-off, touching a fixed point with one hand (cm)				Vertical jump with take-off, touching a fixed point with both hands (cm)			
		Initial	Final	Dif.	Dif. (%)	Initial	Final	Dif.	Dif. (%)
	Arithmetic mean	306.08	308.92	2.83	1.17%	298.67	301.25	2.58	1.25%
	Standard deviation	8.21	8.17			6.77	6.52		
	Maximum value	318	323			308	310		
	CV	2.68	2.63			2.26	2.15		

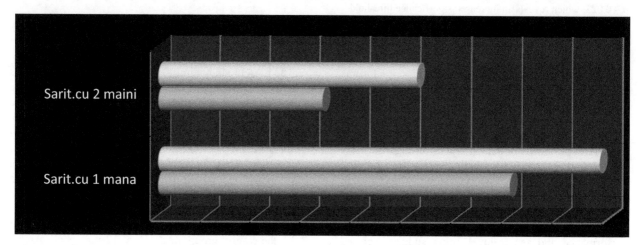

Chart 1. Arithmetic means for the vertical jump, touching a fixed point with one or both hands – the experiment group

Control Group

Table 2. Data registered by the control group when performing the vertical jump with take-off, touching a fixed point with one or both hands on control group

No	Parameters	Vertical jump with take-off, touching a fixed point with one hand (cm)				Vertical jump with take-off, touching a fixed point with both hands (cm)			
		Initial	Final	Dif.	Dif. (%)	Initial	Final	Dif.	Dif. (%)
		301.33	303.08	1.75	0.66%	293.5	295.08	1.5833	0.62%
	Standard deviation	7.31	7.5			6.73	6.7		
	Maximum value	314	317			304	306		
	CV	2.42	2.46			2.29	2.26		

For the vertical jump with take-off, touching a fixed point with one hand, the difference between the two groups to the final testing is 5.84 cm, the experiment group having a 3 cm evolution as compared to the score achieved to the initial testing.

When dealing with the vertical jump with take-off, touching a fixed point with both hands, the difference between the two groups registered to the final testing is 6 cm.

Applying the Student test, one may notice that for the vertical jump with take-off, touching a fixed point with one hand or both hands, the difference between the two groups is significant, certifying the value p – 0.023, which reveals an increased significance threshold.

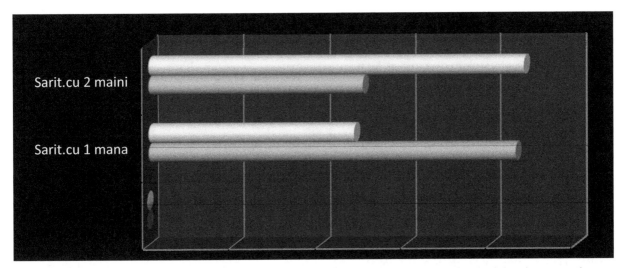

Chart 2. The arithmetic means for the vertical jump touching a fixed point with one hand or both hands – control group

Conclusions

The acrobatic gymnastics consists in a series of spectacular built movements mainly focused on skill, balance and development of the sense of orientation in space. They may be performed individually, in pairs or in group, to the ground or to specific devices, contributing to the improvement of health or to the optimization of the individual's physical and psychical abilities.

The charts of general and specific physical training should be well determined for each stage of training, and indicate obvious objectives in order to achieve an efficient training for the other factors of the sports activity; an efficient physical training is based on technical executions, on the manifestation of tactical resources and psychical education, establishing the interaction with other aspects of the training activity. Considering the means applied to the experiment group, we have observed certain problems in the execution of

acrobatic elements, fact which determines us to reevaluate the means applied for the present research. The tests applied for assessing the level of physical training to junior volleyball players submitted to the preliminary study, have confirmed the role of gymnastic and acrobatic elements performed by the subjects of the experiment group, the differences between the arithmetic means being considerable ($p < 0.05$).

Reference

1. Cosma A., (*2012), Studiu interdisciplinar de evaluare a nivelului de pregătire fizică a voleibaliştilor juniori,* Second report PhD Theses, UNEFS, Bucharest
2. Dragnea A, (1996), *Antrenamentul sportiv (Sports Training),* Didactică şi Pedagogică Publisher, R.A., Bucharest, p.163
3. Trajković N and al., (2012), The effects of 6 weeks of preseason skill-based conditioning on physical performance in male volleyball players,J Strength Cond Res. 2012 Jun;26(6):1475-80

25

Study of neurophysiologic pattern at handball and volleyball athletes

Enescu-Bieru Denisa[1], Călina Mirela Lucia [1,2], Brăbiescu Călinescu Luminița [1], Kese Anamaria[1], Neamțu Oana [1], Neamțu Marius Cristian [3], Cosma Germina [1]

[1] *Faculty of Physical Education and Sport, University of Craiova, Romania*, [2]*Polyclinic of Sports Medicine, Emergency Clinical Hospital Craiova, Romania* , [3]*University of Medicine and Pharmacy Craiova, Romania*

Abstract. Our objective was to identify a possible neurophysiologic pattern associated to the practiced sportive activities, by studying the electroencephalographic activity of handball and volleyball athletes. The study was realized on a group of 20 male professional players, 11 handball players and 9 volleyball players (different stress degrees of the upper members), active for between 5 and 12 years exclusively in either handball or volleyball. Using Nihon-Kohden EEG-9200 device, was recorded EEG line during some activities (relaxation-contraction), which can emphasize possible characteristic cerebral patterns, EEG analyze was made by assessing the classic rhythms. In order to perform spectral analyze was used fast Fourier transformation and for waves values comparison was used Pearson correlation coefficient. For handball players was remarked a high degree of correlation for theta and beta indexes and also a correlation in the dominant hemisphere for alpha1 and 2 waves, accompanied by a slight increase of theta waves values, in comparison with the volleyball group where the theta waves had the highest values and the correlation of EEG indexes was small. EEG complex testing of professional sportsmen, as well as the outlining of an EEG pattern specific to studied sportive discipline, represent an original aspect of this study.

Key words: *neurophysiologic pattern, electroencephalography, handball, volleyball.*

Introduction

Electroencephalography (EEG) represents the technique of cerebral electrical activity acquisition during a period time, through electrodes placed on the scalp and offers only partial information about the functional state of the central nervous system. According to frequency, one of the EEG specific parameters, were identified four types of waves (rhythms): alpha 8-13 Hz, beta 14-30 Hz, theta 4-7 Hz and delta 0,5-3,5 Hz.

Our object was to study the electroencephalographic activity of both professional handball and volleyball players, to compare the obtained data and to identify a possible neurophysiologic pattern, associate to the professional sportive activity which can objectify the athletes' selection and the efficiency of the training specific to the studied sportive disciplines, thus emphasizing the inter-sports differences.

Material and method

The study was realized on a group of 20 male athletes, 11 handball players, which use intensely both the upper limbs (with enhanced stress on one of them) and also, the lower ones and 9 voleyball athletes which use both upper limbs, active for between 5 and 12 years exclusively in either handball or volleyball, with average ages, heights and weights alongside the standard deviation presented in Table 1.

Table 1. Average ages, heights and weights for the studied groups

	Whole group males	Handball males	Volleyball males
Age years	20.06	22.00	21.83
Standard deviation	3.11	2.45	1.33
Height cm	183.81	188.25	191.83
Standard deviation	10.44	5.65	8.04
Weight Kg	75.65	78.75	87.67
Standard deviation	15.13	12.40	12.58

By analysing the age histogram for the whole male group, the age homogeneity of the group is noted.

Although there are characteristic weight differences between the selected sports, the analysed group is homogenous both from the point of view of weight and height and training regime. Taking into account the fact that the investigations took place in equivalent conditions for all subjects, we can state that the determining factor for the different behaviour of the administered tests were the changes induced by the practiced sports.

The studied sports were chosed, taking into account the more extensive representation of the upper limbs in the motor cortex, thus, a higher number of plastic changes are possible to appear as a result of repeated complex movements performed during specific training.

Our studies aimed to compare the two groups of sportsmen without including a sedentary subjects sample group, as the motor cortex did not display significant differences between professional sportsmen and sedentary groups (1).

The testing was performed under current ethical rules, each participant being informed of the experimental processes. All the investigated sportsmen have been subjected to electric-neuro-physiological investigations by measuring the EEG waves, using Nihon-Kohden EEG-9200 device. The EEG response was registered with surface electrodes which have a letter to identify the lobe (F frontal, T temporal, P parietal, C central, O occipital) and a number to identify the hemisphere location (even numbers refer to electrode positions on the right hemisphere, odd numbers to those on left hemisphere), placed on the scalp according to the electroencephalography 10-20 system (Figure 1), bipolar acquisition, 16 channels, the reference being the two ears (A1, A2), using a time constant of 0,3 seconds and a filter below 50 Hz. In consideration of the study objective, we recorded the EEG line during some activities which can emphasize the possible characteristic cerebral patterns.

So, the activities followed during EEG recording were: first relaxation time ((R1), right fist contraction (A), left fist contraction (B), right fist contraction order without performing the move (C), left fist contraction order without performing the move (D) (Figure 2). After every mentioned moment was recorded a relaxation time (R1-R5).

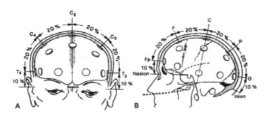

Figure 1. 10-20 electrode placement system

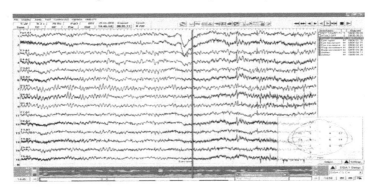

Figure 2. Modification of EEG line by changing an activity to another and the electrodes position

The EEG analyze was made by assessing the classic rhythms: Theta [4-8Hz], Alpha1 [8-10Hz], Alpha2 [10-13Hz], Beta1 [13-20Hz], we, also, used FFT (fast Fourier transformation) on periods of 10 seconds, for spectral analyze, thus, obtaining information about the whole frequency spectrum.

For wave values comparison was used Pearson correlation coefficient.

Results

For handball group, was remarked a slight increase of the theta wave values, during entire recording, as showed in Table 2.

Table 2. Theta values at handball group for every studied moments

channel	R1	A	R2	B	R3	C	R4	D	R5
T5-A1	0.275	0.582	0.511	0.597	0.263	0.189	0.330	0.252	0.504
T3-A1	0.787	0.681	0.786	1.334	1.259	1.119	0.665	0.739	0.602
F7-A1	0.328	0.237	0.261	0.359	0.285	0.232	0.329	0.254	0.281
O1-A1	0.789	0.700	0.869	1.014	1.263	0.974	0.731	0.670	0.627
P3-A1	0.446	0.445	2.652	0.478	0.531	0.420	0.505	0.444	0.475
C3-A1	0.549	0.546	0.581	1.271	0.736	0.663	0.527	0.641	0.533
F3-A1	0.477	0.373	0.540	0.414	0.654	0.394	0.500	0.489	0.475
Fp1-A1	0.585	0.629	0.912	1.104	0.981	0.748	0.533	0.583	0.619
Fp2-A2	0.428	0.365	0.790	0.576	0.700	0.426	0.445	0.425	0.396
F4-A2	0.512	0.391	0.514	0.423	0.630	0.403	0.520	0.440	0.485
C4-A2	0.391	0.449	0.486	0.523	0.447	0.387	0.399	0.400	0.449
P4-A2	0.362	0.355	0.380	0.349	0.318	0.266	0.345	0.320	0.311
O2-A2	0.273	0.207	0.332	0.261	0.300	0.235	0.262	0.266	0.204
F8-A2	0.452	0.359	0.406	0.376	0.498	0.415	0.488	0.407	0.359
T4-A2	0.216	0.157	0.258	0.187	0.278	0.202	0.229	0.181	0.194
T6-A2	0.551	1.165	0.741	1.142	0.506	0.555	0.607	0.520	0.675

At volleyball players our study emphasized the biggest values for theta waves, in comparison with the handball ones, as in Table 3.

Table 3. Theta values at volleyball group for every studied moment

channel	R1	A	R2	B	R3	C	R4	D	R5
T5-A1	0.325	0.293	0.35	0.565	0.3	0.24	0.29	0.412	0.453
T3-A1	0.748	0.721	1.23	3.696	0.84	2.126	0.87	0.939	1.6
F7-A1	0.188	0.206	0.17	0.534	0.16	0.152	0.15	0.148	0.151
O1-A1	0.845	1.696	2.87	2.379	0.81	1.332	1.91	1.127	1.3
P3-A1	0.57	0.554	2.74	0.634	0.74	0.624	0.62	0.589	0.761
C3-A1	0.716	0.775	0.85	1.373	0.7	2.008	0.78	0.841	1.553
F3-A1	0.559	0.487	0.46	0.439	0.5	0.511	0.53	0.457	0.643
Fp1-A1	0.75	1.731	1.54	1.721	0.74	1.228	0.84	0.974	1.048
Fp2-A2	0.39	0.425	0.88	0.537	0.39	0.313	0.37	0.349	0.424
F4-A2	1.491	1.186	1.52	1.496	1.38	1.329	1.6	1.1	1.569
C4-A2	0.352	0.372	2.49	0.424	0.34	0.315	0.42	0.357	0.45
P4-A2	1.208	0.845	1.55	0.997	0.96	1.006	1.27	0.994	1.255
O2-A2	0.268	0.268	0.24	0.665	0.23	0.263	0.27	0.251	0.329
F8-A2	0.577	0.568	0.53	0.667	0.56	0.572	0.57	0.608	0.569
T4-A2	0.264	0.316	0.31	0.772	0.28	0.236	0.25	0.254	0.415
T6-A2	1.012	0.809	0.9	1.049	1.01	1.086	1.07	0.889	1.129

Handball athletes' alpha1 activity was proved to be more homogenous and with classic reactivity, being lower during any active moment and higher during repose moments, regarding alpha1 EEG activity for volleyball players, that one was lower in the dominant hemisphere, as presented in Table 4 and Table 5.

Table 4. Alpha1 values at handball group for every studied moments

channel	R1	A	R2	B	R3	C	R4	D	R5
T5-A1	0.934	0.711	0.97	1.031	1	0.345	0.91	0.520	1.01
T3-A1	0.792	0.519	0.94	0.887	1.39	0.806	0.8	0.595	0.813
F7-A1	0.661	0.407	0.74	0.675	0.72	0.409	0.91	0.338	0.695
O1-A1	1.085	0.934	1.26	0.865	1.58	0.912	1.44	0.677	1.366
P3-A1	1.717	1.057	2.65	1.293	2.54	1.087	2.5	1.340	1.915
C3-A1	0.313	0.314	0.33	0.609	0.48	0.408	0.35	0.320	0.347
F3-A1	2.093	2.209	4.68	2.174	3.09	1.858	3.45	2.260	1.931
Fp1-A1	0.334	0.323	0.4	0.586	0.45	0.429	0.31	0.312	0.366
Fp2-A2	0.685	0.309	1.11	0.489	1.09	0.447	1.06	0.451	1.054
F4-A2	2.681	2.348	2.46	2.082	2.12	1.706	2.6	1.568	1.793
C4-A2	0.57	0.275	0.71	0.404	0.93	0.414	0.76	0.601	0.664
P4-A2	1.505	1.213	1.61	1.385	1.38	0.854	1.5	0.976	1.159
O2-A2	1.803	2.685	3	1.478	2.24	1.805	2.34	1.836	1.467
F8-A2	1.304	0.979	1.03	0.932	0.94	1.024	1.07	0.906	0.699
T4-A2	1.067	0.757	1.88	0.783	1.66	0.69	1.58	0.893	1.251
T6-A2	2.282	4.076	0.74	1.876	1.68	1.711	1.61	1.581	1.034

Table 5. Alpha1 values at volleyball group for every studied moments

channel	R1	A	R2	B	R3	C	R4	D	R5
T5-A1	2.298	2.210	1.72	1.765	1.46	1.321	1.47	1.504	2.67
T3-A1	1.412	1.166	0.88	1.492	0.9	1.564	1.1	0.963	1.54
F7-A1	0.34	0.353	0.33	0.445	0.36	0.363	0.36	0.358	0.436
O1-A1	0.641	0.568	1.18	0.867	0.57	0.992	1.89	0.858	0.855
P3-A1	5.043	5.418	2.74	3.812	4.14	3.818	4.17	3.302	5.034
C3-A1	0.542	0.540	0.5	0.591	0.58	1.399	0.63	0.55	0.968
F3-A1	1.817	1.411	1.66	1.289	2.24	1.752	1.78	1.716	2.221
Fp1-A1	0.486	0.562	0.71	0.638	0.51	1.129	0.65	0.58	0.729
Fp2-A2	0.41	0.271	0.63	0.362	0.35	0.291	0.37	0.271	0.441
F4-A2	11.92	10.668	10.6	5.542	16	24.13	17.4	8.718	16.61
C4-A2	0.381	0.324	1.14	0.380	0.34	0.328	0.42	0.311	0.452
P4-A2	7.878	8.182	6.49	4.316	7.58	9.223	9	5.108	9.865
O2-A2	0.67	0.514	0.89	0.814	0.98	0.616	0.95	0.658	1.04
F8-A2	5.035	4.832	4.23	4.971	4.76	3.54	4.36	3.509	4.232
T4-A2	1.983	1.484	0.85	0.704	1.29	1.593	1.77	0.935	1.669
T6-A2	4.535	5.823	4.2	2.764	5.04	5.429	6.08	3.871	7.207

Alpha2 values are lower for handball players in comparison with the volleyballs' ones, that are also characterised by a small activity of the left hemisphere, reflecting a "quiet" conduct, aspect revealed in Table 6 and 7.

Table 6. Alpha2 values at handball group for every studied moments

channel	R1	A	R2	B	R3	C	R4	D	R5
T5-A1	0.522	0.401	0.7	0.618	0.61	0.469	0.52	0.393	0.577
T3-A1	0.732	0.413	0.75	0.747	1.24	0.616	0.69	0.494	1.202
F7-A1	0.608	0.458	0.73	0.692	0.78	0.613	0.68	0.548	0.736
O1-A1	0.62	0.328	0.9	0.511	1.37	0.719	0.82	0.532	1.412
P3-A1	1.767	0.913	2.52	1.829	2.43	1.881	2.42	1.457	1.973
C3-A1	0.255	0.218	0.35	0.454	0.42	0.425	0.37	0.341	0.429
F3-A1	2.114	1.460	3.64	2.967	2.77	1.783	2.63	2.037	3.363
Fp1-A1	0.232	0.229	0.37	0.381	0.41	0.354	0.25	0.224	0.37
Fp2-A2	0.625	0.243	0.95	0.846	1.33	0.594	0.81	0.490	1.216
F4-A2	2.402	1.679	3.08	2.799	3.02	2.798	2.7	1.860	2.597
C4-A2	0.667	0.394	0.87	0.961	1.13	0.691	0.78	0.498	1.152
P4-A2	1.086	0.752	1.52	1.637	1.3	1.101	1.19	0.883	1.382
O2-A2	0.749	0.527	1.38	0.868	0.85	0.52	1.04	0.827	1.263
F8-A2	2.233	1.531	2.55	2.128	2.62	3.046	2.9	1.629	2.046
T4-A2	0.404	0.216	0.78	0.510	0.59	0.339	0.71	0.419	0.807
T6-A2	1.778	1.814	2.6	2.171	2.4	2.26	2.18	1.354	1.459

Table 7. Alpha2 values at volleyball group for every studied moments

channel	R1	A	R2	B	R3	C	R4	D	R5
T5-A1	1.381	1.585	1.79	1.518	1.96	2.178	2.05	2.254	1.67
T3-A1	0.788	0.731	1.01	1.121	1.11	1.357	1.04	1.121	1.206
F7-A1	0.447	0.490	0.53	0.597	0.62	0.558	0.65	0.57	0.66
O1-A1	0.678	0.667	0.91	0.739	0.78	0.813	1.13	0.971	1.016
P3-A1	1.875	1.454	2.41	1.724	4.45	4.502	3.87	3.406	2.717
C3-A1	0.333	0.300	0.29	0.335	0.4	0.692	0.43	0.431	0.652
F3-A1	1.279	1.087	1.59	1.086	2.31	2.102	2.32	1.74	1.938
Fp1-A1	0.317	0.427	0.41	0.385	0.33	0.423	0.41	0.465	0.456
Fp2-A2	0.414	0.251	0.51	0.337	0.46	0.432	0.52	0.337	0.577
F4-A2	6.534	5.684	5.89	5.505	8.16	9.659	7.96	8.247	7.353
C4-A2	0.341	0.238	0.62	0.324	0.41	0.46	0.44	0.385	0.482
P4-A2	5.629	5.701	5.81	4.705	6.44	7.759	7.36	6.811	7.326
O2-A2	0.568	0.556	0.71	0.631	0.72	0.59	1.14	0.743	0.818
F8-A2	4.206	4.408	4.52	3.970	5.99	6.184	5.59	4.931	4.346
T4-A2	0.817	0.704	0.85	0.729	1.03	0.971	1.11	0.965	1.011
T6-A2	4.317	3.899	4.61	3.161	5.08	6.43	4.79	4.458	5.167

Regarding beta band power spectrum was observed a perfect synchronization of both beta frequencies, connected to the analyzed moments, both for dominant and non-dominant hemisphere at handball athletes, for volleyball ones, this beta characteristic is valid only for the non-dominant one, as showed in Tables 8, 9.

Table 8. Beta1 values at handball group for every studied moments

channel	R1	A	R2	B	R3	C	R4	D	R5
T5-A1	0.12	0.178	0.17	0.196	0.13	0.104	0.14	0.134	0.159
T3-A1	0.263	0.209	0.28	0.402	0.31	0.255	0.2	0.213	0.244
F7-A1	0.121	0.120	0.12	0.136	0.11	0.085	0.12	0.090	0.11
O1-A1	0.232	0.187	0.24	0.211	0.3	0.206	0.19	0.201	0.236
P3-A1	0.289	0.280	0.42	0.279	0.11	0.34	0.33	0.268	0.307
C3-A1	0.149	0.132	0.15	0.221	0.17	0.145	0.12	0.132	0.141
F3-A1	0.272	0.223	0.31	0.239	0.38	0.286	0.31	0.274	0.237
Fp1-A1	0.143	0.145	0.18	0.180	0.17	0.132	0.1	0.108	0.143
Fp2-A2	0.137	0.096	0.21	0.125	0.16	0.105	0.11	0.107	0.15
F4-A2	0.291	0.256	0.3	0.297	0.35	0.286	0.27	0.298	0.256
C4-A2	0.145	0.109	0.17	0.135	0.16	0.112	0.12	0.123	0.149
P4-A2	0.147	0.227	0.16	0.168	0.16	0.117	0.12	0.134	0.13
O2-A2	0.127	0.133	0.16	0.120	0.15	0.112	0.14	0.146	0.12
F8-A2	0.413	0.328	0.43	0.415	0.58	0.513	0.5	0.527	0.308
T4-A2	0.106	0.093	0.11	0.088	0.12	0.093	0.1	0.088	0.099
T6-A2	0.309	0.534	0.5	0.553	0.41	0.364	0.36	0.288	0.312

Table 9. Beta1 values at volleyball group for every studied moments

channel	R1	A	R2	B	R3	C	R4	D	R5
T5-A1	0.125	0.151	0.129	0.133	0.152	0.136	0.129	0.325	0.188
T3-A1	0.174	0.196	0.197	0.254	0.176	0.301	0.205	0.196	0.290
F7-A1	0.057	0.064	0.051	0.072	0.054	0.060	0.047	0.047	0.065
O1-A1	0.142	0.259	0.306	0.233	0.149	0.197	0.208	0.223	0.217
P3-A1	0.198	0.185	0.176	0.158	0.101	0.194	0.211	0.171	0.192
C3-A1	0.106	0.112	0.119	0.129	0.115	0.245	0.140	0.116	0.224
F3-A1	0.142	0.119	0.149	0.107	0.149	0.143	0.170	0.123	0.143
Fp1-A1	0.121	0.216	0.181	0.142	0.117	0.148	0.168	0.146	0.143
Fp2-A2	0.062	0.055	0.106	0.063	0.061	0.050	0.069	0.056	0.062
F4-A2	0.486	0.451	0.417	0.365	0.505	0.513	0.492	0.390	0.503
C4-A2	0.059	0.053	0.205	0.054	0.055	0.050	0.075	0.060	0.065
P4-A2	0.344	0.377	0.361	0.310	0.361	0.310	0.947	0.276	0.380
O2-A2	0.112	0.105	0.090	0.100	0.115	0.089	0.109	0.102	0.104
F8-A2	0.323	0.331	0.282	0.273	0.285	0.260	0.272	0.290	0.292
T4-A2	0.117	0.149	0.117	0.102	0.126	0.125	0.112	0.090	0.145
T6-A2	0.394	0.464	0.331	0.315	0.337	0.423	0.394	0.474	0.378

The statistic analyzes (Pearson correlation coefficient) emphasized the presence of some correlations between the waves offered by the spectral analyze realized through FFT (Table 10).

Table 10. Pearson correlation coefficient values between EEG wave values

Handball					
channel	theta-beta	beta-alfa1	beta-alfa2	alfa2-theta	alfa1-alfa2
T5-A1	0.9608635	0.5324221	0.3479288	0.3171618	0.7405733
T3-A1	0.8335601	0.5532527	0.3614415	0.2296869	0.7797635
F7-A1	0.6875358	0.5663743	0.1793132	0.404506	0.7418648
O1-A1	0.6556294	0.6064433	0.7437811	0.2794794	0.8079079
P3-A1	0.5524751	-0.0304525	0.0580903	0.4703894	0.8616823
C3-A1	0.9286536	0.9059936	0.5051707	0.5304877	0.6924991
F3-A1	0.8608326	0.5950598	0.258417	0.5069357	0.568636
Fp1-A1	0.84843	0.7234934	0.6937507	0.7877677	0.7590493
Fp2-A2	0.8207278	0.7522409	0.6797538	0.5723488	0.8336191
F4-A2	0.6399374	-0.0516744	0.480521	0.5516581	0.1425279
C4-A2	0.4269137	0.6751589	0.7072291	0.4439933	0.6107754
P4-A2	0.5363437	0.2451065	-0.2197973	0.1842602	0.4791343
O2-A2	0.7632224	0.7399968	0.4612652	0.4053844	0.1613303
F8-A2	0.7604668	0.2167896	0.5148729	0.6197465	0.2905145
T4-A2	0.9037122	0.8333468	0.4688858	0.5678533	0.7911052
T6-A2	0.8369329	0.3405259	0.5510039	0.0511357	-0.2161857
Volleyball					
channel	theta-beta	beta-alfa1	beta-alfa2	alfa2-theta	alfa1-alfa2
T5-A1	0.2582091	-0.0768146	0.4939092	-0.3645368	-0.7540847
T3-A1	0.6519118	0.7540958	0.7283511	0.4944922	0.2751812
F7-A1	0.7001795	0.7101558	-0.0290752	0.0172719	0.5934066
O1-A1	0.8393633	0.2510353	0.1944004	0.1627211	0.7709
P3-A1	-0.0441773	0.2247836	-0.2418007	-0.1261327	-0.3417795
C3-A1	0.9076206	0.9549176	0.9447176	0.7963528	0.9164743
F3-A1	0.46821	0.6073983	0.768484	0.3249752	0.7266626
Fp1-A1	0.6653416	0.0800388	0.5060266	0.3196749	0.4137965
Fp2-A2	0.9275772	0.919325	0.4256794	0.1921761	0.6129242
F4-A2	0.2677948	0.869208	0.5542217	-0.1975302	0.7858313
C4-A2	0.9921712	0.9909946	0.7517197	0.7212396	0.7603832
P4-A2	0.2937318	0.3877208	0.342871	0.0742323	0.6747052
O2-A2	-0.093662	0.2434962	0.2490772	-0.1443276	0.6417043
F8-A2	-0.1500796	0.5035175	-0.5332899	-0.3480164	-0.4781295
T4-A2	-0.149585	0.4944788	-0.0852356	-0.4938668	0.3223887
T6-A2	-0.4125542	0.2781336	0.172456	0.4224447	0.5407628

For handball players, was remarked a high degree of correlation for theta and beta indexes and also a correlation in the dominant hemisphere for alpha1 and alpha2 indexes. At volleyball athletes the correlations were not structured equally

and were smaller.
Discussions
Because our study aimed the identification of neurophysiologic patterns specific to a long sportive activity, the attention was directed towards athletes of whom the initial cerebral plasticity process stopped and the morphologic differences are born especially in M1 (primary motor) area.

Was suggested the importance of theta and beta waves, in order to understand, evaluate and measure the motor memory processes, but especially, for improving the motor performances, in our case, the sportive ones (2,3). Thus, is considered that a decrease of alpha activity (non-synchronization) and an increase of theta one (synchronization), reflects a high capacity of memorization (4). Following during our study, the electroencephalographic activity of each studied sportive discipline, we observed different response patterns, but constant for the same group of athletes, specific changes being reported by Pearce in 2000, by using magnetic stimulation (5). At the beginning of the recordings, neither of the studied sportive disciplines presented theta power spectrum activity. The same moment of recording showed for handball group an alpha frontal-occipital activity, followed by beta rhythm, with a larger spreading but a smaller power, as for volleyball players, is recorded a frontal-occipital activity for alpha and beta waves, but only for the non-dominant hemisphere, aspect described by Andrew and Pfurtscheller in 1997. The dominant hemisphere presented only an occipital activity at handball group, aspect reported by Klimesch in 1998 and Babiloni in 2009. The right fist contraction moment produces spectacular EEG modifications in comparison with initial moment ones.

Volleyball players presented an increase of the theta band activity, so the theta band was very well represented in left frontal, parietal and occipital-temporal, well outline areas, while the theta band for the right hemisphere was not systematized, as was in the dominant hemisphere. The handball group did not show the same theta activity during right fist contraction.

Group of volleyball athletes presented minor right frontal modifications for alpha2 bands. Is sustained the affirmation that for volleyball players, the changes during right fist contraction were mostly in theta band, having a long duration motor memory for the performed move (6,7).

For handball alpha1 and 2 and beta decreases were obvious during this action, showing a high attention (Klimesch, 1998), so another EEG feature was outlined, that emphasize the difference between the two sports.

During relaxation moment R2, theta activity is constant or increases at volleyball group and alpha2 activity presents a slightly increase in parietal area, for handball, the frequencies bands had an increased activity in the areas where these frequencies already existed, characteristic for these is an alpha2 increase,

more difficult to explain. The left fist contraction determined the same changes for alpha and beta frequencies bands as the right one, additionally appearing little left frontal-temporal-occipital areas that presented minimum increase of theta spectrum at handball players.

The changes find until now at the two sportive disciplines can not be totally explain by the literature, there are maybe the final result of an intermediary processes pointed out by other authors.

From this moment, the EEG characteristic patterns of the two sports, remain constant, being a small theta increase for handball in the left hemisphere and a alpha, beta majority for both hemispheres at the same sport.

Alpha 1 activity is not higher in the right hemisphere at volleyball athletes, instead, alpha2 activity is higher in the left parietal area. The last recording moments are not so different from the initial moments at handball players, but for volleyball athletes the theta activity remains dominant for temporal and central areas.

Because of the particularities of each sportive discipline, is outlining the idea of some sportsmen presenting a performed movement imagination bigger than the one of other tested sport, which is produced by structural changes, signaled by Pearce in 2000.

The whole EEG testing aimed to emphasize the classic rhythms power spectrums modifications, produced by different orders (fists successively contractions, movement thinking without perform it), in comparison with the relaxation moments between actions. The literature describes many observations regarding the motor memory, our objective study was to emphasize the differences inter-sports, an original aspect enough conspicuous outlined by the previous affirmations.

Conclusions
The identification of some neurophysiologic patterns specific to long period sportive activities through electrophysiological tests is imposed as a viable method and easy to use for cerebral electrogenesis appreciation, in presence of functional plastic changes determined by the training.

By processing the results recorded at handball group, was remarked the presence of classic rhythms specific to wakeful state at adult, both during relaxation moments and activity, with a diminution reaction characteristic to each rhythm, depending on relaxation-activity moment.

Volleyball players, unlike handball players, presented both during relaxation and movement thinking, theta band activity, aspect mentioned in literature as accompanying the motor memory process, which dominates at volleyball players(7,8).

Complex testing through EEG and automatic analyze of EEG waves lines at professional sportsmen from handball and volleyball, as well as the outlining of an EEG pattern specific to each studied sportive discipline, represent an original aspect of this study.

References

1.Thomas, N.G., Mitchell D., 1996, Somatosensory-evoked potentials in athletes, *Med Sci Sports Exerc,* 4(28): 473-481

2. Aglioti, S.M., Cesari, P., Romani, M., Urgesi C., 2008, Action anticipation and motor resonance in elite basketball players, *Nature Neuroscience,* Volume 11, pp. 1109-1116

3. Babiloni, C., Del Percio, C., Paolo, M., Rossinib, D.F., Marzanog, N., Iacobonig, M., Infarinatoc, F., Lizioc, R., Piazzah, M., Pirritano, M., Berlutti, G., Cibelli, G., Eusebi, F., 2009, Judgment of actions in experts: A high-resolution EEG study in elite athletes, *NeuroImage,*Volume 45, Issue 2, pp. 512-521

4. Tianbao, Z., Hong, Z., Zheng, T., 2008, Revelations of the new developments of brain science on early education, Computer and Inormation Science, No. 3, Vol. 1

5. Pearce, A.J., et al., 2000, Functional reorganisation of the corticomotor projection to the hand in skilled racquet players, *Exp Brain Res* 130, pp. 238-243

6. Andrew, C. and Pfurtscheller, G., 1997, On the existence of different alpha band rhythms in the hand area of man, *Neurosci Lett* 222, pp. 103-106

7. Klimesch, W.M., Doppelmayr, H., Russegger, T., Schwaiger, J., 1998, Induced alpha band power changes in the human EEG and attention, *Neuroscience Letters*, Volume 244, Issue 2, pp. 73-76

8. Doppelmayr, M.P., Doppelmayr, H., 2008, Modifications in the human EEG during extralong physical activity, *Neurophysiology*, Number 1/January.

26

Sociological Study Concerning the Role of Physical Training in Volleyball Players' Activity

Cosma Alexandru[1], Orţănescu Dorina[2]

[1] *National University of Physical Education and Sport, Bucharest, Romania*
[2] *University of Craiova, Faculty of Physical Education and Sport, Romania*

Abstract. The research aims at revealing the role of gymnastic elements in physical training to volleyball juniors, therefore, we have considered as necessary the achievement of a sociological inquiry applying the questionnaire method meant to analyze the trainers' opinions concerning the use of working methods, a compulsory approach which provides accurate data on the current methodology applied in volleyball. The questionnaire addressed to trainers (no 50), included a number of 15 questions having one possible answer, each question having an objective, namely, the achievement of certain real data on the way in which the physical training is performed at the level of junior volleyball players. The questions refer to the physical training of volleyball players and the lot includes trainers performing within several sports clubs and high schools in the country, responsible for the junior volleyball players' training. A large number of trainers wish to train multilateral players, though, none of them apply acrobatic drills within the training program. Because of the poor material conditions registered in the sports high schools from Romania, none of the trainers apply the modern technology as an evaluation means during the physical training of junior volleyball players, however, 90% of them would be interested in considering the information provided by these testing instruments.
Key words: volleyball, physical training, gymnastics

Introduction

The sport of volleyball has continued to increase in participation since its inception over one hundred years ago. Volleyball has become one of the most widely played participant sports in the world with over 200 million players (Aagaard et al., 1997; Briner and Kacmar, 1997). (1)

The level reached nowadays by the development of sports practice, as any activity involving interdisciplinary features, is constantly submitted to an alert dynamics, putting aside training techniques and means which do not comply anymore with the requirements for achieving high performances. (2). Through the required level of training, through the body coordination and self-control in motion, through the force and the endurance developed in training and through their effect on the general health condition, the acrobatic drills are also useful for other sports branches representing additional means in achieving the general physical and psychological training. (3)

Method

The research aims at revealing the role of gymnastic elements in physical training to volleyball juniors, therefore, we have considered as necessary the achievement of a sociological inquiry applying the questionnaire method meant to analyze the trainers' opinions concerning the use of working methods, a compulsory approach which provides accurate data on the current methodology applied in volleyball.

The questionnaire addressed to trainers included a number of 15 questions having one possible answer, each question having an objective, namely, the achievement of certain real data on the way in which the physical training is performed at the level of junior volleyball players. The questions refer to the physical training of volleyball players and the lot includes trainers performing within several sports clubs and high schools in the country, responsible for the junior volleyball players' training.

Among the 50 trainers submitted to the research, 7 register a teaching seniority which does not exceed 10 years (20%), 15 have a seniority varying between 5 and 10 years of activity (30%) and 25 register a teaching seniority of over 10 years (50%), all of them training juniors aged between 15 and 16 years.

Results

To the first question, concerning the physical training to junior volleyball players on international level, 56% of the responders consider this sports training component as being very good, 10% believe that it is good, 4% classify it as being ordinary and, unfortunately, 30% are unaware of the volleyball status on international level.

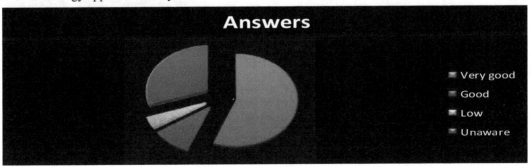

Chart no 1. Trainers' answers concerning the physical training of junior volleyball players on international level
(Answers: Very good; Good; Low; Unaware)

To the second question regarding the physical training of junior volleyball players on national level, 13% of the responders confirm a very good level of physical training, 40% consider it as being good, 20% believe that it is ordinary and 14% classify it as being low

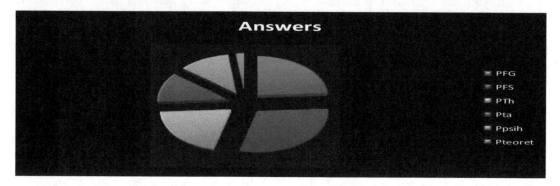

Chart no 2. Trainers' answers concerning the physical training of junior volleyball players on national level (Answers: Very good; Good; Ordinary; Low)

According to the responders, 30% consider that specific physical training prevails in the training process, 24% consider that the general physical training is highly important, 20% agree on the importance of technical training, 12% on the importance of tactical one, 12% focus on psychological training and only 2% on the theoretical one.

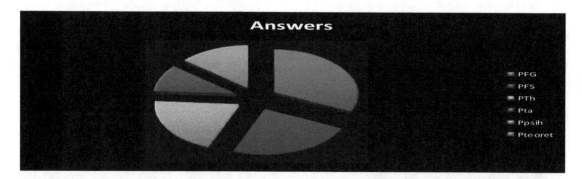

However, questioned on which of the sports training factors they should focus on junior level, 32% agree that the general physical training is an important aspect of the sports activity, 20% consider that the specific physical training essential, 24% focus on the technical one, 10% on the tactical one and 14% prefer the psychological one.

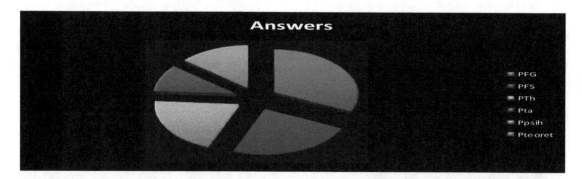

All the interviewed trainers (50), agree that the physical training has great value in junior volleyball players' sports activity.

To the question referring to the current level of physical training possessed by their trainees, 45% of the trainers consider it good, 35% ordinary, 15% very good and 5% low.

87.5% of the responders state the fact that they are using means focused on the development of the coordination and of the mobility correlated to the playing position within the physical training, while 12.5% do not use such means.

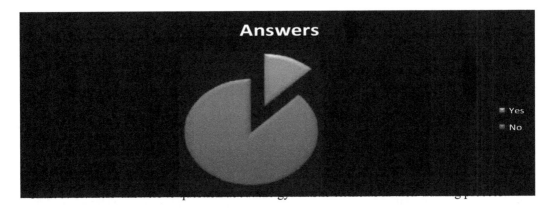

Most of the trainers (94%) confirm that the training activity planning does not include gymnastic and acrobatic elements, while 6% claim that they use such means. However, none of the responders include these element on a weekly basis. Even though they do not apply gymnastic and acrobatic elements in the physical activity, 84% of the trainers agree on the fact that junior volleyball players should benefit from a multilateral training. Unfortunately, till present, none of them have applied acrobatic features in the sportsmen's training, 64% considering them not so important and 36% applying them for lack of time.

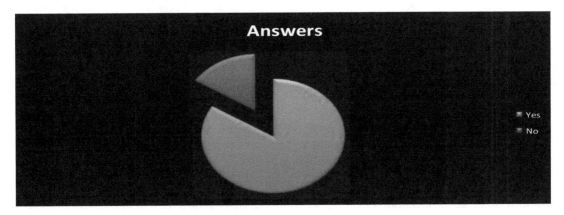

While performing the sportsmen's evaluation, trainers do not apply instruments for movement analysis, though, 90% of them recognize that if they had the opportunity to apply such instruments, they would do this analysis as it could provide important information.
Almost all of the trainers (94%) agree on a reevaluation of the physical training process to the level of junior volleyball players.

Conclusions
Following the analysis of the questionnaire, we may conclude that:
The inquiry based on the questionnaire reveals the opinions of the trainers charged with the physical training of junior volleyball players (aged between 16 and 18 years) from Romania.
Most of the responders (32%) consider the fact that the general physical training plays an important role in the junior players' formation and the focus should be on this type of training at the level of junior volleyball players. A large number of trainers wish to train multilateral players, though, none of them apply acrobatic drills within the training program. Because of the poor material conditions registered in the sports high schools from Romania, none of the trainers apply the modern technology as an evaluation means during

the physical training of junior volleyball players, however, 90% of them would be interested in considering the information provided by these testing instruments. The physical training in high performance volleyball represents the basis for optimizing all the other factors of the sports training. It has a special role to each level of training.

References
1.Tillman M. and al., Jumping and landing techniques in elite women's volleyball, *Journal of Sports Science and Medicine (2004) 3, 30-36*
2.Simion, Ghe., Mihăilă I, Stănculescu G., (2011), *Antrenament sportiv. Concept sistemic* , University Press Publisher, Constanța, p.118
3.Pascu, D., (2007), *Optimizarea modelării, pregătirii şi concursului în voleiul de performanţă cu ajutorul unor tehnici de obiectivizare matematică a eficienţei acţiunilor de joc,* Doctoral dissertation, N.A.P.E.S., Bucharest, p.85

27

Role of physical therapy in improvement spasticity in children with cerebral palsy

Anghel Mihaela [1,2], **Rață Gloria**[1]

1University "Vasile Alecsandri" FȘMSS, Bacau, Romania
2 National University of Physical Education and Sports PhD Student, Romania

Abstract: In cerebral palsy, spastic form, mobility and flexibility are influenced by central factors. Spastic muscles are affected with muscle hypertonic (abnormal resistance expressed by the execution of passive movements) predominantly flexor muscles of the upper limb and lower limb extensor muscles, especially in distal muscles (biceps elbow, fist, finger flexors, ankle –triceps sural) characteristic is, the phenomenon of knife blade. "Hypertonic condition - muscle contracture may evolve in time by fixing the advent retraction become permanent muscle can generate retraction posture abnormalities and deformities of the affected limb (foot equine, equine varus) or spine (scoliosis). „Infantile cerebral paralysis (ICP) describes a group of permanent disorders of the development of motor skills and posture, causing activity limitation or causes that are attributed to non-progressive damage occurring in developing fetal or infant brain. These motor disorders of cerebral palsy are often accompanied by sensory disturbances, perceptual, cognitive, communication and behavior, epilepsy and secondary musculoskeletal impairment " (Rosenbaum P, colab.2007).
Keywords: *improvement, spasticity, cerebral palsy*

Introduction

Cerebral palsy is a neurological disorder involution which is the main manifestation of spasticity, coordination problems accompanied by the emergence of involuntary movements, sinkinezii, and balance disorders. [1]. There are three degrees of PC: spastic (the most common), athetosis and ataxia. Spastic form corresponds to an exaggeration of the stretch reflex, hypertonic are conserved from birth. This is seen for clinical examination by osteo-tendon reflexes acute (strong), Babinski reflex to stop expansion and joint amplitude for rapid mobility in functional terms so that voluntary movements can not escape from stereotyped motor schema, for example scheme is the most classic walking with hip adductor, turning inward flexion knee and foot sharks or upper limbs, an object near the flexion elbow, wrist pronation and flexion.

Objectives should follow child psycho-motor behavior modification, adjustment and control of your own body in various environmental conditions. Thus, the study of psycho-motor is paramount in organizing educational-rehabilitation for all ages and types of impairments, as for ordinary people.

Child with cerebral palsy use their opportunities within his motor, but recording stability problems of the upper limb and lower develop a scheme very static, little separated and symmetrical. Qualitative development remains delayed motor skills trunk (rotation and balance) and probably fixing activities are negatively influenced. Hand crossing the midline can not be adequately developed place having trunk rotations. Motor activity of the trunk will develop further in a very limited extent, with obvious consequences on the quality of balance and movement variability.

Material and methods

Aim and hypothesis

Based on the cases seen and treated for a long time, but also from literature that reflected in the bibliography attached to follow how the various paralysis, especially of the legs, can affect balance, standing and walking, has been followed up on cases, installing different attitude data spasticity, and their treatment. This research presents the particular measures that physical therapy is done functional recovery; normalize muscle tone, balance, standing and walking. Important goal is to improve spasticity play functionality to play in the best possible conditions.

The research hypothesis

It is assumed that by applying the optimal intervention program can improve spasticity in children with cerebral palsy.

Place and duration of research

The research was conducted in the research center of the University "Vasile Alecsandri" Bacau on a group of 3 children with cerebral palsy aged 2 to 6 years for a period of 14 months.

Table no. 1. Sample of subjects

No.	Name	Age	Sex	Diagnosis
1.	L.P.	2 years	M	Spastic tetraparesis
2.	R.I.	3 years	F	Spastic diplegia
3.	G.I.	5 years	F	Spastic paraplegia

The methods used in the study were: bibliographic documentation, observation, testing method.
Spasticity assessment was performed using Tardieu scale [2]
0 - does not appear spasticity during passive movement;
1 - slight spasticity during passive movement;
2 - marked spasticity, a well-defined angle;

3 - clonuses occurs at a well defined angle (clonuses duration is less than 10 seconds);
4 - clonuses, lasting more than 10 seconds;
5 - joint is stiff, can not be mobilized.
I used to assess gait "Get up and go" this is a test commonly used to quantify neurological patients 0, 1, 2, 3 scale:
0 - unable;

1 - done with difficulty and help from physiotherapist;
2 - done only with difficulty;
3 - done without difficulty.

Methodology

Following assessment has been aware of spasticity in all three cases, which lead to postural instability affecting motor performance tasks and activities of daily life. This gave the possibility of targeting the program in the context of motor behavior:
- improving spasticity;
- increased stability and balance in various positions;
- rehabilitation of walking.

Program aimed at inhibiting abnormal activity, normalization of postural tone, improving resistance to muscle hypotonic and activation recovery reactions and balancing that by aligning and correcting segment in a sitting position to obtain a better quality of voluntary movements. [3]

The head and trunk alignment improved functional capacity in the upper hand. For increased stability, the balance was chosen closed kinetic chain exercise conducted by posts carrying out co-contraction, because in addition to use its own muscle load, place also load on bones, joints, tissues. Changed position so that weight bearing segments, which is a resistive force (quadruped, sitting with hand support, standing on the hands, standing completely) [4,5].

That the method used to describe communication, correct, explain, encourage, stimulate, motivate them to perform certain tasks, touch to stimulate the execution of a movement for the purpose of facilitating post-inhibitory reflex, I used the key points to inhibit pattern sites of abnormal posture and movement, relaxation techniques, automatic deco traction techniques, passive mobilization techniques, sensor motor stimulation techniques, demonstration accompanied by an explanation of how to do the work, practical work (Method exercise), imitation by demonstrating action Whereas some do not fully understand verbal images using symbols and psychic color therapy with somatic influences.

Throughout the therapeutic recovery program was taken into account intervention individualization according to the present deficit, the level of neurons motor development, the level of cognitive, affective emotional condition, the form of verbal communication and nonverbal (kinesthetic, emotional).

In the rehabilitation program was necessary stability and balance in sitting position, quadruped, and standing on her knees. During game programs were used whose functions have contributed to remedy or even normalization of deficient motor acts, the formation of basic skills and motor skills (grip strength, walking, running), the formation of appropriate conduct and behavior of some positive attitudes to language development etc.

Results

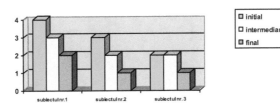

Graphic no. 1. Evolution of subjects Tardieu Scale

Following application of the intervention program has seen an improvement in psychomotor behavior against the normalizing tone movement tasks which enable children to act with efficiency, speed, spontaneity, under any circumstances, based on their own decisions. For all subjects observed real progress, if we consider the initial and final values. It can be seen that subject 1 has a much better due to age and precocity treatment versus subject 3.

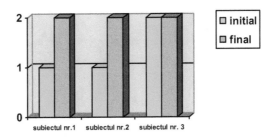

Graphic no. 1. Evolution test subjects "get up and go"

We can see improvement in all parameters included in the test: if at first they were dependent on others there is now a noticeable favorable managed to move them even if they do with difficulty.

Following implementation of the program have been positive children in three areas: self-care (personal hygiene), mobility (travel, transfers) and social (recognize of sounds, words, family member), managing to behave near age. So we could see all the dynamics of parameter includes in the test: some children have been passed from food to cut food pieces, if at first failed to grasp fork initiates movement, now have a better seat of stabilities managed to maintain position at different external stimuli travel through the house are made more easily, interaction better with family members, a part of them even managing to participate in various games.

Programs have been used for a period determined by the particular age, sex, education, short and long term objectives, and priority issues. During a meeting was between 35-70 minutes in the 2-3 sessions a week.

Conclusions

Physical therapy in children with cerebral palsy applied as early as possible to optimize the tonic function, static and dynamic child to better organize their gestural behavior in time and space.

Individualization intervention characteristics looked adapted age and level of each child's behavior, the latter feature is crucial in determining the therapist-patient communication.

Psycho-motor education the child with cerebral palsy becomes increasingly imperative for a better integration in schools and society.

Thinking the child with cerebral palsy in the education and development is a task of psychomotor existential retroaction system by which children are given problems in relation to its ability to timely and heuristic thinking.

References:

1. Robanescu, N. și colab. (2001). *Reeducarea neuromotorie*, Ed. Medicala. P 133-38, 224-243,271-76.

2. Tardieu C., et. al.(1982), Muscle hypoextensibility in children with cerebral palsy: clinical and experimental observation, Atch phys Med Rehab: 63; 97-102.

3. Robănescu, N. (1992), *Reeducarea neuro-motorie*, ed. Medicală, București;

4. Berard, C. et al.(2008), *La paralysie cérbrale de l'enfant.* Sauramps med. p. 79-81.

5.Bobath K, Bobath B., (1964), *Physiotherapy,* p.1, 8.

28

Somatoscopic and somatometric evaluation at a group of volleyball women athletes

Călina Mirela Lucia [1,2], Enescu-Bieru[1]Denisa, Dinu Valentina [2], Stanomirescu Ana Maria [1,2]

[1] *Faculty of Physical Education and Sport, University of Craiova, Romania*
[2] *Polyclinic of Sports Medicine, Emergency Clinical Hospital Craiova, Romania*

Abstract. Introduction. Aim of actual paper is to analyze the physic development and the state of nutrition corresponding to age at a group of junior women athletes that practice volleyball, by determining and evaluating the morpho-anthropometric parameters, in order to improve their performer biotype. **Material and method.** Growth and physic development evaluation was performed at Biometric Explorations Cabinet of Polyclinic of Sports Medicine Craiova, on a group of 20 women athletes that practice volleyball, with ages between 12 and 14,5 years. Women athletes' exam was made during periodic examination, in order to estimate the physic development and state of nutrition level, to compare the constitutional biotype of examined athlete with the one of biological model corresponding to the practiced sport, to establish some indications referring to worsening prevention or correction of possible observed physic deficiencies. **Results.** The data obtained after the measurements for physic development and state of nutrition evaluation were realized on the 20 studied women athletes and were compared them with the ones of the biologic micromodel characteristic to volleyball. **Conclusions.** The biologic model must constitute for the selection an objective that have to be reached and even exceeded by the future performers from all sportive disciplines. The biologic model of the studied athletes is not superposable to the one appertaining to volleyball performer for all investigated biologic parameters; but junior women athletes are during the primary or secondary selection stage and there are not yet changes of the morphotype according to effort solicitation type.
Key words: *volleyball, somatoscopic, somatometric evaluation*

Introduction

Human body dimensions have great importance to establish sportive performances and represent even, for some sportive disciplines, indispensable factors to obtain high results. Comparing the data obtained after the evaluation of the examined subjects with the ones of the biologic model of the performer, characteristic to each sportive discipline, can be drawn conclusions over the level of concordance between his growth and physic development and the requirements of the sport he practices.

Exam of growth and physic development interpretation includes also the diagnosis of possible physic deficiencies and their level and the obtained data are synthesized through somatoscopy and somatometry (1,2).

Final stage of the interpretation of the data offered by growth and physic development exam is represented by the elaboration of the indications and contraindications of sports and physical education practice, concretely specifying the measures and ways adequate to each case (3).

Aim of actual paper is to analyze the physic development and the state of nutrition corresponding to age at a group of junior women athletes that practice volleyball, by determining and evaluating the morpho-anthropometric parameters, in order to improve their performer biotype.

Material and method

Growth and physic development evaluation was performed at Biometric Explorations Cabinet of Polyclinic of Sports Medicine Craiova, on a group of 20 women athletes that practice volleyball, with ages between 12 and 14,5 years.

Women athletes' exam was made during periodic examination, in order to estimate the physic development and state of nutrition level, to compare the constitutional biotype of examined athlete with the one of biological model corresponding to the practiced sport, to establish some indications referring to worsening prevention or correction of possible observed physic deficiencies (4).

For this purpose were performed the following examinations:

➤ **somatoscopic exam**, clinic method representing the visual observation of the subject from frontal plan (from face to back), from sagittal plan (from profile), during repose, walking or specific movement, in order to realize a global and segmental appreciation (harmonious body develop, physic deficiencies diagnosis, comparison with the practiced sport somatic biotype (1,2);

➤ **somatrometric exam**, paraclinic, objective method, evaluates the physic development and the state of nutrition, based on measurement of some tees and calculation of anthropomorphic indexes; were made the following anthropometric measurements, using taliometer, metric rib, anthropometric compass, human scale and palmar and scapular force dynamometer (1,2):

• **height (H) (cm)**, interpreted for female, as:
- **small** : under 150 cm;
- **medium**: over 160 cm;
- **high:** over 170 cm;

• **bust (B) (cm)**, interpreted through index **B x 100 / H**, with values of 53 – 54 %, for female;

• **weight (W) (kg)**, whose values are interpreted in correlation with height, according to the formula **Brugsch: - W = H - 100,** for H ≤ 164 cm;
  - W = H - 105, for H = 165- 174 cm;
  - W = H – 110, for H ≥ 175 cm;

• **diameters (cm)**: biacromial (D_{BA}), bitrohanterian (D_{BT}), transvers of thorax (D_T), during maximum inspiration and forced expiration, anteroposterior of thorax (D_{AP}), during maximum inspiration and forced expiration;

• **perimeters (cm)**: of thorax (P_T), during respiratory repose, maximum inspiration and forced expiration; the thorax elasticity is appreciated by the difference between: P_T maximum inspiration - P_T maximum expiration, with normal values over 6 cm;

➤ **dynamometric exam,** method of measuring and recording the force of some muscular groups during flexion and extension, using some special apparatus (dynamometers), whose dimensions, strength and shape are adapted to the muscular groups that follow to be tested; thus we determined (1,2):

- **palmar flexors force** (F_{pr}, F_{pl}) **(kgm)**, its normal values for female are about 50% of body weight;

- **scapular region muscle force** (F_{scp}) **(kgm)**, its normal values for female are about 40% of body weight;

These measurements were used to calculate the following indexes (1,2):

✓ **BMI (Body mass Index)** = **W** (kg) / **H^2** (m), with the following interpretation: < 18,5 = underweight; 18,5 -24,9 = normal weight; 25-29,9 = overweight; >30 = obeses;

✓ **of proportionality**:

▪ **Giufrida Ruggeri index:** I_{GR} = **B x 100 / H,** with normal values of 53 %, for female;

▪ **Adrian Ionescu index:** $I_{A.I}$ = **B – H / 2,** with normal values of 4-5 cm, for female;

✓ **of harmony:** Erismann: I_E = $P_{T(repose)}$ – **H / 2,** with normal values of 6 cm;

✓ **thorax elasticity:** $P_{T\ maximum\ inspiration}$ - $P_{T\ maximum\ expiration}$, with normal values of ≥ 6 cm;

✓ **palmar force index:** I_{FP} = (F_{pr}+ F_{pl}) / **2W x 100,** with normal values of 50%, for female;

✓ **scapular force index**: I_{Fscp} = F_{scp} x 100 / **W,** with normal values of 40%, for female.

The results obtained from somatoscopic and somatometric exams, as well as from the calculation of anthropomorphic indexes, were written for each athlete on an individual sheet, beside the medical and sportive indications adequate to each case.

Graphic representations were realized using the **arithmetic mean** of a values series.

Results

Analyzing the data obtained after the measurements for physic development and state of nutrition evaluation were realized on the 20 studied women athletes and comparing them with the ones of the biologic micromodel characteristic to volleyball, we discovered the following aspects:

- medium values of **height** on groups of age at the studied women athletes, overlapped the standard values presented by the literature and showed thier increase with every age group: **12-12,5 years** (7 athletes): H medium (cm) = 158,1; **13-13,5 years** (5 athletes): H medium (cm) = 166,3; **14-14,5 years** (8 athletes): H medium (cm) = 168,9;

- regarding the **weight** of the studied women athletes, we recorded the following results:

- 10 cases (50%) of normal weight sportive, with a BMI having an average value of 20,51 kg/m^2, 8 cases (40%) of underweight sportive, with a BMI having an average value of 17,65 kg/m^2 and 2 cases (10%) of overweight sportive (a case of obesity level I/II), with a BMI having an average value of 28,35 kg/m^2. (figure 1).

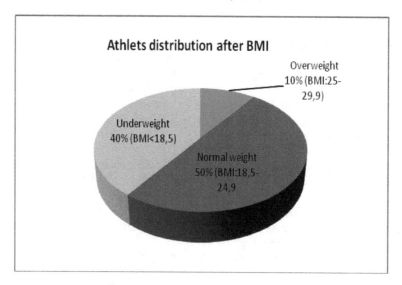

Figure 1 Athletes distribution after BMI

- **the scale** had low values (S < H) at 12 (60%) of the studied athletes, representing a limiting factor of the sportive performance;

- regarding the **proportionality indexes**, Giufrida Ruggeri index presented an average value of 52,1%,

being in normal limits of 52-54% for female, while Adrian Ionescu index had ideal values at 5 (25%) athletes (an average of 4,6 cm) and values over the ideal ones (an average of 7 cm) at 6 (30%) athletes, which indicates a concordance between the growth in length of the trunk and the limbs one, favorable to sportive performance; values under the ideal ones (on average 2,19 cm) were found at 9 (45%) from the studied athletes. (figure 2)

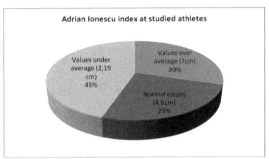

Figure 2 Adrian Ionescu index at studied athletes

• **Erismann harmony index**, important for establishing the constitutional type and to appreciate the biologic performances of respirator and cardiovascular apparatus, at child has negative values, reaches zero at age between 16-28 years and becomes positive at adult age; at 12 (60%) of the studied athletes, this index presented values under the mean corresponding to age (unfavorable to performance), signifying a thorax insufficiently developed, asthenic, aspect showed also by the somatoscopic exam (fig 3);

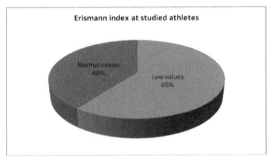

Figure 3 Erismann index at studies athletes

- **thorax elasticity** (cirtometric index), presented very good values (+ 6, +10 cm) at all 20 studied athletes;
- **segmental force indexes**, with average values of 31,7% for palmar force and of 29,25 % for scapular force, were under the ideal values at all 20 studied athletes;
- **somatoscopic** exam emphasized the following defects of posture and physic deficiencies:
→ deviations of spine in **sagittal plan** at 6 athletes (30%), from which:
- 3 cases with cifolordosis attitude;
- 3 cases with lordosis attitude;
→ deviations of spine in **frontal plan:** 2 cases (10%): one case with dorsolumbar scoliotic attitude and a case with dorsolumbar scoliosis grade I/II;
→ deviations of spine in **sagittal and frontal plan:** 6 cases (30%): 4 athletes with dorsolumbar cifoscoliosis attitude, from which 2 presented also lordosis attitude, a case of lumbar scoliotic attitude with the physiologic lumbar lordosis pronounced and a case with dorsolumbar cifoscoliosis grade I/II;
→ 6 athletes (30%) presented normotone posture;
→ asthenic thorax, with sequel of rickets, found at 7 (35%) of the athletes, in correlation with negative values of Erismann index present at these athletes, while at 4 of the sportive we discovered a hypotonia of the abdominal wall muscles, associated with lordotic attitude (fig. 4, 5).

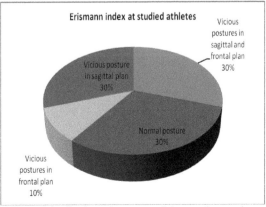

Figure 4 Distribution of postures vicious and normal

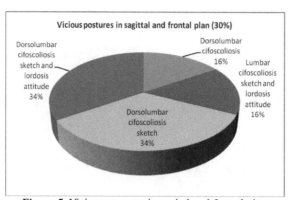

Figure 5 Vicious postures in sagital and frontal plan

Conclusions

➢ The present study was performed on a group of 20 junior women athletes, with ages between 12-12,5 years, that practice volleyball, sport characterized by a mixed type of effort, aerobe-anaerobe. The athlete's examination was realized at Biometric Explorations Cabinet of Polyclinic of Sports Medicine Craiova, during periodic examination, in order to estimate the physic development and state of nutrition level and to compare the constitutional biotype of examined athlete with the one of biological model corresponding to the practiced sport.

➢ Reporting of the studied athletes anthropometric parameters values (height, weight, bust, thorax perimeter, nutrition and harmony indexes) to the national standard values of the age group 7-18 years, offered by the Hygiene and Public Health Institute Bucharest, leads to the conclusion that these values exist into the limits of maximal values presented by the reference tables and their increase is according to age group.

➢ The biologic model of the studied athletes is not superposable to the one appertaining to volleyball performer for all investigated biologic parameters; but junior women athletes are during the primary or secondary selection stage and there are not yet changes of the morphotype according to effort solicitation type. A limiting parameter of performance for volleyball is represented by the scale, that had low values (A < I) at 12 (60%) of the studied athletes.

➢ Erismann index, that appreciates the thorax robustness had normal values at 40% of the studied group athletes, 60% had values under average; from this point of view, the thorax robustness must be considered as a perfectible parameter that should be in the attention of medical-sportive equip.

➢ A special attention must be accorded to the correction of spine vicious postures. Cifotic, lordotic or scoliotic deviations discovered at all studied athletes, represent in the majority of cases, the accentuation of normal physiologic curves and are produced by the insufficient toning of abdominal muscles in comparison to the paravertebral muscles. That is why we consider the introduction of muscles toning exercises into the training programme, beneficial, in order to realize an equilibrium between the paravertebral and abdominal muscles, allowing the correction of these vicious postures, unfavorable to performance.

➢ The biologic model must constitute for the selection an objective that have to be reached and even exceeded by the future performers from all sportive disciplines.

References

1.Drăgan, I. și colab., 2002, *Medicină Sportivă*, 215-224, Ed. Medicală, București
2.Drăgan, I. și colab., 1994, *Medicina Sportivă aplicată*, 230-243, Ed. Editis, București
3.Dinu, V., Călina, M.L., Enescu-Bieru, D., 2010, Aspects of anthropometric and morphofunctional cardiac parameters at a lot of junior football players, *2end Congress of European College of Sport and Exercise Physicians and 12th Scientifics Conference in SEM, Centre for Sport and Exercise Medicine, Queen Mary,* University of London
4.Dinu, V., Călina, M.L., Enescu-Bieru, D., 2010, Body composition assessment methods, A XXIV-a *Conf. Naț. a Soc. Rom. de Științe Fiziologice, Oradea,* Băile Felix

29

Self-Esteem and professional formation in physical education and sports

Raţă Gloria, Raţă Bogdan Constantin, Raţă Marinela

"Vasile Alecsandri" University of Bacău

Abstract. This paper represents an observational study conducted on 60 graduate students. The study has been organized and conducted in January 2013, within the Faculty of Movement, Sports, and Health Sciences, at the "Vasile Alecsandri" University of Bacau, aiming to highlight the manifestation of self-esteem in the graduate students enrolled in the following master's programs: Curricular and leisure time motor activities, Athletic high performance, and Physical Therapy in functional education and reeducation. In order to know the subjects' level of self-esteem, the "Self-esteem Test," presented by the Quebec Psychologists Association, was used as an assessment instrument. The test comprises 20 questions that allowed the creation of a diagram of the graduate students' self-esteem. We used as research methods: the study of the professional literature, the testing method, the statistical-mathematical method, the graphical representation method. The results showed that 25% of the 30 male and 30 female students that were questioned have a high self-esteem, and that 75% have a medium-level self-esteem. The hypothesis stating that "the physical education and sports graduate students' level of self-esteem is above medium level in most cases," as well as the one stating that "the female students have lower self-esteem than the male students," has been confirmed.

Key words: self-esteem, professional formation, graduate students

Introduction

The human beings' behavior, manifested through conceptions, motivations, attitudes, beliefs, opinions, mentalities, traditions, states of mind, feelings, can be seen in the respect for other people, and in their self-esteem. Self-esteem is not an action of egotism or narcissism, but recognition of the feeling of believing in your own capabilities, a confidence that allows people to have a positive behavior. Psychosociology analyzes the people's psychological particularities, as socio-cultural beings, it analyzes the people's behavior within their social groups, but also the group behavior particularities that "manifest themselves in common feelings and behaviors" (*Dicţionar de psihologie socială*, Dictionary of Social Psychology, 1981) M. Epuran (2005, p. 4.) thinks that the "psychological-behavioral phenomena presented by the people's participation in activities" are concretized in the "social impact on the individual behavior and the personal relations in accomplishing certain social actions" (Epuran M., Holdevici I., Toniţa F., 2008). The manifestation of certain behaviors determines the individual's development and place within the inter-individual relationships, and group manifestations that can have repercussions on personal development, and on professional integration. The self-perception of one's social ambiance "determines the individual to make an effort to adapt and to influence it" (Golu, P., 2004, as cited in Dragnea, C.A., 2006, p. 7), an aspect which influences the professional activity in a positive way. Any group activity presupposes "a certain personal control over the other" (Newcomb, Turner, Conners, 1965, as cited in Dragnea, C.A., 2009, p. 72), but also "preferential relationships" (highlighted by Rioux şi Chappuis, as cited in M. Epuran, 2005, p. 69), of an affective and operational type, mutual esteem and respect.

Researches have led to the idea that the inclusion of young people in the professional formation programs favors the framing and consolidation of self-esteem, and the appearance of a confidence feeling that is based more on personal resources, developed within the working groups. Self-esteem constitutes a condition for personal development, and is formed of a feeling of confidence, self-knowledge, a feeling of belonging (to a family, a group, a socio-professional category, etc.), and a feeling of competence. The feeling of self-confidence is decisive in obtaining results during the learning process, and during the action of confronting the fundamental difficulties of life. As a pure and essential aspect of an individual, self-esteem is perceived as a psycho-dynamic development, or/and as a psychological state. Each individual tries very hard to materialize his/her aspirations, to develop, to progress, to arrive at a certain level, and this depends on his/her high self-esteem, on his/her confidence to succeed. "The road to knowing yourself and the others around you implies sincerity, perseverance, spontaneity..., but also an appeal to the instruments of scientific knowledge, mainly the psychological tests" (Calancea A., 1997, p. 302), with the help of which one can assess a small part of the human behavior. Self-esteem represents a support that contributes to the positive personal and professional development of individuals.

Material and Methods

The "Self-esteem Test," presented by the Quebec Psychologists Association, was applied in order to reveal the level of self-esteem of the second level of professional formation (master's degree). The test comprised 20 questions through which one can assess the graduate students' self-esteem. Each assertion is marked using three numerical values (A = 4, N = 2, and C = 0 points), according to the subject's answer. The results were interpreted based on an assessment scale (60-80 points = high level of self-esteem; 40-59 points = medium level of self-esteem; and below 39 points = low level of self-esteem). The information gathered from the results calculated from the answers recorded for the self-esteem test can be useful in creating a psychosocial profile of the future teachers, as this can influence, in a positive or negative way, their behavior in the various situations they will be confronting in their professional activity (teaching). This transversal study started from the hypothesis stating that "the physical education and sports graduate students' level of self-esteem is above medium level in most cases," and from the hypothesis stating that "the female students have lower self-esteem than the male students." The study has been conducted in January 2013 (Faculty of Movement, Sports, and Health Sciences, the "Vasile Alecsandri" University of Bacau), comprising 60 graduate students (30 females and 30 males). For this study, the research methods were: the study of the professional literature, the observation, the statistical-mathematical method, and the graphical representation method.

RESULTS

The results from the tests have been recorded and organized in the two following tables (Table 1 and Table 2).

Table 1 - Test results for the males group

I.	Sum of the points	Test items - points																			
		1	2	3	4	5	6	7	8	9	10	11	12	13	14	15	16	17	18	19	20
BA	52	4	0	4	4	4	2	2	2	4	0	2	4	2	4	4	4	0	4	0	2
BT	42	2	2	4	0	2	2	2	0	4	0	2	4	4	4	0	2	4	2	0	2
DM	42	2	0	2	0	4	2	4	0	4	0	2	4	2	4	2	4	0	2	0	4
SS	54	4	0	2	4	4	4	2	4	4	4	2	4	4	2	0	2	4	2	0	2
AA	54	4	2	0	4	2	4	4	0	4	0	4	4	4	4	0	4	4	2	0	4
DR	44	4	0	4	0	4	4	4	0	4	4	2	2	2	0	4	0	0	2	4	0
MG	64	4	0	4	4	2	4	4	4	4	4	2	4	2	4	2	4	4	4	2	2
NM	64	4	0	2	4	4	4	2	4	2	4	4	4	4	4	0	4	4	4	2	4
PC	42	4	0	2	4	4	2	0	0	4	2	2	4	2	4	0	2	0	2	0	4
RR	58	4	4	4	2	2	2	0	0	4	4	4	4	2	4	4	4	4	2	0	4
ZC	56	2	4	4	2	2	2	0	0	4	4	4	4	2	4	2	4	4	2	2	4
MS	58	4	0	4	4	4	2	2	0	4	4	4	4	4	4	2	4	4	2	0	2
IG	48	4	0	4	2	2	2	4	4	4	2	2	4	4	2	4	2	0	0	0	2
MM	58	4	4	4	4	2	2	2	2	4	4	2	4	2	4	4	2	0	4	0	4
AA	60	4	4	4	4	4	2	4	4	4	4	0	4	4	4	4	0	4	2	0	0
AC	56	2	4	0	4	4	4	4	4	4	4	4	2	4	2	4	2	0	2	0	2
VC	56	4	2	4	2	2	2	4	4	4	2	2	4	4	0	4	2	4	4	0	2
DD	62	4	4	0	4	4	4	4	0	4	4	4	4	4	4	2	2	2	4	0	4
RT	64	4	4	2	4	4	4	4	0	4	0	4	4	4	4	0	2	4	4	4	4
MR	46	2	4	0	4	4	4	4	0	2	0	4	4	4	0	2	0	2	2	2	2
I C	54	4	2	0	2	2	4	4	4	4	4	2	4	4	4	0	4	0	2	0	4
MA	60	4	4	2	2	4	4	0	4	4	4	2	4	4	4	2	2	2	4	4	0
AS	52	4	0	4	2	4	2	4	4	2	2	2	4	4	4	4	2	0	2	0	2
MN	62	4	2	4	4	2	2	4	2	4	4	2	4	4	4	4	2	2	4	0	4
AT	60	4	2	4	4	4	2	4	4	4	4	2	4	4	4	4	0	4	2	0	0
AC	56	2	4	0	4	4	4	4	4	4	4	4	2	4	2	4	2	0	2	0	2
CM	56	2	2	4	2	2	4	4	4	2	2	2	4	4	0	2	2	4	4	2	2
DM	58	2	4	0	4	4	2	4	0	4	4	4	4	4	4	2	2	2	4	0	4
RR	58	4	4	4	2	2	2	0	0	4	4	4	4	2	4	4	4	4	2	0	4
MZ	56	2	4	4	2	2	2	0	0	4	4	4	4	2	4	2	4	4	2	2	4
X	55.07	3.40	2.20	2.60	2.93	3.13	2.87	2.80	1.93	3.80	2.87	2.73	3.80	3.33	3.33	2.33	2.53	2.27	2.67	0.80	2.67
S	6.55	0.93	1.77	1.75	1.36	1.01	1.01	1.63	1.93	0.61	1.63	1.11	0.61	0.96	1.32	1.67	1.28	1.87	1.09	1.35	1.42
VC	11.90	27.42	80.43	67.45	46.46	32.17	35.16	58.12	99.76	16.06	57.01	40.69	16.06	28.77	39.65	71.48	50.50	82.69	41.00	168.67	53.34

*Legend: I= subjects' initials , X = mathematical mean, S = standard deviation, and VC = variability coefficient.

As one can see in Table 1, the arithmetical mean of the individual sums (the third vertical column) recorded by the graduate students is of 55.07 points, which is an average situated in the superior side of the medium level of self-esteem. The average values for 18 assertions are between 2.20 and 2.80 points, meaning above half of the average value, and for only 2 assertions we have values under the average of two: 1.93 and 0.80 points. The standard deviation and variability coefficient values are high, this showing the group's lack of homogeneity, which is normal, considering that the 22-28-year old students have different goals, aims, and behaviors.

Table 2 - Test results for the females group

I.	Sum of the points	Test items - points																			
		1	2	3	4	5	6	7	8	9	10	11	12	13	14	15	16	17	18	19	20
FF	52	4	4	4	4	4	2	2	4	2	2	4	4	2	2	0	2	0	4	2	0
GA	58	4	4	4	4	4	2	2	4	2	2	4	4	2	4	0	4	4	2	2	0
IM	72	2	4	4	4	4	2	4	4	4	4	4	4	4	2	4	2	4	4	4	4
RM	48	4	2	0	4	4	4	0	0	4	4	4	4	2	4	0	2	0	2	2	2
PA	52	4	2	4	4	2	2	0	0	4	4	2	4	4	4	0	2	4	2	0	4
FM	58	4	2	4	4	4	2	4	4	0	4	4	4	2	4	0	2	4	2	0	4
MR	56	4	2	4	4	4	2	4	0	4	0	2	4	2	4	2	0	4	4	2	4
AA	52	4	2	4	4	4	2	2	4	2	2	4	4	2	2	2	2	0	4	2	0
DG	58	4	4	4	4	4	2	2	4	2	2	4	4	2	4	0	4	4	2	2	0
BA	68	2	4	2	4	4	2	4	4	4	4	4	4	4	2	4	2	4	4	4	4
HA	46	4	2	0	4	2	4	0	0	4	4	4	4	2	4	0	2	0	2	2	2
LC	52	4	2	4	4	2	2	0	0	4	4	2	4	4	4	0	2	4	2	0	4
NA	58	4	2	4	4	4	2	4	4	0	4	4	4	2	4	0	2	4	2	0	4
ZA	54	4	2	4	4	4	2	4	0	4	0	2	4	2	4	2	0	4	2	2	4
MM	54	2	4	4	4	4	2	2	4	4	2	4	4	2	2	0	2	2	4	2	0
RA	58	4	4	4	4	4	2	2	4	2	2	4	4	2	4	0	4	4	2	2	0
RZ	74	4	4	4	4	4	2	4	4	4	4	4	4	2	4	2	4	4	4	4	4
PM	48	4	2	0	4	4	4	0	0	4	4	4	4	2	4	0	2	0	2	2	2
PC	52	4	2	4	4	2	2	0	0	4	4	2	4	4	4	0	2	4	2	0	4
FA	60	4	2	4	4	4	2	4	4	0	4	4	4	2	4	0	2	4	2	2	4
BA	58	4	2	4	4	4	2	4	0	4	2	2	4	2	4	2	0	4	4	2	4
CE	52	4	4	4	4	4	2	2	4	2	2	4	4	2	2	0	2	0	4	2	0
DM	58	4	4	4	4	4	2	2	4	2	2	4	4	2	4	0	4	4	2	2	0
AM	70	2	4	4	4	2	2	4	4	4	4	4	4	2	4	2	4	4	4	4	4
RA	50	4	2	2	4	4	4	0	0	4	4	4	4	2	4	0	2	0	2	2	2
SF	52	4	2	4	4	2	2	0	0	4	4	2	4	4	4	0	2	4	2	0	4
ZT	58	4	2	4	4	4	2	4	4	0	4	4	4	2	4	0	2	4	2	0	4
UN	60	4	2	4	4	4	2	4	0	4	0	4	4	2	4	2	2	4	4	2	4
FD	50	4	4	4	4	2	2	2	4	2	2	4	4	2	2	0	2	0	4	2	0
LN	56	4	2	4	4	4	2	2	4	2	2	4	4	2	4	0	4	4	2	2	0
UB	68	4	4	4	4	2	2	4	4	4	4	2	2	4	2	4	2	4	4	4	4
PS	50	4	2	0	4	4	4	0	0	4	4	4	4	2	4	0	2	0	4	2	2
X	56.63	3.75	2.81	3.38	4.00	3.50	2.31	2.25	2.38	2.94	2.94	3.50	3.94	2.56	3.38	0.94	2.13	2.81	2.88	1.88	2.44
S	7.12	0.67	1.00	1.48	0.00	0.88	0.74	1.67	2.00	1.44	1.34	0.88	0.35	0.91	0.94	1.52	1.01	1.82	1.01	1.24	1.81
VC	12.57	17.92	35.48	43.72	0.00	25.14	31.91	74.03	84.04	48.87	45.70	25.14	8.98	35.65	27.91	173.57	47.44	64.77	35.06	66.02	74.3

*Legend: I= subjects' initials , X = mathematical mean, S = standard deviation, and VC = variability coefficient.

As one can see in Table 2, the arithmetical mean of the individual sums (the third vertical column) recorded by the graduate students is of 56.63 points, which is an average situated in the superior side of the medium level of self-esteem (considering the medium level to be between 40 and 59 points). The average values for 18 assertions are between 2.13 and 4.00 points, meaning above half of the average value, and for only 2 assertions we have values under the average of two: 1.88 and 0.94 points. The standard deviation and variability coefficient values are high, this showing the group's lack of homogeneity, which is normal, considering that the 22-28-year old students have different goals, aims, ways of feeling and maturing.

Discussions

The people's development is determined also by how they perceive themselves, by the trust and esteem that they enjoy from themselves and from those around them. The lack of self-esteem provokes numerous psychological problems that can have negative repercussions on the young generation's professional development. Considered to be a connecting science, psychosociology studies psychosocial aspects of individual and group behavior that arise from the communication and interaction between people, and in the communication and interaction with the "self" in all activities.

The "Self-esteem Test," presented by the Quebec Psychologists Association, was applied in order to highlight the level of self-esteem of the second level of professional formation (master's degree). These informations are useful in creating a psychosocial profile of the graduate students, the projection and accomplishment of their personal development, as the level of self-esteem can influence, in a positive or negative way, their behavior in the various situations they are confronting.

As one can see in Table 1, and Figure 1, out of the 30 male graduate students, 8 are situated between 60-80 points, and 22 between 42 and 58 points. A percentage of 26.67 of the total number of male subjects have a high self-esteem, meaning that they have confidence in their own abilities, and have the appreciation and respect of their colleagues. A relatively high percentage, 73.33, of the male graduate students is situated at a medium level with regards to self-esteem, meaning they have self-respect and self-esteem, but not that much.

The results presented in Table 2, and Figure 1, show that out of the 30 female graduate students, 7 are situated between 60-74 points, and 23 between 46 and 58 points. A percentage of 23.33 of the total number of female subjects have a high self-esteem, they have confidence in their own abilities, and have the appreciation and respect of their colleagues. A relatively high percentage, 76.67, of the female graduate students is situated at a medium level with regards to self-esteem, meaning they have self-respect and self-esteem, but not completely.

According to the results presented above, the studied graduate students show, on average, a medium level of self-esteem, which is advantageous for their professional formation. The fact that 75% of the graduate students perceive their self-esteem level as being medium can be due to a too high self-criticism, or the way in which their professional formation was not sufficiently encouraging. If the same perception is maintained, with regards to the self-esteem of those students, their will and desire to get completely involved in the improvement process of professional formation can be diminished. Of course, there are students whose score positions them at a higher level on the self-esteem scale. If to the 25% of the graduate students whose score is between 60 and 74 points, one would add another 21.66% (meaning 13) graduate students with a score in the immediate proximity of 60 points (meaning 58 points), the percentage of graduate students with a high self-esteem becomes higher for this group of subjects, meaning 46.66%.

Figure 1 The percentage expression of the graduate students' self-esteem for the "Self-esteem Test"

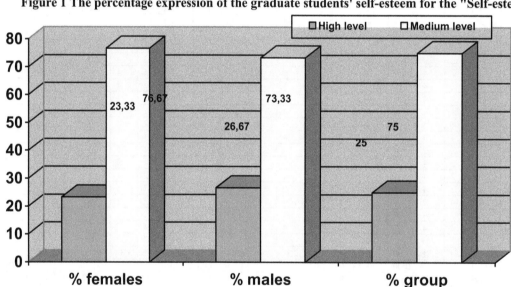

The value of the arithmetical mean, as it can be seen in Tables 1 and 2, is over 2 points for 18 assertions, which shows that the group of subjects has a good perception of their self-esteem level.

Conclusions

This study allowed the drawing of a series of conclusions with regards to the manifestation of self-esteem in the 22-26-year old graduate students.

One can see that 26.67% of the male subjects have a high level of self esteem, and 73.33% of them have a medium level self-esteem, while 23.33% have a high level, and 76.67% have a medium level self-esteem. These values confirm the hypothesis stating that "the physical education and sports graduate students' level of self-esteem is above medium level in most cases."

Also, one can observe that the high self-esteem percentage value in male students (26.67%) is higher than the female students' (23.33%), which confirms the second hypothesis, stating that "the female students have lower self-esteem than the male students."

None of the 60 subjects has recorded the maximum value of 80 points, or a value below 40 points.

There are 3 persons in the female graduate students group that have a score over 70 points, considered to be close to the maximum of 80 points, meaning they have a high self-esteem, an aspect that stimulates them in the activity of learning professional skills.

References
1. *** *Dicţionar de psihologie socială,* 1981, Editura Stiinţifică şi enciclopedică, Bucureşti
2. Epuran. M., 2005, *Elemente de psihosociologia activităţilor corporale,* Editura Renaissance, Bucureşti
3. Epuran M., Holdevici I., Toniţa F., 2008, *Psihologia sportului de performanţă,* Editura Fest, Bucureşti
4. Dragnea, C.A., 2006, *Elemente de psihosociologie a grupurilor sportive,* Editura CD Press, Bucureşti
5. Calancea, A., .1997, *Cunoaşterea de sine şi a celorlalţi, Psihoteste,*Edit. Ştiinţifică şi Tehnică, Bucureşti, România
http://www.scritube.com/sociologie/psihologie/Testul-pentru-evaluarea-stimei103812124.php.

30

Study of offence efficiency in conditions of superiority and inferiority at The Handball E.C. 2012, Serbia

Popescu Marius Cătălin, Forțan Cătălin, Mangra Gabriel Ioan, Popa Gabriel Marian

University of Craiova, Faculty of Physical Education and Sport

Abstract. Purpose During handball matches is too often seen that, in the situation of superiority and inferiority of one more or less players, they don't find an appropriate solution for tactical combinations an decide too soon to shot even they don't have perfect position yet. Some tactical solutions enable players to learn how to solve problems with creativity and courage in case of a game with one player more in the offence. A high level of dynamics must be maintained . The interaction with the pivot is very important as it enables the offensive team's numerical superiority to be taken advantage of.

Key word: *handball , offence, player, goals*

Introduction

Obtaining high performance in major competitions has highlighted a number of technical and tactical aspects that characterize current handball game practiced by the best teams in Europe. Competition among the best teams and value changes at European level require improvements of the game and training. Game concept must establish ways of action able to make full availability of performance of athletes.

Training handball players to obtain great performance is based on technical and tactical training focused on preparing both physically and psychologically. Training process can not take place without perspective and current planning, without methodical and scientific approach from the coach. Theoretical training, intelligence and psychological training of the players are factors that should be considered in preparing the current handball players.

Materials and methods

Playing with one player less or more on the court is a very important factor in a handball match with regard to both defence and offence. This is corroborated by data acquired in large competitions. The data in the diagrams below illustrate the importance of that portion of a game played by an unbalanced number of players on the court.

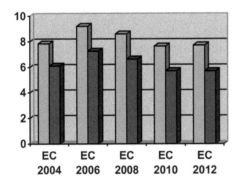

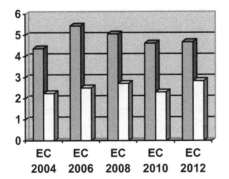

1.Number of offences and goals in case of superiority and inferiority on the court at the European Championships from 2004 to 2012

The above diagrams shows that the number of offences in superiority is slightly higher than the number of offences in inferiority. The number of goals by the numerically superior team is higher – teams with one player more score about 5 goals per match on average and the outnumbered teams slightly less than 3 goals.

Table 1: Average number and time of eliminations per team and match at the EC 2012 in Serbia

European Championship 2012 in Serbia			
Team	No. of matches	2-minute eliminations from the game	Average elimination time (mins)
Germany	6	34	10
Denmark	8	33	8
Hungary	6	27	8.5
Macedonia	7	34	9.3
Slovenia	7	27	8.1
Spain	8	18	4.2
Poland	6	20	6.7
Norway	3	21	12.3
Croatia	8	38	9.7
Iceland	6	27	8.7
Serbia	8	36	8.9
France	6	33	11.0
Sweden	6	28	9
Czech Rep.	3	17	12
Russia	3	16	10.6
Slovakia	3	15	10
TOTAL	94	424	9.15

Table shows that the average playing time per match by teams that were one player short is slightly less than 9 minutes for all teams. What is striking is the large number of eliminations in some national teams whose competitive performance was poorer – Norway and Czech Rep.

Table 2: Total number of attacks, number of attacks in superiority and inferiority and the efficiency of completed attacks at the EC 2012 in Serbia

European Championship 2012 in Serbia				
Team	No. of matches	Total no. of goals/offences	Goals/offences in superiority	Goals/offences in inferiority
Germany	6	182/344 (53%)	26/38 (69%)	20/43 (48%)
Denmark	8	205/395 (52%)	43/66 (66%)	16/36(47%)
Hungary	6	173/356(49%)	25/37(68%)	15/35(43%)
Macedonia	7	194/367(53%)	35/52(67%)	14/36(39%)
Slovenia	7	211/392(54%)	29/59(52%)	18/39(48%)
Spain	8	223/449(50%)	40/62(65%)	10/23(46%)
Poland	6	155/337(46%)	25/43(59%)	11/28(41%)
Norway	3	78/167(47%)	11/22(50%)	9/27(33%)
Croatia	8	247/457(54%)	47/76(62%)	20/45(44%)
Iceland	6	170/348(49%)	36/58(62%)	15/30(50%)

Serbia	8	222/463(48%)	32/63(51%)	13/46(28%)
France	6	176/353(50%)	28/48(58%)	25/46(54%)
Sweden	6	184/381(49%)	28/41(68%)	14/38(38%)
Czech Rep.	3	82/160(52%)	9/18(50%)	12/26(48%)
Russia	3	75/167(46%)	14/23(63%)	9/24(38%)
Slovakia	3	86/180(48%)	11/23(48%)	6/21(29%)
TOTAL	94	**2663/5350(50%)**	**439/729(60%)**	**226/542(42%)**

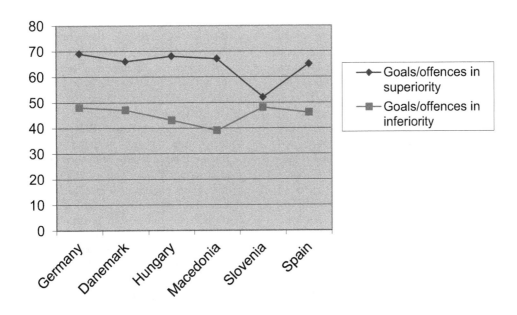

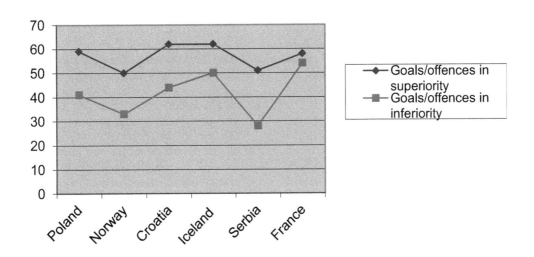

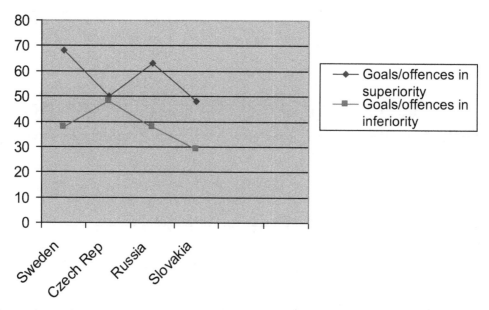

The study above shows that about one-quarter of all offences during handball matches are played while one team outnumbers the other. Nearly 14% of all offences are played when one player more is on the court. This is certainly a high percentage and shows that an important part of a handball match is played in superiority or inferiority. The data which substantially negatively deviate from the average are coloured red and those substantially positively deviating are coloured green. The blue colour indicates the France national team where the share of goals scored in superiority or inferiority is nearly the same. This is undoubtedly because coaches often fail to dedicate enough time to tactical preparations for this part of the game. The tactical problems players face during a game when a team has one player more or less are very specific in many respects. The defence usually adapts to the new situation and tries to counter the offensive activities using specific tactical methods.

Offence in superiority

From the tactical point of view, the advantage of having superiority on the court in handball is big, although this advantage diminishes substantially with other factors, primarily psychological ones. Most high-quality teams follow a specific concept during an offence whereby they outnumber their opponents by one player, and this concept focuses mostly on the pivot positioning.

1. The pivot stands between the half and the centre defender when the offensive players start attacking the goal. In this method, the left back and the pivot try to cover the half and the centre defender. The left back then continues the game by passing the ball to the pivot, the centre back or any other free player. If the defensive players react inappropriately, the left back can also take a shot at the goal.

2. The pivot stands between the half and the centre defender on the side without the ball i.e. the opposite side from where the offensive players start attacking the goal. The offensive players' basic tactical purpose is to take advantage of the pivot's block on the centre

defender. Accordingly, the centre back, after receiving a pass from the left back, takes a running start passing by the blocked defender and tries to take advantage of the culmination of events or to in any other way create a situation to continue the game

The defensive players try to hinder the classical offence by three back-court players by penetrating deeply into the area of action of the three offensive players. They thereby limit their manoeuvring area for offensive actions. The offensive players thus have difficulties receiving a passed ball during a running start and also with passing it on. The defenders offer the offensive players solutions which are tactically less appropriate and more risky. One of the possibilities for the offensive players to avoid the traps set by the defenders is to move one of the offensive players to the position of the second pivot. This transition can be carried out from the position of wing or a back-court player. It can be spontaneous, depending on the development of the playing situation, or planned as part of a tactical combination. The figure shows an example of repositioning the centre back to the position of the second pivot. The centre back runs along the goal line at the time the right back receives the ball from the right wing. The centre back tries to block the left half, whereas the right back – with a running start – tactically correctly takes advantage of the set block and tries to continue with the game.

The described tactical solutions must of course be adjusted to the team's structure or the quality of the players in individual playing positions. It is too often seen during matches at different levels that players cannot find an appropriate solution in the framework of well-conceived tactical combinations. One of the biggest problems is that players decide too soon to take a shot even if their position is not yet perfect. The offensive players are too impatient when preparing appropriate positions for shooting. The game is characterised by an insufficient number of adequately prepared dangerous running starts and passes without any interruptions due to breaches of the rules. The defenders can often easily anticipate the course of action from the initial position of the pivot and the initial development of the tactical situation – the offensive players' action becomes too predictable and thus facilitates the defender's response.

An appropriate choice of tactical solutions enables players to learn how to dynamically and creatively solve problems encountered during the game with one player more in the offence. Most of all, a high level of dynamics must be maintained together with an adequate sequence of running starts, all of which must be in line with the depth and width of the play. The interaction with the pivot is very important as it enables the offensive team's numerical superiority to be taken advantage of. The pivots must take the opponents by surprise in their play – they must position themselves and get open in various ways. The blockades must efficiently break up a homogeneous defence and thwart the anticipatory action of the defenders.

Offence in inferiority

By attacking with numerical inferiority, opponents defending system should be taken into consideration. Usually teams use two different tactical approaches when defending against attack with a player less:

• teams remain in the same defence formation as they use by numerical equality (for example 6:0, 5:1 and only adept basic principles of defending – for example „doubling—against attacker with a ball;

• teams change basic defense system – usually into combined 5+1 defense or in an aggressive and deep zone defense.

Certain tactical principles have to be followed when attacking in inferiority. It is particularly important that the offence players in their game look for the possibilities to create such situations, where there are equal in or have a higher number of players on some part of the field. Forward runs towards the goal area line can help this if they are performed suddenly or inside some particular combination. Such run in could be spontaneous (improvisation) or as a part of the certain tactical combination.

It is also important that opportunities are created for the most dangerous attackers, as defenders wish to cut them off the game. In the last years some teams try to attack with an additional offence player who substitutes a goalkeeper. Thus risk a lot but with a good collaboration among players it could be the way to overcome the opponents.

Players can also use other solutions which are difficult for the defenders to recognise and react to:

• an exchange of places between the centre back and the left back after the pass from the centre back to the right back and then the switching of places between the left back and the right back or the transition of the left back or even the centre back to the place of the second pivot;

• the switching of places between the centre back and the right back and then the transition to the place of the second pivot or without a transition;

• a return pass from the centre back to the left back who cuts towards the middle and overtakes the half;

• indicated wide switching of places between the right back and the centre back and passing of the ball between the right back and the left back who again cuts towards the middle.

Conclusion

A target-oriented and tactically correct offence in superiority or inferiority is certainly extremely important for a successful offence. A specific tactical concept must be employed, enabling the players to be very creative and choose activities the defenders find difficult to anticipate. Thus, the offensive players exploit the advantages given by their numerical superiority or to hide the disadvantages of player less in a more controlled way. The methodology is extremely important as it gradually introduces the players to correct tactics. Work with young age categories of players is very important as it enables them to upgrade their knowledge in absolute terms.

References

1. Dragnea , Adrian, Antrenamentul sportiv, Editura Didactică şi Pedagogică, Bucureşti ,1996;
2. Ortanescu Corneliu, Popescu Catalin, Handbal – Teoria şi metodica jocului, Editura Universitaria , Craiova, 2011;
3. Kunst-Ghermanescu, Ioan – Handbal – Teoria şi tactica jocului, Editura Sport Turism, Bucureşti, 1978.
4. http://www.frh.ro
5. http://www.ehf.com

31

Theoretical and Conceptual Arguments Regarding the Research on the Quality of Life at the level of students

Dumitru Roxana, Cosma Germina

University of Craiova, Faculty of Physical Education and Sport

Abstract. The purpose of this paper is to identify a number of existing concepts currently focused on improving the quality of life by means of aerobics. The environment and, particularly the democratization of social life - act on the body's health through public hygiene practices and human interrelations, depending on the significance attributed to motor values (physical), of accessibility and the universalisation of exercise and sports and of growth in the level of demand from them. Research in recent years layed great emphasis on the quality of life with increasingly more information on the impact of physical activity on it. Rigorous research attests also a positive influence of exercise and sport on well-being. It was shown that the 'balance' model works for aerobics "" in the sense that negative psychological states (depression, anxiety, confusion, fatigue, moodiness generally) turn into relaxation and fun after.
Key words: quality of life, student, review.

Introduction

Physical education and sport is a pedagogical act approach concerning all human ages, in response to a double necessity: a social and an individual one, namely: the health of human body, its normal development and the extension of human life. In a society's system of values, biological health with its indicators - tone and physical strength, harmony and beauty of body, bio-psychic vigor and psychosomatic equilibrium - is one of the vital values, that intersect with the health of nature (the environment) and the mental health of humans. The World Health Organization defines quality of life as the perception that an individual has a place in life in the context of culture and value systems in which they live and in relation to its goals, expectations, standards and concerns. The quality of life concerns the subjective experience of our perceptions and of our spiritual needs first, and the objective conditions of life remain in the background. It reflects the perception of the degree to which a person is able to satisfy his psycho-physiological needs. Some international studies (Singer et al., 2001) regarding the quality of life suggest the need to assess a complex set of variables focused on the person's subjective well-being, his emotional state, the persistency of mood, the values and skills of the individual, the socio-cultural context, the sport activity and the physical wellbeing (1).

Method

The purpose of this paper is to identify a number of existing concepts currently focused on improving the quality of life by means of aerobics. The environment and, particularly the democratization of social life - act on the body's health through public hygiene practices and human interrelations, depending on the significance attributed to motor values (physical), of accessibility and the universalisation of exercise and sports and of growth in the level of demand from them. This form of training involves a systemic approach (neglected in may works of "pedagogy" school.)

Calin M (2). distinguishes a system of physical education and sport, consisting of:
• the enhancement of physical education curriculum, divided by age and educational levels both for adolescents with a normal physical development, and those with motor impairments (eg, paralysis of limbs, spinal deformity, uncertainty static equilibrium, creating social adjustment problems);
• the enhancement of military physical education and sports (practiced in aviation, marine, infantry etc.).
•preventive or curative physical education (to maintain the bio-psychic condition of adult generation); medical physical education and health, etc. Through these subsystems physical education and sports show its importance:
• in relation to the development and improvement of the quality of the body.
•in relation to the existence of a category of professions (physical education teacher, sports coach in various sports, arbiter, sports doctors, researcher in physical education and sports administrator or sports manager etc.).

D. Ionescu, quoted by Orțănescu D. (3) appreciates the fact that gymnastics is moving, movement is health and the health of a nation is the greatest gain for the benefit of mankind.

The discipline of "Physical education" and sport is present in all curricula of all faculties and higher education profile as being mandatory or optional, being recognized as part of the educational process for the preparation of students.

Thus, we can point out a number of objectives of physical education and sport activities:

a) objectives with health-genetic functions aimed at the continuous improvement of health, physical, mental vigor, a well as the harmonious physical development, ensuring compensation effects on intellectual activity, treatment of sedentary lifestyle, stress, fatigue.

b) objectives with educational functions, which determine the raising of the general level of motility and the learning the basics of the practice of some sports branches, the forming and strengthening of a system of theoretical and practical knowledge (hygienic, physiological, educational, methodical, organizational), the modeling of behavioral and psychological states and their implementation in the practice of life (responsibility, perseverance, confidence, self-discipline, teamwork, fair play).

c) objectives with social function, one that aims to cover all subjects in practicing systematic and organized physical exercise and favorite sports, the development of beliefs and habit formation of independent practice of sports activities, with hygienic purposes, leisure and sports education

d) objectives that aim at furthering sports performance destined to students with some training and sports classification, those who are part of representative teams.

The interest given to aerobic gymnastics in recent years, the objective requirements for continuous improvement of this activity among students, as an efficient and accessible means in the multilateral training, of preparation and education of younger generations are enough reasons for today's aerobics to be on top of the preferences of students, and particularly female students regarding the physical education classes. (4).

Aerobics covers a wide range of media, taken from basic gymnastics, other sports branches, from classical and modern dance, performed and adapted on musical background, resulting rhythms, amplitudes and different positions in which effort is conducted under aerobic regime .

Combining aerobic gymnastics maintenance means with the acquiring of specific items and motor structures specific to aerobic sports, resulted in larger, richer and more attractive gymnastics lessons. Thus, in addition to the general objectives aimed at forming a proper body attitude, we obtain the toning of muscles, the establishing and maintaining of an optimal body weight, which facilitate the execution of a lesser difficulty elements, constructions or pyramids between executing parties, etc..

Due to the fact that aerobic exercise is accompanied by music, it determines and transmits a certain emotional state in students, leading to increased interest in practicing sports. Among the many contributions aerobics brings, the most important one is the harmonious physical shape and the acquisition of some feminine traits to the female students.

In recent years, research in the field have shown the lack of full health is closely linked to sedentarism and inactive lifestyle in terms of sports. Knowledge of these correlations, associated with a better awareness of what health care means and how it can change his lifestyle and to turn it into an active one, based on systematic practice of physical exercise.

Thus, the current enthusiasm towards physical activities is not only a matter of fashion, motor activities are those that refine movement and transform the need for movement in internal motivation, making it an activity that provides high intensity emotional satisfaction.

Those responsible for promoting active and healthy lifestyle always recognized the educational potential of sport and they exploit it, integrating it into education policies and actions to improve the quality of life, including in terms of health (5).

On quality of life, this implies a theory of human nature, of the system of human needs, the factors that govern their dynamics. (6).

Thus, Amza L. (7), certifies the previously said through a study applied to a group of 20 students who have performed for 10 weeks work programs that included means of aerobic gymnastics in physical education classes that proved that the motric level of the subjects has changed considerably as a result of a systematic and regular practice of this type of exercise.

In Romania, Stoenescu G., gave special attention to training exercises for a suitable posture, to combat obesity and improve the motric expressiveness. Since 1973 this has made an important contribution to the sports development by publishing a series of editorials, structured to be useful to a large number of readers. M. Stancu (8), establishes a correlation between motor activity and state of health of respondents by applying self-assessment questionnaires, to a sample of 312 women over 18 year swhich resulted in sports being not among their priorities , 52.6% practicing them occasionally, while 37.8% not practicing at all. S. Popescu (9), after the application of work schedules based on specific means of aerobic gymnastics for a period of 1 year observed radical changes on the group of female students who do not practice or practice aerobics occasionally (73%), so the number of female students engaged in aerobic exercises covers almost the entire lot of research (96.5%), reflecting the author's approach efficiency.

Gagiu M. (10), in his comparative study on the effectiveness of different types of aerobics programs in developing motor capacity, based on over 20 years experience in the of aerobic gymnastics finds that the issue of these activities is open to changes and additions to substance and form. Thus he considers that remaining dependent on traditional aerobics only means limiting its effectiveness in driving capacity development. The author makes some changes in content and certain details about the methodology of this activity through the development of type "callanetics", "cardio" or aerobic dance, choreography block form. The study undertaken, the author concludes that the practice of aerobic gymnastics after a certain rigorously developed program , with the inclusion of "cardio", "calistenics" and dance aerobics exercises led to the development of motor capacity higher values.

Fitness achieved by practicing systematic exercise translates on an individual plane through increased performance, confidence, independence physically and psychologically, contributing to perceived quality of life. (11). Although many trainees have general knowledge about the importance of exercise, their beneficial effects for the body, they can not clearly define the concept of "active lifestyle". The incentives to support the activity represent knowledge and beliefs of an aesthetic order . The fact that through physical exercise cumulative effects can be achieved, although it is not clearly stated, appears from the responses. Though most answers are satisfactory from the point of view of the specialist we should not neglect the fact that the sample chosen has as a feature the homogeneity of of social class, level of education.

Below this reserve it should be emphasized that we see a lack of concern from other social categories for leisure physical activities. Popa F. (12) argues that improving the quality of life of many people is the main benefit that you can make exercising one or more forms of movement. Underlying this goal there is the notion of perceived health by each individual. It Is the first step in order to identify the consequences of not practicing physical movement, which can affect the quality of life, on some levels: the physical ability, the existence of pain, sleep quality, social integration, the energetic ability to solve daily activities etc..

Regarding the effects of practicing sports as exercise (exercise, in English) on the psyche itself, it has been shown that aerobic and fitness activities primarily , but also competitive sports such as tennis, volleyball and football , reduce short-term anxiety and depression (of longer term) (13). Tucker (1990) shows that a good physical condition can significantly reduce the risk of psychological disturbance in adults of both sexes. Exercise practiced regularly can stimulate emotional functioning so that stress factors are more easily tolerated. As a consequence, social contacts are positively affected. (14).

A division of the United Nations released a top according to the human development index (HDI) and, as in 2011, our country was ranked 50th with a score of 0.781 (15). According to studies, the term "quality of life" and specifically, "health related quality of life" refers to the physical, psychological, social and health domains, seen as distinct areas that are influenced by people's experiences ,beliefs, expectations but also by the perceptions that the individual has on his own "health". (16,17,18).

Most research analyses the quality of each field of the quality of life separately by specific questions regarding its most important components. Most often they ask the respondents a question such as "Please rate the quality of life and overall health on a scale from 1-10," which may provide a useful overall assessment on "the quality of life" and "the overall health." This research provides subjective data though. On the other hand, relying solely on data indicating health as a goal, such as medical reports, they omit a number of relevant factors such as a person's threshold for tolerance to discomfort. (19)

Because many of the components the quality of life can not be directly observed, they are usually evaluated according to the classical principles of the theory. The measuring instrument assumes that there is a true value the quality of life noted by the authors ,Q, which can not be measured directly, but can be measured indirectly by asking a series of questions known as "elements" each of which truly measure the same concept or construct. These questions are addressed to the subject and the answers are converted to numeric scores, which are then combined to obtain "scale" scores that can also be combined to obtain domain scores and other scores calculated statistically by the summary. (20)

Rejeski and all analyzes critically the literature on physical activity and quality of life in older adults. In this regard, attention is given to the quality of life as a psychological construct represented by life satisfaction, as well as a geriatric clinical outcome represented by the basic dimensions of health or health-related quality. Literature is also examined to identify potential mediators and moderators of physical activity and quality of life relationship. (21)

The issue is whether there is a dose-response relationship between these concepts and the extent to which physical activity is associated with important aspects of cognitive, physical, and psychosocial function. Finally, they proposed a multidimensional model to examine potential mediating and moderating factors in physical activity and quality of life and the practical implications of such a model for practitioners (23).

Conclusion

Research in recent years layed great emphasis on the quality of life with increasingly more information on the impact of physical activity on it. Rigorous research attests also a positive influence of exercise and sport on well-being. It was shown that the 'balance' model works for aerobics "" in the sense that negative psychological states (depression, anxiety, confusion, fatigue, moodiness generally) turn into relaxation and fun after. Aerobics classes should arouse interest and pleasure of movement, providing disconnection and active rest, relaxation and recreation, as required by the program rather busy student training, which involves prolonged static postures . Regarding the effects of practicing sport as exercise (exercise, in English) on the psyche itself they have shown that aerobic and fitness activities first, but also competitive sports such as tennis, volleyball and football reduce short-term anxiety and depression (of longer term). Provided that the exercise should take place at least twice a week regularly and for more than six weeks. Even presently media spots urging people to take exercise at least 30 minutes are presented every day.

References

1. http://www.sportscience.ro/html/articole_conf_2007_-_46.html Singer, - accessed on 30.05.2012
2. Calin M., (2003), Theory and meta-theory of the educational action, Aramis Publishing House, Bucharest, p.39
3. Orţănescu D., Nanu C., Cosma G., (2007), Aerobics, Universitaria Publishing House, Craiova, p.103
4. Nanu C., (2009), Aerobics, fitness optimization tool, Universitaria Publishing House, Craiova
5. The Official e E.U., 2012, C 9/75
6. Zamfir C., (1998), Dictionary of Sociology, Babei Publishing House, Bucharest, pp.79
7. Amza L., 2008, Contribution regarding the improvement of the mobility training using exercises from aerobic gymnastics in the physical education lesson of the female students from faculties without a physical education profile, *Proceeding International Conference Physical Education, Sport and Helth, nr.12 (1/2008)*, Editura Universităţii din Piteşti, pp. 51
8. Stancu M., 2008, The comparative analysis of the helth condition perception of the women practicing physical exercises during their spare time and women who don`t,

Proceeding International Conference Physical Education, Sport and Helth, nr.12 (1/2008), Editura Universității din Pitești, pp. 149-150

9. Popescu S., 2009, Ways and attractive means for promotion of the principle of active life among female students, PhD Thesis, UNEFS, Bucharest, p.198

10. http://www.sportscience.ro/html/articole_conf_2004_-_22.html - accessed on 20.06.2012

11. Popescu S., 2009, Ways and attractive means for promotion of the principle of active life among female students, PhD Thesis, UNEFS, Bucharest, p.198

12. http://www.sportscience.ro/html/articole_conf_2002_-_52.html - accesssed on 20.06.2012

13. http://www.sportscience.ro/html/articole_conf_2004_-_53.html - accesssed on 20.06.2012

14. Sabau Ghe, 2010, Effects of organized physical movement practice on the quality of life, PhD Thesis, University "Babes-Bolyai" Cluj-Napoca, p.8http://web.ubbcluj.ro/ro/pr-acad/rezumate/2010/sociologie/sabau_gheorghe_ro.pdf

15. CCPS, 1996, The significance of sport for society. The impact of sport on health, Bucharest, p.30

16. http://www.ghimpele.ro/2011/11/studiu-calitatea-vietii-in-romania-un-pic-mai-buna-decat-cea-din-cuba/

17. Brook RH, Ware JE Jr, Davies-Avery A, Stewart AL, Donald CA, Rogers WH., 1979, *Conceptualization and measurement of health for adults in the health insurance study.* Vol. VIII, overview. Santa Monica, Calif.: Rand Corporation, 1979. (Publication no. R-1987/3-HEW.)

18. Patrick DL, Bush JW, Chen MM., 1973, Toward an operational definition of health. *J Health Soc Behav 1973;14:6-23*

19. Brook RH, Ware JE Jr, Rogers WH, et al., 1983, Does free care improve adults' health? Results from a randomized controlled trial., *N Engl J Med 1983;309:1426-1434*

20. Anderson RB, Testa MA. Symptom distress checklists as a component of quality-of-life measurement: comparing prompted reports by patient and physician with concurrent adverse event reports via the physician. *Drug Inf J 1994;28:89-114*

21. Ware JE, Kosinski M, Keller SD. 1994, SF-36 Physical and mental health summary scales: a user's manual. Boston: The Health Institute, New England Medical Center

22. W. Jack Rejeski, Shannon L. Mihalk, 2001, Physical Activity and Quality of Life in Older Adults, *J Gerontol A Biol Sci Med Sci (2001) 56(suppl 2): 23-35 doi:10.1093/gerona/56.suppl_2.23, pp.23-35*

23. Sarah F. Griffin and all, 2010, Results from the Active for Life process evaluation: program delivery fidelity and adaptations, *Health Educ. Res. (2010) 25(2): 325-342*

32

The effects of psychological training on the anger-hostility mood states generated by competition stress

Alexe Cristina Ioana[1], Alexe Dan Iulian[2]

[1] "Stiinta" Bacau Sports Club, Bacău, România,
[2] "Vasile Alecsandri" University Of Bacău,[1] Department of Physical Therapy and Occupational Therapy

Abstract. The attitudes, the behavior and the personality of professional athletes, as well as the complexity and diversity of the factors that generate stress during competitions, are still far from being completely clarified. The increased states of psychological tension, accumulated throughout the days and hours prior to competitions, as well as the tensions accumulated during them, condition, usually, the quality and the success of the athlete's psycho-motor performances. **The purpose** of this research envisaged the analysis of the manifestation of the anger-hostility mood states in the professional middle distance and long distance runners, during stress-generating competition situations. **Methodology.** The research envisaged the dynamics of the manifestation of the anger-hostility moods, in three different stages, over a 6 month period (February-August 2011), in 12 subjects with various experience in professional track and field, and in their particular event. The athletes, under their freely expressed consent, were subjected to three psychological tests, in three different stress situations: before two major competitions (national championships - selection competitions), and at the middle of the period between the two important competitions. The research instrument was the P.O.M.S. test (by McNair, 1971). **Results.** The subjects have gained the most in their way of approaching the competition, and controlling their negative, intense psychological tensions before an important competition, a fact highlighted by the statistically calculated significant differences. Finally, they managed to lower them considerably, thus developing their ability to regulate their reactions of hostility, generated by competition stress. **Conclusions.** The lack of a specially adapted psychological training envisaging the control of the anger-hostility moods might increase the risk of the athletes not recognizing the models for comparing the different psycho-affective moods, a fact that could generate confusion, which does not necessarily affects negatively the athletic performance, but it does not stimulate it, either.

Keywords: competition, stress, anger-hostility, athletes, performance

Introduction

Defining stress as a "stimulus with a strong psychological-affecting signification" (1), and affectivity as the "relation of concordance or discordance between the dynamics of internal events (one's own states of motivation) and the dynamics of external events (the surrounding situations, objects, persons) (2), the professional literature highlighting the psychological implications that stress determines in one's individual life, permanently modifying his/her psycho-affective mood states. The modifications of psycho-affective moods can determine, according to psychologists, positive or negative states, reflecting, in the opinion of P.Popescu-Neveanu (3), the relationships between the subject and the ambiance.

Regarding the relationships between the ambiance and the professional athlete (as a subject), the studies from the last several years have clearly highlighted a higher intensity of the states of psychological tension experienced by the athletes, especially during competition periods (unanimously recognized as stress-generating factors). This aspect is also due to the fact that professional athletes react differently to the pressure exerted by the complex situations to which they are subjected during training and during competitions, based on a whole series of factors.

The dynamics of the manifestation of the various psychological states of professional athletes is determined (4,5,6,7,8) also by the subjective way of perceiving the result. According to the above-mentioned specialists, the perception of the result, as an inherent factor, is tied to the subjective probability of success. Thus, the professional athlete will adjust his/her attitude according to the chances that he/she is giving himself/herself in reaching the desired result. This adjustment can determine an increase in the different states of psycho-affective tension, among which the states of anger, hostility (with regards to the people around them, and their own person).

With regards to one specific sports branch or event, numerous studies have emphasized the fact that some professional athletes react differently, compared to others, to the same stress factor, a reaction highlighted in the manifestations of the psycho-affective states analyzed in this paper. Thus, regarding the professional athletes, the studies of Morgan and Pollock (9) have highlighted the fact that they have a distinct profile of psychological moods, especially during competitions. After applying certain psychological tests (among which the one used in this study - P.O.M.S.), the above-mentioned specialists stated that the athletes are under the normal average with regards to tension, depression, fatigue, and confusion; around average regarding anger, fury, hostility; and above average regarding activeness, vigor, mental energy.

Material and Method

Research Hypotheses

- the application of a psychological training program specially adapted to the specifics of the training and of the competition system, can diminish the moods of anger-hostility generated by the competition stress in the middle distance and long distance runners;

- the anger-hostility moods generated by the competition stress in the middle distance and long distance runners can highlight a significantly decreasing dynamics when the training includes specific psychological training techniques.

The research envisaged the analysis of the psycho-affective moods of *12 professional middle distance and long distance runners* (Table 1), from 5 Romanian sports clubs, with an average age, at the beginning of the experiment, of 22 (minimum 18, maximum 28), with an experience in track and field between 5 and 14 years, and a specialization in the middle distance and long distance events of minimum 4 years. The subjects' athletic performances are from good to very good (from nationally medaled to multiple national and Balkan champions, participants and medaled in various international competitions).

Table 1 - The subjects (identification data at the beginning of the research)

No.	Subject	Age	Experience in Track & Field	Event the athlete is specialized in	Experience in event
1	G.I.	23	9 years	3000m stc	6 years
2	S.A.	20	5 years	5000 m, 10.000m	4 years old
3	I.C.	26	11 years old	5000 m, 10.000m	8 years old
4	C.V.	20	7 years	800m	5 years old
5	P.G.	21	8 years old	800m, 1.500m	7 years old
6	G.A.	23	11 years old	3000m stc.	8 years old
7	Z.I.	28	17 years old	800m, 1.500m	12 years old
8	M.I.	19	8 years old	800m, 1.500m	4 years old
9	F.C.	23	9 years old	5000m, 10.000m	4 years old
10	B.C.	19	6 years old	800m, 1.500m	4 years old
11	B.A.	24	14 years old	1500m, 3000m stc	8 years old
12	C.I.	18	5 years old	800m, 1.500m	4 years old

Legend: m = meters; stc. = steeplechase

The research instrument we used was an adapted form of the P.O.M.S. test (the Profile of Mood States, McNair, (10). This test was applied as a questionnaire. Based on indications, the obtained scores were transfered on a specific test profile chart, comprising T-scores for each factor. The graphical representation of the data shows "iceberg"-type diagrams, considering the visible side as being delimited by a line found at the 50 point mark. The variables subjected to the POMS analysis usually are: tension-anxiety, depression-dejection, anger-hostility, vigor-activity, fatigue-inertia, and confusion-bewilderment.

This paper focuses on the variable *A-H* **(anger-hostility)**, which expresses:

• dispositions of anger and dislike toward other persons, toward self, or toward certain situations ("angry, furious, ready to fight");

• feelings of intense and visible anger ("irritated," "upset");

• lighter/reduced feelings of hostility ("indignant," "malicious");

In order to determine the manifestation dynamics of the anger-hostility moods under different conditions of psychological stress, we applied the tests in 3 moments of major importance for the subjects' professional activity (3 major competitions, at different times in the competition season, each with a different meaning for the subjects):

• the initial testing (February 2011, National Senior Championship, indoor, goal - medal);

• the intermediary testing (June 2011, International Championship, outdoor, goal - time);

• the final testing (August 2011, National Senior Championship, outdoor, goal - medal);

The determination of the psycho-affective moods appearing before the athletic competitions was done in the first day for each of the three competitions, in the morning, after the athletes woke up and served breakfast, the testing being supervised by a psychologist.

The utilized means system

We specify that the research was conducted through a specific psychological training program, over the course of 6 months. We applied 30 means destined for a specific psychological training, in 48 lessons, throughout 24 weeks (6 months). The specificity of the lessons was adapted, mainly to regulate the dispositions generated by the 6 variables evaluated through the POMS test. We must mention that the athletes' training before the three envisaged competitions (the final 6 days before entering the competition) din not include anymore high levels of intensity or volume, the runners performing standard training sessions, specific to the week before the competition. These training sessions have subjected no longer the body to new adaptations or stimuli, having as main goals: the active rest, maintaining the obtained energy to an optimal level, the psychological and tactical preparation for the competition.

Results

The data recorded after the 3 assessments regarding the anger-hostility moods in all the professional athletes subjected to this analysis are shown in Table 2. That table also presents a minimum of statistical data (for a general view over the studied phenomenon).

After transforming the obtained points in T scores (Table 2), according to the chart, and taking into account the value-imposed limitation of 50 (mark), the application of the POMS test, regarding the moods of anger and hostility experienced by the subjects before the competition has presented interesting results, recorded during the *initial testing.* Thus, the analysis of the *A-H variable* shows that all of the subjects, with

the exception of the subject G.I. (47 value), have recorded individual scores above the mark value of 50 (the average value being of 63.00), a fact that has determined the orientation of the peak of the "iceberg" profile toward this variable (Figure 1), highlighting moods of hostility - anger - irritation - increased psychological tension before starting the actual competition.

Table 2 - Data recorded by the subjects during the POMS test, variable A-H

No.	initials	gender	age	A-H			Average
				t1	t2	t3	
1.	G.I.	M	23	47	45	48	46.67
2.	S.A.	M	20	64	60	57	60.33
3.	I.C.	M	26	62	56	54	57.33
4.	C.V.	M	20	51	54	52	52.33
5.	P.G.	M	21	80	74	66	73.33
6.	G.A.	M	23	63	42	48	51.00
7.	Z.I.	M	28	66	66	38	56.67
8.	M.I.	M	19	65	64	53	60.67
9.	F.C.	F	23	54	52	49	51.67
10.	B.C.	F	19	70	51	49	56.67
11.	B.A.	F	24	64	39	47	50.00
12.	C.I.	F	18	70	70	51	63.67
		Average	22.00	**63.00**	**56.08**	**51.00**	**56.69**
		S	3.05	8.96	11.08	6.65	
		Cv	13.84	14.23	19.76	13.03	

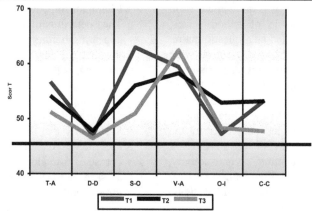

Figure 1 - Comparative analysis regarding the profile of the psycho-affective dispositions in all three tests

The highest value was recorded by the subject P.G. - T-80 score, which indicates a very high level of anger, hostility, and discontent. Trying to understand the causes for this disposition, we later had a conversation with the subject, during which he revealed that his mood is caused by his financial situation related to the track and field section that he represents in competitions, as well as by the low rewards he gets for his efforts. We also noticed two relatively high values in two other subjects (B.C. – 70, C.I. -70, Figure 2). The comparative analysis of the individual values in relation to the other variables of the POMS test presents some extremely interesting aspects of the profile of the two middle distance and long distance runners: if in C.I. the *A-H* (anger-hostility) value is high (70), and in V.A. the value is low (54), in B.C. the

values for both variables are high, showing anger - irritation - tension, but also, at the same time, high vigor, activeness, and mental energy values.

The analysis of the data recorded during the intermediary testing (transforming the obtained points in T scores, according to the chart, taking into account the value-imposed limitation of 50) before the second competition, gave the following results:

• the standard deviation (S) and the variability coefficient (Vc) show a relative homogeneity in the values recorded by the subjects (between 10% and 20%)

• the average values show that the A-H variable recorded values over the chart mark (Table 2), highlighting dispositions of anger and "ready to fight" attitudes (*a positive aspect, in our opinion, before a competition*);

• 9 of the 12 subjects (75%) recorded values over the limit of 50 points. The subject P.G. is still the one recording the highest value for this variable, just like during the initial testing (albeit slightly lowered, from 80 to 74);

• for the *A-H variable*, compared to the first testing, when only one subject recorded positive values (under 50 points), during the intermediary testing, 3 subjects recorded values below the limit, and the average value dropped with 6.92 points (from 63.00 to 56.08). This aspect makes us believe that the program applied so far was effective with regards to regulating the disposition of anger, irritation, nervousness, before the competition.

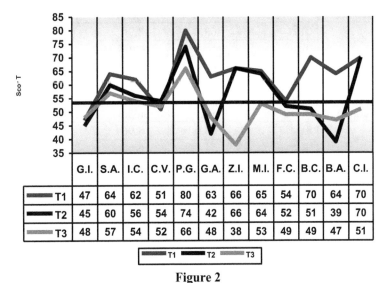

Figure 2
Development of the values for the *A-H variable* in the three moments of the testing
(initial test – T1, intermediary test -T2, final test -T3)

For a much more eloquent scientific and statistical argument, the Student's t-test was applied, to determine the significant differences between different variables, at the significance threshold of p < 0.05. In order to verify the existence of significant differences regarding the psychological dispositions of anger and hostility of the subjects, determined by competition stress during the first two tests (initial and intermediary), the t-test for paired samples was applied, having as independent variable the variable *test* (*test_1* versus *test_2*), and as dependent variable, the *A-H* variable, specific to the psycho-affective moods profile (POMS).

Thus, in the case of the *A-H variable, there are significant differences* between the results for test_1 and test_2 [t (11) = 2.5666, p < 0.05]. If one looks at the averages, one can see that after the psychological training program, the results for the A-H variable have significantly decreased between test 1 and test 2 (Table 3). This aspect highlights the significant decrease in the moods representing irritation, anger, moods with which the subjects approached the previous competitions.

The ending of the period of application of the psychological training program has imposed the last testing (*the final testing*), to determine the modifications in the subjects' behavior. Synthesized, the results are as follows:

• the average values of the *A-H* variable (51.00) indicate a low level of irritation, anger, nervous tension. This can be interpreted as the subjects having optimally regulated their moods. The analysis of the individual values shows 5 values (41.67%) over the 50 points mark, but these values are not high (with the exception of the subject P.G.), and when analyzed together with the values from other variables, they indicate an optimal level of the psycho-affective moods before the August 2011 competition, when this research came to an end;

• the values of the *A-H* variable during the final testing (characterized by irritation, negative psychological tension, hostility) decreased from 56.08 (slightly high and negative value during the intermediary testing) to **51.00** (close to the limit of 50, thought to be optimal for controlling these moods);

• after analyzing in comparison to the initial testing, one can observe that in the final testing, the level of hostility, anger, irritation (toward colleagues, coach, opponents, competition, etc.) is much lower, descending from 63.00 points to 51.00 points; this decrease can be viewed as an improvement of the subjects' psycho-affective moods, as an adaptation of their attitude to the moods generated by competition stress;

• the comparative calculation of the individual values recorded by the subjects for the psychological variables during tests T2 and T3 shows that for the *A-H* variable, compared to the intermediary testing, when 9 subjects recorded values over 50 points, during the final testing only 5 subjects have recorded again negative values, these being visibly lower than the ones in the intermediary testing. This aspect, together with the decrease in the average value by 5.08 points, makes us believe that the program applied so far was effective with regards to regulating the disposition of anger, irritation, nervousness, before the competition;

In order to verify the existence of significant differences regarding the psychological dispositions of anger and hostility of the subjects, determined by competition stress during the last two tests

(intermediary and final), the t-test for paired samples was applied, having as independent variable the variable test (test_2 versus test_3), and as dependent variable, the *A-H* variable, specific to the psycho-affective moods profile (POMS). In the case of the A-H variable, there are no significant differences (Table 3) between the results for test 2 and test 3 [t (11) = 1.716, p = 0.114].

Table 3 - The t test for comparing the average values between the situations *test_1, test_2, and test_3*

Variable	Test	Average	St.Dev	t-test results
A-H	Test_1	63.00	8.96	t (11) = 2.566,
	Test_2	56.08	11.08	p = 0.026
Variable	Test	Average	St.Dev	t Test results
A-H	Test_2	56.08	11.08	t (11) = 1.716,
	Test_3	51.00	6.65	p = 0.114
Variable	Test	Average	St.Dev	t Test results
A-H	Test_1	63.00	8.96	t (11) = 4.723,
	Test_3	51.00	6.65	p = 0.001

The psychological training program applied between February 2011 (initial testing) and August 2011 (final testing) on a group of 12 subjects, middle distance and long distance runners, had as an effect a decrease by **12 points** in the moods of hostility, irritation, anger toward the competition situation (the *A-H* variable) Thus, the psycho-affective states specific to this variable have recorded the highest drop. On a practical level, the subjects have gained the most in their way of approaching the competition, and controlling their negative, intense psychological tensions before an important competition. Finally, they managed to lower them considerably, thus developing their ability to regulate their reactions of hostility, generated by competition stress.

The verification of the existence of significant differences regarding the psychological dispositions of anger and hostility of the subjects, determined by competition stress between the initial test (T1) and the final test (T3), the t-test for paired samples was applied again, having as independent variable the variable *test* (test_1 versus test_3), and as dependent variable, the *A-H* variable, specific to the psycho-affective moods profile (POMS). In the case of the *A-H variable, there are significant differences* between the results for test 1 and test 3 [t (11) = 4.723, p < 0.05] (Table 3).

A comparative analysis of the average values allows us to see that after the psychological training program was applied, the moods of hostility, irritation, anger 9the A-H variable) before the actual start of the competition have significantly dropped between test 1 and test 3 (Figure 2).

The qualitative analysis of the statistical correlations regarding the sense of modifications in the values for the psychological variables throughout this applicative intervention has emphasized the following aspects:

- the A-H variable, although it initially correlated positively and weakly with the score recorded by the subjects during the initial testing (T1, February 2011), after the intervention program was applied, it comes to correlate negatively with the score obtained by transforming the athletic performance recorded during the final testing (T3, August 2011, Table 4);

- as the A-H variable signifies anger- hostility and is a negative dimension, and the correlation has become negative, one could estimate that as the subjects tend to record lower T scores for this variable, they will tend to obtain higher performances during the important competition they are participating in (and this happened, in our opinion, only after the application of the special psychological training program);

Table 4 - The Pearson r correlation coefficients between the values of the psychological variables and the values from the students' points recorded during the analyzed track and field competitions

Variable	Score 1 (N = 12)	Score 2 (N = 12)	Score 3 (N = 12)
A_H1	r = 0.155 p = 0.631		
A_H2		r = − 0.198 p = 0.536	
A_H3			r = − 0.365 p = 0.243

Discussions

The simple visualization of the average values recorded for the *A-H* variable during the initial and final tests (the variable describing complex reactions that a professional athlete can manifest in his/her attitude) shows us that the psychological training program applied in this research (based on various ways of communication, suggestion, and autosuggestion, self-awareness, biofeedback, developing self-esteem, coping, neuro-psychological recovery, activeness optimization strategies, pep talks, using posters etc.) has determined significant decreases in the states of anger, irritation, hostility, moods that influence negatively the behavior of an athlete before a very important competition.

This observation is useful for the practice of professional track and field, emphasizing the importance that the specialists in this discipline should give to the creation of a specific psychological training that would optimally undermine and control the moods of hostility and anger, and to orient the athlete's behavior and psychological energy toward achieving the main goal - a top performance.

Conclusions

The first hypothesis, stating that "the application of a psychological training program specially adapted to the specifics of the training and of the competition system, can diminish the moods of anger-hostility generated by the competition stress in the middle distance and long distance runners" was confirmed. The second hypothesis, stating that "the anger-hostility moods generated by the competition stress in the middle distance and long distance runners can highlight a significantly decreasing dynamics when the training includes specific psychological training techniques" was also confirmed.

In our opinion, in professional track and field the moods of anger, fury, hostility can have effects that are positive (mobilization, "ready to fight" attitudes, etc.), but especially negative (useless energetic discharges, unfavorable to the performance, blocking the constructive psychological processes, limitation). From this perspective, considering the specifics of professional track and field and the characteristics imposed by the particularities of the effort, as well as the results of this research, we think that the relationship between a specific psychological training and the dynamics of the psycho-affective moods (anger-hostility) must be a directly proportional one, but must be permanently controlled.

In other words, a specific psychological training for the middle distance and long distance events should permanently try to maintain the psycho-affective moods of anger-hostility within a neutral area that is optimal for the manifestation of high athletic performance (if the level of the hostility moods are too low, there could be a chance to diminish the fighting attitude of the athletes).

Also, the lack of a specially adapted psychological training envisaging the control of the anger-hostility moods might increase the risk of the athletes not recognizing the models for comparing the different psycho-affective moods, a fact that could generate confusion, which does not necessarily affects negatively the athletic performance, but it does not stimulate it, either.

References

1. Holdevici, I., (1993), Psihologia succesului, Editura Ceres, Bucureşti, p.34;
2. Golu,M., (2000), Fundamentele psihologiei. Volumul I, Ed. Fundaţiei România de Mâine, Bucureşti, p.79;
3. Popescu-Neveanu, P., (1977), Curs de psihologie generală. Vol.II, Editura Universităţii din Bucureşti, Bucureşti;
4. Martens, R., (1987), Coaches Guide to Sport Psychology, Human Kinetics USA, Champaign-IL;
5. Delignieres, D., (1993), Anxiété et performance, în „Cognition et performance" (1993) sub îndrumarea Famose, J. P., INSEP, Paris;
6. Hanin, Y., L., (1999), Emotion in Sport, Human Kinetics Books, Champaign, USA;
7. Stevens, M., J., Lane, M., A., (2001), Mood-Regulating Strategies Used By Athletes în revista Athletic Insight – The Online Journal of Sports Psychology, Volum 3 Issue 3, U.K.;
8. Delignieres, D., (2008), L'Anxiété compétitive. Chapitre II dans le livre Psychologie du sport. Press Universitaires de France, Paris;
9. Morgan W.,P., Pollock, M., (1977), Psychologic characterization of the elite distance runner, în Annals of the New York Academy of Sciences, Volume 301/ oct 1977 (The Marathon: Physiological, Medical, Epidemiological, and Psychological Studies), p.382–403;
10. McNair, D., M., Lorr, M., Droppleman, L., F., (1971), Manual for the Profile of Mood States, CA: Educational and Industrial Testing Services, USA, San Diego;

33

The importance of kinetic profilaxy in harmonious development of the somatosensory parameters to preschoolar

Cristuţă Alina Mihaela[1], Raţă Gloria[1], Lupu Gabriel[2]

[1] *„Vasile Alecsandri" University from Bacău, Bacau, Romania*
[2] *National University of Physical Education and Sport, Bucharest, Romania*

Abstract. The concept of a "harmoniouschild's development" has been studied a long time by the representatives of the most advanced educational and is of the utmost importance to the family and in school,for parents who grants a attention problems of education. This concept is great and full of meaning, as it incorporates all facets of life a child and the holistic approach we are working toward the need planting all their skills contained in it.A common concern in the field of the child's harmonious development is represented by delays in development consisting of the retard in the purchasing age specific skills in step of development. The purpose of research has been the importance of kinetic profilaxie application of harmonious development of the parameters in somatomotor to preschoolars. The means for the exploration and evaluation, used in the research to assessing the development of preschoolar children, are relevant and gives the necessary information to highlight role of kinetic prifilaxie to this category of age. Kineticprofilaxy may constitute an earlyoperation and welcome to the problems of delay in development, and knowledge and its application on a large scale it should be a special concern of parents and those working in mass caterers of prescoolar.

Key words: *development, kinetic profilaxie, preschoolar*

Introduction

Over the last few years, the activities carried out at home and in physical mass caterers have never known a rapid development. Attention was also directed to the need to provide fresh air children, to learn correct ways to make the movement, to make the sequence correct between study and rest - all of which are a subject much discussed by those working with children. The importance of gymnastics has been removed from the crowd as being particularly important, in the same way as games carried out in the open air, the activities manual and trips, (4).

Obtaining a kept soft curves of the body can be achieved by active participation by the child, and it is necessary as he was to be directed in this respect by both the rescuer and the permanent operation to their family. The harmonious development of preschoolars is always current becausthe man goes through the same processes of growth and development, training of attitude of body and of the trend of fact during his life. The concern on the problem development and to keep correct attitude of the body may be seen in the literature especially in the medical field and educational purposes.

Increased interest and number in the research on this field, have brought to the foreground new theories and strategies with wide applicatins in practice, that helps promote application of the methods kinetoprofilactice to the level of all mass caterers (1).

Material and methods

A common concern in the field of the child's harmonious development is represented by delays in development consisting of the retard in the purchasing age specific skills in step of development.

Kineticprofilaxie may constitute anearly operation and welcome to the problems of delay in development, and knowledge and its application on a large scale it should be a special concern of parents and those engaged in mass caterers of preschschoolars.

Knowledge and information on stages of development of the children give parents and educators an opportunity to work on preventing the occurrence of various shortcomings of the body and of the effects of their parameters on the somatomotor body functional

Currently in the research, we suggest checking the work of the two assumptions, that is, if the means for the exploration and evaluation used in the research to assessing the development of preschoolar children ,are relevant and gives the necessary information to highlight role of kineticprifilaxiei in this age category.; the exercise can improve physical somatomotor to preschoolarparameters, If it is carried out in a form prepared and closely observed?

The methods of research I used: The theoretical investigation method, the method of observation, the methods of exploration and assessment, the method of recording and processing of the data, thegraphics method.Numeric values obtained from statistical tests have been processed, both in the initial phase, as well as in the final to emphasize how much more clearly the level at which it has gone.

Research has been carried out for a period of 6 months (december 2010 - May 2011), in which we have made initial and final assessments from the subjects, and the implementation of programs of kineticprofilaxy, which have had a frequency of 2 sessions/week.

Research consists in carrying out specific tests for measuring the parameters somatici (weight, the length of the body and the segments, the perimeter chest, abdominal perimeter) and operational (respiratory rate, heart rate, arterial blood pressure) in patients included in researchGrowth was monitored by comparing weight and length or height standard child with the references provided by maps of growth (graphic appearance - age, weight, height, weight, age, body mass index - age).

Were calculated and the indices of development corresponding somatic (the index of proportionality - Adrian Ionescu, the index thoraco-Erissmann, body mass index) (3).

Developing functional parameters has been observed by making recordings initial (at the beginning implementation of the program of kinetoprofilaxie) and end (at the end of the period of application ofPrograms of kinetorpfilaxie), to which is added calculation of indices for assessing physiological growth and development (lung index of resistance-Demeney).

To develop this work, I noticed 3 subjects with ages between 5 and 6 years.

The program of kinetoprofilaxie pursued objectives:
- development of the entire, of the body to create balance, and coordination between agonistă and opposing muscles of the segments of body and of the organism as a whole;
- drive improvement of big organic functions (circulation, Respiration, metabolism);
- learning correct skills drive base;
- learning a breaths correct, and complete;
- by preventing respiratory buccal;
- development interest for performing physical exercise;
- ensuring proper physical preparation in relation to age specific features;
- formation of a correct attitude of the body;
- getting started with pursuit of sports activities (e.g. ,

swimming).

Used means consisted in exercises in their mattresses in prone or supine, sitting, on his knees; games with variousobjects; exercises for the development and consolidation of the basic skills drive (walking, running, his leap, climbing up, throwing and catching objects) - waveforms applicative; exercises and games in the water (1).

Results obtained

From the program of kineticprofilaxie applied, have been influenced in a positive way and physiological indices anthropometric growth two children included in research. It has improved and the general condition of health of subjects.

The graphs below shows the comparison between the level of the indices of the three subjects development from initial testing and final. Also are presented and the values obtained from the two ratings on nomographs for growth and development when compared to standard values of the tables correctly.

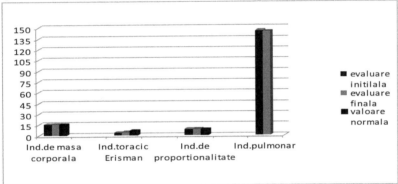

Graph no. 1 dynamics somatic and functional indices obtained initial assessment and final, compared withnormal values, on the subject no 1 P.A.

The graph no. 1 shows dynamic somatici and functional indices obtained initial assessment and final no. 1 to the subject matter, compared with normal values, for the age appropriate. It should be noted that the index of bw maintains values approximately equal to both assessments, because initially, it fit into normal values graph of growth and development. The index of proportionality and pulmonary shows normal values, and the index chest shows a value slightly low.

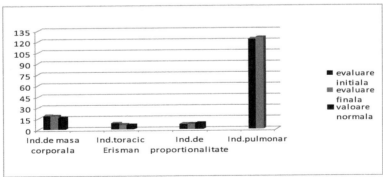

Graph No. 2 The value indices and functional somatic obtained initial assessment and final, compared withnormal values, on the subject no. 2 A. A.

No. 2 shows the graph dynamics somatici and functional indices obtained initial assessment and final no. 2 to the subject matter, compared with normal values, for the age appropriate. It is noted that body mass index is greater than the values normal age appropriate, and it has a lower value to final assessment, apropiidu to normal values. The index of proportionality and pulmonary shows normal values, and the index chest has a lower value to final assessment, aproaching to the normal

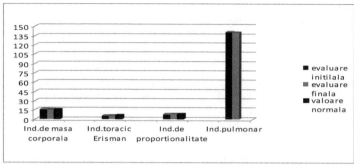

Chart No. 3 The value indices and functional somatic obtained initial assessment and final, compared withnormal values, on the subject no 3 S.A.

On the graph no. 3 is observed somatici dynamics and functional indices obtained initial assessment and final patient no. 3, compared with normal values, for the age appropriate. It should be noted that all indices show values that fall within normal.

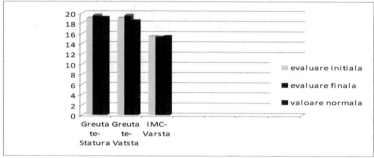

Chart No. 4 the values obtained on nomographs to increase (High, weight and age, body mass index and age) at initial assessment and final, compared with normal values on the subject no 1 P.

In the graph of no4, are given the values on nomographs weight depending on the dapper, of the weight according to age and body mass index as a function of age, in the initial and final assessments.

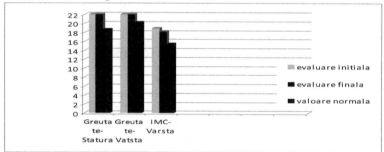

Chart No. 5 the values obtained on nomographs to increase (High, weight and age, body mass index and age) at initial assessment and final, compared with normal values on the subject no. 2 A.

On the graph no 5,Which is represented dynamic values recorded on nomographs weight depending on the dapper, of the weight according to age and body
mass index according to age, it is observed that the final assessments, the patients moved closer to normal values, recorded in nomograph of growth and development.

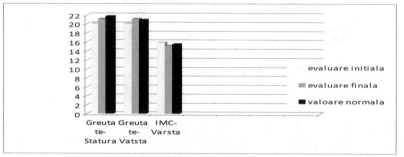

Chart No. 6 the values obtained on nomographs to increase (High, weight and age, the index ofbody table grapes-age) at initial assessment and final, compared with normal values on the subject no 3 S.

In the graph no 6 What is dynamic values recorded on nomographs weight depending on the dapper, of the weight according to age and body mass index depending on age, it should be noted that the final assessments, the patients moved closer to normal values, recorded in nomograph of growth and development.

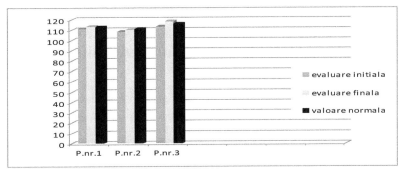

Chart No. 7 the values obtained on nomographs of growth (dapper-age), oninitial assessment and final, compared with normal values in the 3 subjects

On the graph showing the values obtained on nomographs of growth (dapper-age),the initial assessment and final, compared with normal values in the 3 subjects, you can see a change in a positive direction of the values that is close to normal.

Discussions and conclusions

The harmonious development of the children represents a chapter particularly important of human pathology, which should be given due attention. Its importance is due to both frequency and the consequences as well as the development deficit may have on organism and on the integration and acceptance of social.Incorrect posture of the body young children in nursery, in both ortostatism, in travel and in the framework of the achievement of various physical activities, leads to the appearance changes in functional parameters the heart, lungs, metabolism, as well as to the level of the others systems of the body.

By the means and methods of assessment i could analyze the development of the patient's systemic and operational table of contents in the study.After study, I came to the conclusion that it is of the utmost importance implementation of a program of kinetoprofilaxie preşcolari to groups of children to help them to the strengthening of health, the increasing resistance of natural body as agents of external environment, establishing a balance physical and mental stress normally between body and environment.

Via kineticprofilaxie, can be achieved one of the most important objectives in the harmonious development of children, which is to ensure that conditions for normal growth and development of the organism, and default prevention physical deficiencies and illness which could affect their optimal development.

Kineticprofilaxie may constitute an early and well intervention arrived to the problems of delay in development, and knowledge and its application on a large scale it should be a special concern of parents and those engaged in mass caterers of preschoolars.

References
1. Balint, T. , (2007), *Kineticprofilaxie –Note progress for students of physical education and sport;*
2.Mârza, D. , (2005). *Kineticprofilaxie through tangible activities and free time* - Note progress, Bacau;
3.Raţă, G. , (2006), Skills in the motor activity, Ed. EduSoft, Bacau;
4.http://en.wikipedia.org/wiki/Child_development
5.http://www.merckmanuals.com

34

The popularization of certain sport games as key factor to improve the health state and to attract young students towards an active life during their free time

Constantinescu AnaMaria

Motor Activities and University Sport Department, Petroleum and Gas University from Ploieşti

Abstract We live in a society filled with inactivity, stress and aggression, in a world too hasty as to practice sport activities, dominated by cardio-vascular, pulmonary diseases and osteo-articular pain, where every day, unconsciously, we take a fight of survival with ourselves. Lack of sports culture leads to poor motor and body development. Regarding physical education, we notice rigid programs, out of age materials and old ways of working and evaluation, leading to capping and lack of interest towards the sport phenomenon. Through this project we aim to offer the possibility to each student to maintain or improve health independently through the practice of sports like football, handball, basketball, volleyball. It aims at attracting an active life of young students for a good economic and social efficiency, having a continuity even after completing their studies. It aims to permanently maintain a state of optimal health, problem that each of us should reach. It is much healthier "to prevent than cure", maybe that's why we should be more responsible in life and hence with our health.

Key words: games, students, life, free time.

Introduction

We live in a society filled with inactivity, stress and aggression, in a world too hasty as to practice sport activities, dominated by cardio-vascular, pulmonary diseases and osteo-articular pain, where every day, unconsciously, we take a fight of survival with ourselves. Lack of sports culture leads to poor motor and body development. Regarding physical education, we notice rigid programs, out of age materials and old ways of working and evaluation, leading to capping and lack of interest towards the sport phenomenon. To these there are added a small number of minutes (100 minutes) allocated to physical education and sport, every two weeks. The lack of free time activities, in which practicing sport activities should occupy an important role, leads to an increase in sedentary and promotes contemporary society's illnesses, the prompt resolution of opportunities by being able to initiate long-term strategic programs for sports activities to combat physical inactivity, obesity, fatigue, stress, various cardiovascular, respiratory, osteo-articular diseases. The development of the individual from the bio - psycho – social point of view needs to create preferential programs aimed primarily to improve and maintain the health and quality of students' life. Another problem would be the existence of certain flexible, modern programs and the existence of laws that should clearly define their application. A healthy individual with real meanings to a high quality of life requires a continuity of practicing sport even after graduation.(2). Through this project we aim to offer the possibility to each student to maintain or improve health independently through the practice of sports like football, handball, basketball, volleyball. It aims at attracting an active life of young students for a good economic and social efficiency, having a continuity even after completing their studies. It aims to permanently maintain a state of optimal health, problem that each of us should reach. It is much healthier "to prevent than cure", maybe that's why we should be more responsible in life and hence with our health. Prospects for study and intervention used to improve or maintain health have as main role o diminished or reduce the risk for disease. It follows an interaction between somatic and psychic health maintenance.

Methods

Our research starts from the finding that the physical development of students from technical profile universities and their health is not yet approached at a level where we can say that physical education contributes to improving the quality of life of students. Therefore in the experimental approach we start from the presumption that the elaboration and use of certain basic sport programs is strictly necessary, especially if we consider the relation between the health and the physical education and sport activities content taught to students.

In the operational support we started from the following premises:

➢ health state represents the essential factor in improving the quality of life of students from Petroleum university and not only;

➢ Practicing certain sport games in a systematic way lead to a wellbeing state and to the improvement of life quality of the individual in order to cope with everyday social requirements. The development place of the research was the sport base of the Petroleum and Gas University from Ploiesti. We had available a group of 50 students (boys and girls) divided as follows: 14 students (handball), 10 students (basketball), 10 students (volleyball) and 16 (football). The programs were implemented for a 28 weeks/3 sessions/week period, in their spare time. They were selected by comparison with e witness group formed of 25 students that participate at the classic modules from the physical education classes. We must mention that in our research we used as methods explanation, demonstration and practice. Its purpose is to attract a larger number of students to practice sports games, even in their spare time, improving the health state and the bio-psycho-motor capacity through an active life. We aim the social factor during the sport games by spending the free time in a fun and healthy way and why not selecting the students that are available in order to form the university teams. The time spent/training session is of 90-120 minutes, divided as 15-20 minutes learning – consolidation and 40-60 minutes other activities. We use as psychological resources the competition spirit, integrity, team spirit, adaptability, responsibility and communication. Its purpose is to attract a larger number of students to practice sports games, even when students free, improve health and bio-psycho-motor capacity through an active life. The aim is the social factor in leisure sports game in a fun and healthy and not selecting students to availability, university teams to form. The time spent / training session is 90-120 minutes, divided as 15-20 minutes 40-60 minutes learning-building and other activities. Use as psychological resources spirit of

competition, integrity, teamwork, adaptation, responsibility and communication.

As performance indicators we follow:
➢ Improving and maintain an optimum health state of the students;
➢ Improving the cardio-respiratory system;
➢ Toning and harmonious development of muscular and osteo-articulary systems.

At the testing we used the series of Eurofit tests (3).

Results The most conclusive results will be presented below as follows

Table 1 – Statistic indicators – experimental group

Group	Testing	Statistic indicators								
		Mean	Median	d deviatio	Maximum	Minimum	Amplitude	C.v. (%)	Difference($m_F - m_I$)	Cohen Index
E_1	I	8.63	8.75	1.10	11	7	4	12.70%	-0.35	1.64
	F	8.28	8.35	0.97	10	6	4	11.73%		
E_2	I	7.87	8.05	0.69	9	7	2	8.81%	0.04	0.14
	F	7.91	8.00	0.66	9	7	3	8.30%		
E_3	I	7.91	7.90	1.01	10	7	3	12.73%	-0.14	0.65
	F	7.77	7.70	0.99	9	7	3	12.68%		
E_4	I	9.44	9.35	0.38	10	9	1	4.07%	-0.44	2.72
	F	9.01	9.00	0.26	10	9	1	2.85%		

Table 2 – T test results bilateral dependent – sped run for 50 meters – experimental group

E_1		E_2		E_3		E_4	
t	P	t	P	t	P	t	P
7.33	**< 0.05**	0.61	**> 0.05**	2.90	**< 0.05**	12.17	**< 0.05**

Figure 1 – Speed run for 50 m – experimental groups

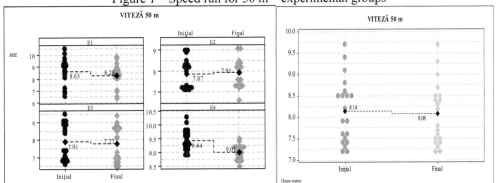

Figure 2 – Speed run for 50 m – witness groups

Table 3 - Statistic indicators at the commute test 1- x 5 meters – experimental groups

Group	Testing	Statistic indicators								
		Mean	Median	Standard deviation	Maximum	Minimum	Amplitude	C.v. (%)	Difference ($m_F - m_I$)	Cohen Index
E_1	I	15.50	15.55	1.54	17	12	5	9.94%	-0.77	1.89
	F	14.74	14.94	1.37	17	12	4	9.32%		

E₂	I	13.69	13.84	0.93	16	12	4	6.79%	-1.10	1.67
	F	12.58	12.56	0.69	14	11	3	5.47%		
E₃	I	13.97	13.66	1.13	16	13	3	8.10%	-0.57	1.20
	F	13.40	13.18	1.00	15	12	3	7.43%		
E₄	I	16.85	16.84	0.93	19	15	4	5.49%	-1.30	1.75
	F	15.56	15.61	0.72	17	14	3	4.60%		

Table 4 – T test results bilateral dependent – commute test – experimental group

E₁		**E₂**		**E₃**		**E₄**	
t	P	t	P	t	P	t	P
8.43	**< 0.05**	7.46	**< 0.05**	5.34	**< 0.05**	7.83	**< 0.05**

Figure 4 – Cardio –respiratory resistance test – witness group

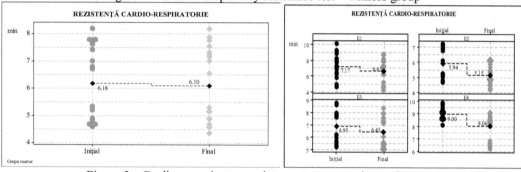

Figure 5 – Cardio – respiratory resistance test – experimental groups

Table 5 - Statistical indicators for the Cardio – respiratory resistance test – experimental groups

Group	Testing	**Statistic indicators**								
		Mean	Median	Standard deviation	Maximum	Minimum	Amplitude	C.v. (%)	Difference ($m_F - m_I$)	Cohen Index
E₁	I	7.17	7.47	1.64	10	5	6	22.85%	-0.52	1.32
	F	7.05	7.10	1.39	9	4	5	20.92%		
E₂	I	6.34	5.67	1.01	7	5	3	16.93%	-0.79	1.83
	F	5.15	5.12	0.71	6	4	2	13.84%		
E₃	I	7.35	6.94	1.33	9	5	4	19.08%	-0.50	1.35
	F	6.45	6.63	1.22	8	5	3	18.88%		
E₄	I	9.00	9.04	0.46	10	8	2	5.06%	-0.93	0.87
	F	8.06	8.40	0.93	9	6	3	11.48%		

Table 6 - The t test dependent for Cardio – respiratory resistance test – experimental groups

E₁		**E₂**		**E₃**		**E₄**	
t	P	t	P	t	P	t	P
5.91	**< 0.05**	8.18	**< 0.05**	6.04	**< 0.05**	3.88	**< 0.05**

Discussions
After applying the series of Eurofit tests we reached the following conclusions
1. There are significant differences between initial and final testing at the crunches over 30 " tests, mobility, speed run of 50 meters, dynamometry test, mobility and especially at the Speed Talk resistance test.

2. There are differences between the two tests for the commute test, Flamingo equilibrium test, and functional strength test by keeping the hanging position.
Table 1 and 2
E1 group: the mean decreased by 0.35 sec, Cohen index (1.64) shows a large difference between the

means from high to very high. The difference reached statistical significance, p <0.05.

E2 group: the mean increased by 0.04 sec, Cohen index (0.14) indicating a very small difference between the means. Difference is not statistically significant, p> 0.05.

E3 group: the mean decreased by 0.14 sec, Cohen index (0.65) expresses the difference between the means medium to high. The difference reached statistical significance, p <0.05.

E4 group: the mean decreased by 0.44 sec, Cohen index (2.72) specifies the difference between the means from high to very high. The difference is statistically significant, p <0.05.

Table 3 and 4

E1 group: the mean decreased by 0.77 sec, Cohen index (1.89) shows a large difference between the means from high to very high. The difference reached statistical significance, p <0.05.

E2 group: the mean decreased by 1.10 sec, Cohen index (1.67) shows a large difference between the means from high to very high. The difference is statistically significant, p <0.05.

E3 group: the mean decreased by 0.57 sec, Cohen index (1.20) expresses the difference between the means from high to very high. The difference reached statistical significance, p <0.05.

E4 group: the mean decreased by 1.30 sec, Cohen index (1.75) specifies a big difference between the means from high to very high. The difference is statistically significant, p <0.05.

Table 5 and 6

E1 group: the mean fell by 0.52 min, Cohen index (1.32) shows a large difference between the means from high to very high. The difference reached statistical significance, p <0.05

E2 group: the mean fell 0.79 min, Cohen index (1.83) shows a large difference between the means from high to very high. The difference is statistically significant, p <0.05.

E3 group: the mean fell by 0.50 min, Cohen index (1.35) expresses the difference between the means

from high to very high. The difference reached statistical significance, p <0.05.

E4 group: the mean fell by 0.93 min, Cohen index (0.87) specifies the difference between the means from high to very high. The difference is statistically significant, p <0.05.

Conclusions

We believe that moving outdoors and sports improve the human condition. The one that practices the activities acquires a set of knowledge and skills beneficial both for himself and the society to which he belongs.

One of the positive elements of practicing physical exercises is the state of health. According to our research it can be traced in terms of factors such as: height, weight, body mass index, heart rate, blood pressure, smoking, alcohol, sleep, etc..

By applying our sport programs on campus the sport activity is animated, seeing a significant increase in the number of students.

Regarding the organizational forms of the activity that may occur in the health improvement we can observe mainly in the side that aims the biological, psychological and social sides, from which we can see the students' preferences for sports games, especially for football and handball.

From the things mentioned above we first notice that sports activities and especially their organization in the form of programs can favorably influence the health state of students, that needs to be tested for the obligatory medical examination, accompanied by the subjective and objective indicators likely to be found in practical lessons.

References:

1. Colibaba Evulet, D., (2007), *Praxiology and curriculum design in physical education and sport*, Craiova: Universitaria Publishing House.

2. Constantinescu, A., (2012), *Improving the quality of students' campus life through physical education and sport specific activities*, Piteşti University, PhD thesis.

3. Eurofit, (1993). *Eurofit Tests of Physical Fitness*, Strasbourg: 2nd edition.

4. Igorov – Bosi, M. (2009). *Handball – methodic*, Moroşan Publishing House, Bucharest.

35

The Aerobics Course Effects on the Students of Physical Education and Sports Faculty of Craiova

Nanu Costin, Cosma Germina

University of Craiova, Department Theory and Metodology of Motor Activity

Abstract. This paper highlights the effects of the aerobics class on 25 students (age 21 ± 2), which were applied for a period of 14 weeks work programs that focused mainly on developing muscle strength and mobility. After applying these programs in the aerobics class, students showed positive differences both in strength testing and in the degree of overall coordination and flexibility.
Key words: *gymnastics, aerobics, students*

Introduction

The association of gymnastics with only professional sports is a regrettable lack of culture in physical education and sports domain, which led, currently, to the rejection of some parts of the contents of this discipline, even by some experts, thus minimizing the formative character of it from the point of view of its specific propelling aspect. However, the importance of gymnastics has been recognized and confirmed through its means effects on the body, gymnastics defining itself, in terms of its psycho-propellent character, as a true "alphabet" of human voluntary movement. (1). The creative character of the exercises structures favors the continuous enrichment of the content, as confirmed by the dynamic development of sports technique in artistic gymnastics but also the detachment of some contents defining new sports and new forms of practicing gymnic exercises for maintenance. Thus, we mention , aerobics, gymnastics in boots, trampoline gymnastics, and jumping in the water, skating, fitness, dance, sports and all extreme sports that require execution of movements rooted in the pool of the art of gymnastics under the strict aspect of groups fundamental movements. As a means of physical education, aerobics covers a wide range of resources taken from basic gymnastics, other sports branches of classical and modern dance, performed and adapted on musical background, mobilising rhythms, amplitudes and different positions, with forms of group and individual performance in which effort is conducted under aerobic regime. (2)

The wide popularity enjoyed by aerobics, especially among females, lies in the availability of the means used, the beneficial effects on body harmony and the psycho-physiological component, which is achieved by the correlation between movement, rhythm and the accompanying methodological line. As a result, in the higher education, aerobics represents an effective form of optimizing the lessons, a means holding multiple valences on the body. Combining the means of maintenance gymnastics with the acquiring of specific items and structures pertaining to performance aerobics led to the delivering of gymnastic lessons with a larger, richer and more attractive content. Thus, in addition to the general objectives aimed at forming a correct body attitude, body muscle toning , establishing and maintaining optimal body weight, increasing body's exercise capacity , developing propellent qualities, they added also some objectives aimed at acquiring and improving some performance aerobics propellent skills, such as the less difficult technical elements, constructions and pyramids made between performers, etc. (3) Many researchers investigate the effects of regular gymnastic activity practice on fitness (4). Appropriate aerobic gymnastics can effectively promote mental health of female university students and simultaneously increase their euphoria from sports. (5). Sports like aerobics reduced fat, weight control,improve the capacity and lower limb movement ability has significant effect; aerobics has decreased thigh girth, improve the body flexibility, shape and size effect.(6)

Material and method

This study aims at quantifying work programs in the aerobics class, a course lasting for a period of 14 weeks, two hours a week and is addressed to students of second year of FEFS Craiova, creating experimental group. Thus we observed the influence of specific means of aerobics on psychomotor ability of subjects with a special view on the overall coordination, the strength of lower limbs and of the abdomen but also the anterior-posterior mobility. The experimental group included 25 subjects (age 21 ± 2) which were subjected to initial tests before the start of the course and to final tests after 14 sessions of aerobics. The tests consisted in:

- the long jump (the lower limbs strength test);
- the Matorin Test (overall coordination);
- Raise the trunk from lying in 30 seconds (strength of the abdomen);
- Bending the trunk forward sitting on a gym bench (anterior-posterior flexibility).

Results

No	Long jump		Matorin		Abdomen 30 sec		Mobil. antpost	
	Ti	Tf	Ti	Tf	Ti	Tf	Ti	Tf
Average	197,21	201,34	371,08	390,21	26,04	28,95	6,04	8,73
Stdev	28,51	29,88	63,97	63,68	4,01	4,72	7,58	7,70
Dif.(T2-T1)	4.13		19.13		2.91		2.69	

Table no.1. Results obtained in the two tests

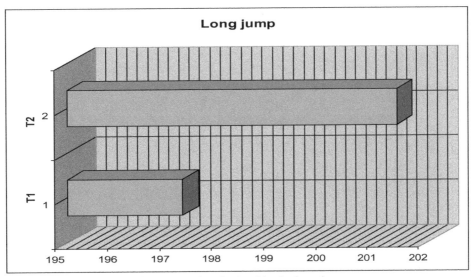

Chart 1 Results obtained in the long jump

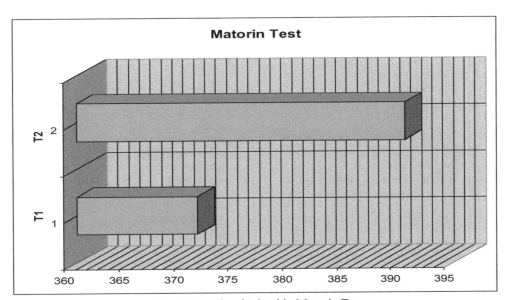

Chart 2 Results obtained in Matorin Test

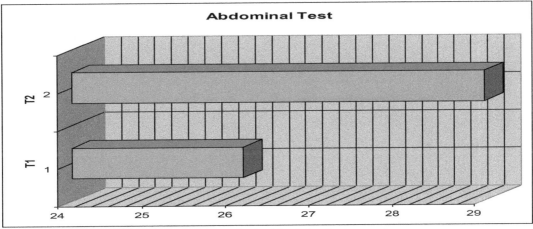

Chart 3 Results obtained in abdominal strength

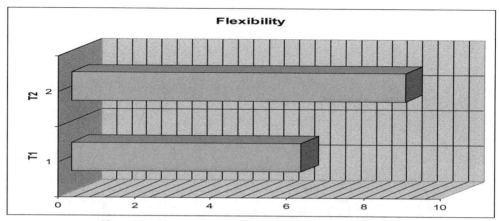

Chart 4 Results obtained in the anterior-posterior flexibility

Disscusion

As shown in Table 1, the application of specific means of aerobics contributed to the upgrading of the tested parameters , the subjects achieving progress in all tests performed as follows:

- 2.09% in the long jump on the spot, where we observed the strength in force lower limbs (chart no.1);
- 5.16% Matorin test, which concerned the general coordination of the students (chart no.2);
- 11.17% to raise the trunk lying meaning improved strength of the abdomen (chart no.3);
- 44.53% bending the trunk forward test that followed the evolution along the anterior-posterior mobility throughout the aerobics class (chart no.4).

The data presented show that aerobics means used led to greater progress in the frame of flexibility and abdominal strength.

Conclusions

Aerobics classes should arouse interest and pleasure of movement, providing disconnection and active rest, relaxation, leisure , much needed by students after the rather loaded program of students , which also implies prolonged static postures. Thus, our approach should arouse students' interest and persuade them to define an active lifestyle through movement, where physical activity be present every day in their independent daily programme.

References

1. Orțănescu D. (2008), *Gimnastica - Componentă a educației fizice școlare*, Publisher Universitaria, Craiova,
2. Nanu M.C., (2009), *Gimnastica aerobică – mijloc de optimizare a condiției fizice*, Publisher Universitaria, Craiova
3. Pruneanu M. (2007), *Gimnastica aerobică în învățământul universitar de neprofil*, Publisher Printech
4. Fabre C., C. Traisnel, P. Mucci (2003), Benefits of gymnastic activity on fitness, cognitive function and medication in elderly women, *Science & Sports, Volume 18, Issue 4, August 2003, Pages196–201*
5. Zhang Chun-mei,JI Liu,XU Bo, (2006), Research of Influences of Aerobic Gymnastics on Mental Health of Female University Students, *Journal of Tianjin University of Sport, 2006-05* [http://scholar.google.ro]
6. Sun Lina, Tan Hua, (2011), Study on Different Sports Courses Influence on College Students, *Procedia Engineering, Volume 23, 2011, Pages 516–520* [http://scholar.google.ro]

36

A twelve-week core exercise program for elite junior tennis players with low back pain

Ilinca Ilona[1], Rosulescu Eugenia[1,2], Zavaleanu Mihaela [1,3], Daian Glicheria[1]

[1]*University of Craiova, Faculty of Physical Education and Sport, Craiova,*[2]*Neuromotor Adults Rehabilitation Center St. Maria, Craiova,*[3]*Sama Medical Center, Craiova*

Abstract. Low back injuries in tennis players are among the most challenging and frustrating clinical situations for sports physicians to diagnose and treat.The purpose of our study was to evaluate the effects of a 12-weeks intensive intervention program on core musculature in elite junior tennis players suffering from non-specific low back pain in order to have a safe and speedy return to high-level sport activities. This core program included different types of exercises aimed to reduce back pain, improve lumbar mobility, increase muscle flexibility, core muscle strength and endurance, and addressed to elite junior tennis players with low back pain. The study concluded that abdominal and low back exercises are important in strength and rehabilitation programs designed for tennis players. We consider that the combined core stability training is a reasonable approach that should result in pain reduction, skill enhancement and a safe return-to-play of a junior tennis player.
Key words: junior tennis players, low back pain, therapeutic exercises

Introduction

The repetitive nature of the tennis swing as well as the constant acceleration, deceleration, and change of direction associated with the game, repeated can result the body susceptible to a variety of sports injuries, both young and old. Back pain is common among those participating in tennis, because of repeated flexion, extension, lateral flexion, and constant rotation of the torso required in this sport [1]. On the other hand, the adolescent athletes are prone to some particular etiologies of back pain which aren't present in the adult athlete due to anatomical and physiological differences between the adolescent and adult spine. A part of these are related to the normal growth process. Lumbar hyperlordosis has been reported as. This condition related to adolescent growth spurts when the axial skeleton grows faster compared to surrounding soft tissue, generating muscular pain. [2]. Although the causes which determined this condition are varied (incorrect body mechanics, poor technique, improper stretching, training strategy, etc., the poorly conditioned athlete places himself at great risk for back injury, especially decreased muscular endurance of the low back musculature. Core stability/strength training has gained wide acceptance as an efficient method of treatment for low back pain rehabilitation, maintenance of a healthy back, and increased sport performance. The core musculature is an important component to the sport of tennis. For tennis athletes the core plays an integral role during specific tennis techniques such as with the forehand drive and volley and during serves and overhead shots. The core is the centre of the functional kinetic chain and a muscular corset that stabilizes the spine, so the limbs can move freely without loss of balance or strength, playing an important role in the transfer of torques and momentum throughout the kinetic chain during sports performance. Any disturbance occurred in this kinetic chain can cause suboptimal performance or injury. [3] Core strengthening and muscular endurance is an essential part of tennis athlete's conditioning/rehabilitation, because increasing strength of the low back musculature provides some protection when greater forces are needed during the performance of specific skills. A stable trunk ensures a solid base for the torques generated by the limbs when hitting a tennis ball therefore spinal stabilization is an important part for physical activity and the rehabilitation of low back pain. Stretching can improve range of motion and reduce high tone in spastic areas. As a conclusion, core strengthening/stabilization and stretching exercises are important in rehabilitation program design for those elite junior tennis players suffering from low back. In order to prevent recurrence of back pain, these exercises should not only be performed following injury but, have to be incorporated into the athlete's normal training schedule. *The purpose* of the current study was to evaluate the effects of an 12-weeks intensive intervention program on core musculature in elite junior tennis players with low back pain in order to have a safe and speedy return to high-level sport activities. We hypothesized that this core exercises program will lead to the improvement in the mobility and endurance of the low trunk muscles among elite junior tennis players diagnosed with low back pain, preventing the recurrence of this condition as well.

Material and Method

In this study were analysed a total of 7 elite junior tennis players (5 girls and 2 boys) from the Tennis Cojan Club (TCC) and Tennis Cofe Club, aged 14-16 years. All players were right–handed, hitting one-handed forehand strokes and two-handed backhands. We included in our study all players that were ranked in the top 50 nationally for the respective age group and trained at these sports clubs. All players were right-handers, hitting one-handed forehand strokes and two-handed backhands, and reported back pain or discomfort during play. Two athletes have a history of repetitive low back pain with associated "muscle spasms" which had required non-surgical intervention and had resulted in time off training and five reported low back pain for the last 6 mounts particularly on execution of a backhand and serve stroke. No sacroiliac involvement, leg length discrepancy or radicular symptoms are noted.The data we collected from the subjects with non-specific LBP included onset time, the nature and location of symptoms, aggravating specific tennis motion, medication, history of back pain or injury, and pain measurements. The study variables and outcome were measure with Visual Analogue Scale, lumbar extension using modified–modified Schober method, movements of the thoracolumbar spine using fingertip-to-floor index and core endurance using McGill protocol. The

Outcome measures of pre and post treatment were subjected to statistical analysis for significance of our program intervention. *Visual analogue scale (VAS).* Pain was assessed using a visual analogical scale (VAS). The VAS consists of a 10-cm line, with the left extremity indicating "no pain" and the right extremity indicating "unbearable pain." The subjects were asked to mark, on this line, between the two extremities, the intensity of the pain which they felt during the sport activity. Higher values suggest more intense pain.*Trunk side bending range* was measured using Fingertips-to-floor distance index. Active movements of the thoracolumbar spine are tested in standing position with the pelvis/iliac crest stabilized. Flexion - patient bends as far forward as possible with knees straight. The distance from the floor to the tip of the middle finger is measured. The amount of forward flexion was recorded to the closest 0.1 cm. The lumbar extension range was measured using the *modified–modified Schober method* [4], in which participants were in neutral standing position. One mark was notice visible at 10 cm superior to lumbosacral junction and another point 5 cm inferior to the junction. Lumbar extension assessed by measuring the attraction of the skin marks, as they approach each other during backward bending. Core endurance was measured with the *McGill protocol* [5], which consists of the right lateral endurance test, left lateral endurance test, flexor endurance test, and a modified Biering-Sorensen back extensor endurance test [6]. Each subject completed a series of 4 static plank holds including: abdominal fatigue; back extensor; right side bridge; and left side bridge. Each subject was instructed to hold each static plank until he chose to stop or proper form was broken. A handheld stopwatch was used to measure the length of time participants were able to hold each isometric position. Subjects were given a minimum of 5 minutes of rest between each test.

Core exercise program (CEP)

The subjects selected participated in 36 supervised exercises sessions, at a frequency of three sessions per week for twelve weeks accompanied by physical and

Results

The descriptive characteristics of the seven subjects who successfully completed the entire study are presented in Table 1.

physical conditioning therapist. Training designed for improving flexibility of the hamstrings, hip extensors and pelvis, and muscle strength targeting core muscle strengthening based on specific stabilizing exercises with co-contraction of deep abdominal (transversus abdominus) and lumbar multifidus muscles. Each season lasted about 45-60 min. The 12 week exercises protocol was divided into 3 phases.

The first level was an four weeks duration period focusing on mobility exercises based on static and dynamic stretching and exercises that promote strengthening the abdominal, low back and pelvic muscles while maintaining neuromuscular control. The dynamic stretching was similar to tennis motion, including hip flexor stretch, hip flexor/quad stretch, hamstring stretch, piriformis/glut stretch. Initial strengthening exercises focused on the training of the deep lumbar stabilizer in isometric and isotonic fashion in a variety of positions and then on superficial global core muscles. The exercises involve exercises promoting voluntarily transversus abdominis, lumbar multifidus, and the pelvic floor muscles contraction, in quadruped, supine, prone, semi-prone, sitting, and standing positions, Prone-Bridge, Side-Bridge, co-contraction of TrA, LM, PF,title left, single leg bridging, supine leg lifts, leg extensions, crunches, clamshell. During the first level the hold time and the number of repetitions were increased every week.

Level two consists from exercises where static contractions will take place in an unstable environment and progress to dynamic movements in a more stable environment. The subjects progressed to the next level of the core training program according to the protocol for that particular day. For this second stage we chose the following exercises: squat with swiss ball, superman, ball prone bridge, shoulder on ball single leg bridging, supine ball hamstring curls, (double leg con progress through single leg) standing wall cross toss, bridge with curl up, diagonal curls on ball, twists on ball.

Level three encompasses resistive exercises that involve medicine ball and resistance bands

All subjects were assigned to a single group. The effects of the 12-week of combined core muscle training program on junior tennis players with non-specific low back pain were analysed.

Table 1. Baseline data for all tennis players who completed the trial

Characteristic	Subjects (n=7)
Age mean (SD)	14,71 (0,75)
Boys/girls%	40%/60%
Height (cm)	175,42
Weight (kg)	61,42
Single/double backhand (%)	100%
Right/left dominance (%)	100%
Play hours per week mean (SD)	15,42 (2,22)
Total play a year hours/yearmean (SD)*	740,57 (106,81)
Years of tennis play mean (SD)	8,28 (0,95)
Pain duration (days)	13,42 (9,36)

Participants were tested before (PRE) and following core exercises program (POST) for severity of back pain (VAS scale), mobility of the lumbar spine (Modified–modified Schober method, Fingertips-to-floor distance index) and core endurance (McGill protocol). Differences in baseline data and post-intervention changes are expressed as mean and standard deviation, (SD) and are presented in Table 2.

Table 2.Changes in flexibility and muscular strength and endurance of Core region in junior tennis player

Variables	Mean (SD)		
	Pre-intervention	Post-intervention	Differences
VAS scale	5,28(±0,75)	1,57(±0,78)	3,71(0,3)
Fingertips-to-floor distance index	7,14(±2,19)	1,57(±1,27)	5,57(0,92)
Modified–modified Schober method	2,92(±0,77)	5,31(±0,37)	2,39 (0,33)
Trunk flexion (s)	131,14 (±13,78)	175,42 (±15,44)	44,28(1,66)
Back extension (s)	112,28 (±15,85)	137,85 (±19,40)	25,57(3,55)
Right flexion (s)	92,28 (±7,52)	118,42 (±8,28)	26,14(0,76)
Left flexion (s)	88,42(±4,89)	114,57(±6,32)	26,15(1,43)
Total McGill core (s)	424,12 (42,04)	546,26 (±49,44)	122,14(7,4)

The pain intensity during the daily sport activities, as assessed with VAS scale, the pain has decrease in intensity after the 3 months period exercises program from the value 6,14 (±1,06) to 1,71 (±0,75).

For assessing the lumbar flexion mobility we used fingertip-to-floor distance index. Before the exercises program the average distance was 7,14 cm (±2,19) and after 12-week period of combined core muscle training program it decrease to 1,57 cm (±1,27) with 5,57(0,92) difference between means. The mean lumbar extension range prior to the intervention was 2,92cm (±0,77) and immediately post intervention it increased to 5,31cm (±0,37). Total McGill core endurance score increased significantly after the 36 weeks program exercise for the group with low back pain. The means difference score between the first assessment and the second was 122,14 s (±7,4).

Discussions

Intensive training during the growth spurt years is linked to injury and different non-systematic musculoskeletal problems. Tennis involves considerably more repetitive and rapid rotation and stretching of the lower spine than other sports. The increased speed and types of strokes used in modern tennis all boost wear and tear on the lower back.

Exercise prescription is one of the most popular approaches in the treatment of patients with non-complicated low back pain because it is documented that exercise speeds up recovery and can even minimize the severity of future episodes of back pain. According to different authors, a specific core exercises program is more effective than classical exercises in reducing pain and disabling the level in a low back pain. From these considerations, the purpose of our study was to evaluate the effects of an 12-weeks intensive intervention program on core musculature in elite junior tennis players suffering from non-specific low back in order to have a safe and speedy return to high-level sport activities. This core program included different types of exercises aimed to reduce back pain, improve lumbar mobility, increase muscle flexibility, core muscle strength and endurance, and addressed to elite junior tennis players with low back pain. After completing the 12-weeks exercises program, a significant difference for lumbar flexion mobility assessed with motion-fingertip to floor method and lumbar extension range evaluated with modified–modified Schober method was found before and after training. A reduction in back pain intensity was recorded as well.

Core endurance was measured with the McGill protocol, which consists of the right and left lateral endurance test, flexor endurance test, and a modified Biering-Sorensen back extensor endurance test. A importance difference for total time was found for pre-intervention and post-intervention within subjects for all tests performed. The 12 weeks' core muscle training, in which flexibility and muscle strength/endurance exercise were combined, helped enhance the flexibility of core regions, muscular strength of the lower back and contributing both to rehabilitation/conditioning the junior tennis players with low back pain as well as preventing the recurrence of this condition.

Conclusion

Pain, and back pain in particular will hinder athletic performance all over the world. The ability to improve this hindered sporting performance in an active natural way is of great importance to all sports area, people, coaches, managers and clinicians. Therefore, by incorporate in the usual training programs some specific exercises for the spine muscles future rehabilitation of athletes suffering from acute low back pain will be more successful, and their training session will be more painless. The study concluded that abdominal and low back exercises are important in strength and rehabilitation programs designed for tennis players. We consider that the combined core stability training is a reasonable approach that should result in pain reduction, skill enhancement and a safe return-to-play of a junior tennis player. This study could have clinical implications for the therapists working with tennis players whose aim is to return the athlete safely to the repetitive demands of their sports training and play, in a pain free state, as quickly as possible.

References

1..Hainline B. (1995) Low back injury. *Clin Sports Med14: 241–266,.*
2. Sassmannshausen G, Smith BG. (2002) Back pain in the young athlete. *Clin Sports Med.;21:121-132.*
3. Press JM. (2009) The importance of core strengthening in back pain management and prevention. *ACSM International Team Physician Course, South Africa; 12 Feb.*
4 Williams, R., Binkley, J., Bloch, R., Goldsmith, C. H., & Minuk, T. (1993).Reliability of the modified–modified Schober and double inclinometer methods for measuring lumbar flexion and extension. *Physical Therapy, 73, 33–44.*
5. McGill SM. (2001) Low back stability: From formal description to issues for performance and rehabilitation. *Exerc Sport Sci Rev 29: 26_31,.*
6. Biering-Sørensen, F. (1984) Physical measurements as risk indicators for low-back trouble over a one-year period. *Spine 9(2),106-119.*

37

The model in playing and training for 16-17 year-old football players

Barbu Dumitru, Stoica Doru, Barbu Mihai, Ciocănescu Daniel
University of Craiova, Faculty of Physical Education and Sport

Abstract. This paper aims to highlight the main aspects of game design and training of football players during one of the most important stages of training (B juniors), a period in which the football player can be recruited among the senior teams, because now there are no game restrictions and training in all aspects of sport training components. Among the important aspects of technical and tactical factors, this paper presents the results obtained in some physical tests, extremely important in the accomplishments of a performer as a future football player.
Key words: *football, model, practice, performance, juniors.*

Introduction

Beyond passions and satisfactions, football is addressed to deeply humane virtues: loyalty, honesty, strength, intelligence, mastery (1,2) These qualities, possessed by almost all great players, make them represent the embodiment of ideals and passions of millions of fans. In football, as in any other sport, the beauty of the game gains value only in relation to its efficiency, when it leads to victory. The game's aesthetic load, whose complexity can satisfy the demands of the finest man of culture, is accompanied perfectly with the intellectual one, in which there are confronted two intelligent tactics, two wishes of winning, in the context of alternating the predictable with the unpredictable, of certitude with probability (3,4).

Materials and methods

In the process of education and instruction of the junior football player with strong personality, an important role is played by the desire of independence, even under the aspect of training. The coach's instructions and criticism regarding their behaviour not only during the game but also outside it, must be carefully done, because they influence the athlete's behaviour, often resuming to giving up on football.

Purpose of research

It is represented by setting the most important aspects related to the B juniors' training (16-17 years old), the methods and specific ways of game and training at this age in football.

Hypotheses of research

1. Knowing the particularities of training the specific age of 16-17 years old will offer the coach a clear image of preparing and leading the future performer.
2. Results obtained at tests with B juniors represent specific indications to the model at the level of the B juniors' age, regarding their selection for professional football.

Methods and techniques of research

To achieve the objectives of this work we have preponderantly used the following methods of research: scientific documentation, statistic method, observation method, experimental method. The results obtained by players will represent landmarks in their training at this level.

Subjects and place of research

Experimental groups consisted of 20 children born in 1996 and 1997, all of them footballers at Gică Popescu Football School in Craiova.

Characterstics of game and training model (1)

The behaviour of the football player is characterized by a critic attitude and the desire to accomplish their tasks. The sphere and character of interests and needs stabilizes, appearing individual characteristics which define their personality. *Juniors no longer distinguish from the seniors, that is why, in this period of time, severity of training in all aspects: physical, technical, tactical, psychological, etc. Reaches the highest level. It is the moment when many juniors take steps to the senior teams.*

Both the team and player model must reflect, at this level, the training content by increasing the number of training sessions per week, requiring increased effort, strengthening, teaching and improving knowledge and skills specific to the training component.

A polivalent player is the football entity who meets the skills on components of training at the highest level, expressed in the game by:

-ability to initiate surprising actions in a smart and effcient way;

-to assume the responsability of achievable actions, not only when there are teammates close in value, but also individually with maximum efficiency, especially in the fourth area of finalization withouth depending on another teammate's support (both in atack and defence).

The player model. Tehnical and tactical skills

To have mastered the basic mechanism of the following components and techniques:

☞   hitting the ball with the string (interior and exterior) and with breadth of foot (standing and moving);

☞   taking the ball with the foot and with the chest by rebound and amortization;

☞   to lead the ball with the interior and exterior of the foot, accompanied by deceptive movements executed while running and protecting the ball with the body and the foot;

☞   hitting the ball with the head from runing and from jump, with range on one or two feet;

☞   throw in on place or momentum;

From the tactical point of view they should master

☞   the skill of using in the game the proper tactics of techniques learned;

☞   the ability to initiate individual actions in attack or defence;

☞   the placement in defense and attack (marking

and demarking);

⚜ collective tactical actions of attack and defense;

⚜ the knowledge of tasks in certain posts, lanes and activity areas;

⚜ book in game tasks of surrounding postions;

⚜ initiating and participating in collective actions for attack and defense of the team in four-defender game system as the game concept;

⚜ strict and aggressive marking in the movement of the ball in front of its box;

⚜ constant battle for a rebound in tackling and interception and return in case of exceeding;

⚜ permanent collaboration in defense by pressing and exchange opponents as well as organisation of the free kick.

Teoretical knowledge. The players should know

⚜ the rules of the game and their interpetation;

⚜ the main problems of and instructive and educational process;

⚜ the main aspects related to the process of instruction and education (requirements, forms of organization, the use of selection and control tests and norms, restoring the body's effort capacity);

⚜ the concept of game (FRF), game dynamics in the game system with 4 defenders (and main variants) and team tactics (own);

⚜ information regarding football events and news.

Psychic qualities: During selection yhey should demonstrat the level of their psychological preparation in terms of their intellect, affective and volitive spheres and the shape of personality.

Goalkeeper model:

⚜ size:180-180 cm;

⚜ flashing:65 cm;

⚜ reaction speed:very good.

Technical and tactical skills for defence:

⚜ managing defence;

⚜ percent placement angle closure;

⚜ promptly getting out of gate;

⚜ safe catch, boxing, blocking and deviation;

⚜ safety clearance kick from outside the penalty area.

Technical and tactical skills for attack:

⚜ rapid throw of hand and foot to opposite direction of the ball;

⚜ long release to counterattack.

Psychic qualities:

⚜ calm, courage;

⚜ power constant concentration;

⚜ risk taking.

The team game model at the end of juniorship B (17 years old)

This doesn't strictly report to the superior mode of global expression and the position of the team in the internal championship, but to each junior's individual abilities and his efficiency to integrate, to attest and to improve in game the inquirements and the habits, with highest coefficients on practice parts. If, in this circumstance, the team built up so – out of gifted and exceptional elements - hit up to range in the top of the internal championship for their age, this approach will prove credibility.

The intermediary game model of a juniors B team, with direct reference to individual and colective actions of the respective player, appears as it follows:

⚜ the players should contribute equally to the two essential circumstances of the game, attack and defence;

⚜ attack actions should evolve cursively, through concomitent and fast demarcations;

⚜ the players should focus on change of attack direction and the game rhythm;

⚜ fixed tacticaly actions should be exploited efficiently (free kicks from 3 and 4 areas, corner, 11m);

⚜ attack actions should be carried on all length and depth of game surface, fast, without uncaused lags;

⚜ the players should move (demarcation) without ball in order to help the player with the ball for creating numerical advantage;

⚜ the game method should be applied flexibly, creatively and adapted to players, according to the acquired knowledge and customs;

⚜ tactical conditions should be provided so as to achieve fast entry from attack to defence and from defence to attack (for retirement in defence using judiciously the pressing, the region and man-to-man defence), as well as the efficient releasing of the counter-attack or the fast attack;

⚜ the defenders redoubling should be ensured permanently;

⚜ the fight for ball and victory should be defined by complete engagement, mobilization ability in hard moments in defence and attack decision in order to reverse some unadvantageous situation.

The exceptional players should be given the possibility to manifest their creativity and fantasy, even while using some technical practices, or some individual tactical actions, accomplishing at the same time the definitive selection of a representative performance team, with a more complex training timetable and maximal exigency.

The balance on practice parts (16 - 17 years)

The physical training	45%
The tehnical training	25%
The tactical training	15%
The theoretical training	10%
The biological training	5%

Acquired results. Tested trials

1. Speed running at 10m

S.R.10m(s)	17 years	16 years
Average	2.0375	2.066
Minimum	1.95	1.93
Maximum	2.17	2.31

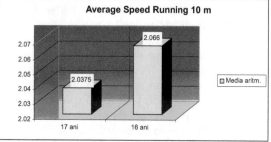

1. Speed running at 10m
- the graph of arithmetic averages
The diference between the twoo groups is 0,0295 s

2. Speed running at 30m

S.R.30m(s)	17 years	16 years
Average	4.399	4.7045
Minimum	4.09	4.47
Maximum	4.9	5.03

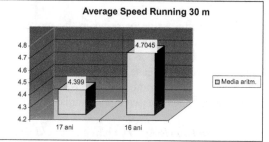

Fig. 2. Speed running at 30m
- the graph of arithmetic averages
The diference between the twoo groups is 0,3055 s

3.Standing in long jump (S.L.J.)

S.L.L.	17 years	16 years
Average	2.275	2.1
Minimum	2	1.7
Maximum	2.45	2.4

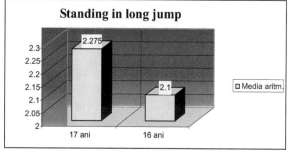

Fig. 3. Standing in long jump
- the graph of arithmetic averages
The diference between the twoo groups is 0,175 cm

4.Abdominal Strength

Abdominal Strength	17 years	16 years
Average	41.4	40.8
Minimum	35	30
Maximum	48	50

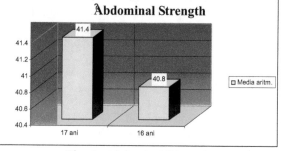

Fig. 4. Abdominal Strength
- the graph of arithmetic averages
The diference between the twoo groups is 0,6 rep.

5.Arms traction force

Traction	17 years	16 years
Average	8.2	5
Minimum	4	1
Maximum	13	8

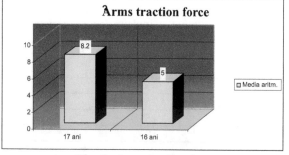

Fig. 5. Arms traction force
- the graph of arithmetic averages
The diference between the twoo groups is 3,2 rep.

6.Running resistance – Cooper Test

Cooper Test	17 years	16 years
Average	3251.5	3000.5
Minimum	2730	2640
Maximum	3800	3750

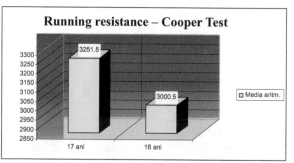

Fig. 6. Running resistance – Cooper Test
- the graph of arithmetic averages
The diference between the twoo groups is 251 m

Conclusions:

1. The results obtained by athletes confirm the biological development and education of motric skills specific for this period.

2. At this age, it is important to work out especially for stamina and strength, two main motric skills required for footballistic accomplishment of young football players.

3. The development process of a polivalent player should become a methodological dominant during the B juniorship (16-17 years old) in such a way that, at the end of this echalon, by promoting to A juniorship (18-19 years old) most of these players are to be requested by senior teams from the 1st, 2nd and 3rd leagues.

4. It would be desirable that the same coach train a children group at least until B juniorship, as it is well-known that coach changing at this age (8-17years old) causes disturbance in the used methods, in the way of organising and developing training sessions, during the showing up of some shorter or longer periods of mutual adaptation (coach-children-juniors).

5. At this junior level, the preparation of advanced players (with remarkable technical and tactical skills and abilities) will continue in every group, using the most complex and most demanding methods. Starting with thislevel, coaches must focus on growing all players' abilities and knowledge required for the function of game coordinator, until perfection has been reached. This means that the capabilities of every player who, if having control over the ball, can and must engage through overrunning with the ball, but also through passing, the most suitable offensive actions (counterattack, quick attack or during positional offensive). These must be surprising, fast and accurate, as a result of tactical thinking, supported by intelligence developed and gained in time. In other words, the possessor of the ball becomes automatically the game coordinator, whose main task is to change tempo and game direction.

6. Both choosing models and preparation itself must be adapted to the characteristics of the area ,as well as to the players's particularities and values, however, without decreasing the demand in training and accomplishing performance objectives.

7. At the age of juniorship, the predilection for certain techniques (the difficult ones) or tactical and more delicate actions are shaped more clearly and more frequently. These must be accepted and carefully cultivated, in order to make sure of their exploitation in the advantage of the team and not personal.

8. The selection of the components of a team (especially of a representative one-no matter the category it belongs to) is made by starting from the players' value first, and then their athletic condition. A player with certain value, even if going through a period of decrease of physical condition,still has a greater eficiency than a player in full perfectioning process who finds himselfs in an optimal state.

References

1.Motroc, I., Motroc, FL., 1996, *Football for children and juniors*, Bucharest, Publisher Didactica si Pedagogica, RA.

2.Barbu,D., 2012, *Theory and practice in high performance football*, Craiova, Publisher Universitaria.

3.Cojocaru,V., 2000, *Strategy in preparation of juniors for high perfomance football*, Bucharest, Publisher Axis-Mundi,.

4.Hahn, E., *Sport training for children*, Bucharest, S.C.J. 104-105, 1996.

38

Aerobic exercise in modulating lipid profile and cardiovascular risk

Macovei-Moraru Mihaela, Luminița Diana Marinescu, Roxana Popescu

University of Medicine and Pharmacy of Craiova, Romania

Abstract: This study analyzes the contribution of aerobic physical exercise in relieving somatic and biochemical parameters in a group of patients with dyslipidemia. In comparison to the control group (n = 20) in the study group (n = 33) we found the resize of abdominal waist (decreased with 6,02%) and body composition (decreased with 8,07%), the decrease of LDL cholesterol with 4,8%, of triglycerides with 3,7%, the increase of HDL cholesterol with 6,8%, improved cardiovascular risk SCORE and the other indexes of risk (Castelli and Reaven).
Key words: *aerobic exercise, dyslipidemia, cardiovascular risk*

Introduction

The World Health Organization has recently issued a warning that physical inactivity is the fourth leading cause of mortality all over the world, meanwhile increasing the risk of cardiovascular disease, diabetes and cancer. Experts endorse this warning but recommendations regarding the amount of weekly physical activity "saving" is incomplete, confusing and sometimes contradictory. It is therefore justified the need for more accurate data on the optimal level of the exercise program, monitoring their effectiveness in accordance with evidence-based medicine, appropriate prescription disease, being outlined such a challenging research topic of this decade.

So far, we have tried, according to personal researches to bring into focus the role of exercise in the treatment of dyslipidaemia, particularly the complex issue and with immediate application in cardiovascular disease prevention.

Epidemiology of dyslipidemia in Romania

Currently, in Romania, more than a third of the population is affected by hypercholesterolemia and this figure is increasing. Through the increased prevalence with clinical or subclinical consequences, despite the costs involved in healthcare, dyslipidemia is an important public health problem. According to the SEPHAR study (2006), the prevalence of mixed dyslipidemia regarding the population of Romania - high cholesterol accompanied by increases in triglycerides - is 46%; in addition, 24% of patients are people in which only total cholesterol levels are increased [1].

Exercise in dyslipidemic diseases

Numerous studies have shown the importance of exercise in improving lipid profile, especially in patients with metabolic syndrome or diabetes. Depending on the type and intensity of physical activity to achieve lower total cholesterol, LDL cholesterol and apolipoprotein B, decreased triglycerides, increased HDL cholesterol and apolipoprotein A1. [2].

The exercise modifies the lipid profile by direct effects on carbohydrate and lipid metabolism and indirect effects, intervening on the risk factors of dyslipidemia (obesity, smoking, diet, stress) [2, 3].

Direct mechanisms (endocrine-metabolic) are represented by [4, 5] and the preferential use of acetoacetate and FFA during sustained exercise with glucose-saving. To restore AGL, chylomicrons and VLDL enzymatic decomposition occurs and thus decreases their serum, stimulation during exercise-adrenergic system catecholaminergic adrenaline generator / noradrenaline resulting acceleration of lipolysis through SS1 receptor, leading to FFA mobilization , increased catabolism of VLDL and LDL cholesterol as a result of activation of the lipases (hepatic lipase, lipoprotein lipase and trigliceridlipase under the impact of stress hormones downloaded during exercise .

Indirect mechanisms relate to improve the risk factors in patients performing physical activity in a regular way. These feel the need to smoke less, to follow a healthy diet, to drink less and are more relaxed [6, 7]. Not to be neglected the role of physical activity in weight loss, a factor of major importance in the treatment of metabolic syndrome [8].

Materials and methods

This study was conducted in the outpatient clinic and Medical Rehabilitation Hospital of Craiova during 2010-2011.

Prospective study was observational and was conducted on a total number of 53 patients with detected dyslipidemia of varying degrees and severity. Patients were diagnosed six months prior to the date of enrollment by conducting common analyzes among the above mentioned patients, which showed altered lipid profile especially in the way of increased atherogenic lipids and decreased protective lipid fractions.

Study objectives

The entire study was aimed to achieve the following objectives:

Designing and implementing exercise programs that are specifically addressed to patients with mixed dyslipidemia for rebalancing the serum lipoprotein levels.

Quantifying the modulating effect of exercise on lipids and establishing a correlation between the type of exercise performed and dynamics of the anthropometric, biological, psycho-emotional and functional patient's dyslipidemia.

Defining the optimal parameters of the therapeutic efficiency that characterize the type of physical training suitable for the dyslipidemic patient .

Comparisons between unique therapeutic interventions (diet only) and complex variant of combination therapy (diet and exercise).

Identifying ways to motivate and stimulate the subject to accept and continue the exercise both during and after completion of the study, involving the research team and the patient,by giving him an active role.

Implementing a periodically follow-up algorithm to reduce the postresearch dropout rate and preserve the adherence to treatment.

Assessment methodology and monitored parameters

Patients included in the study lots were evaluated in accordance with medical ethics, with the consent of each of the subjects, both initially, at the enrollment for achieving precise framing as severity of disease, and in a class SCORE cardiovascular risk and end exercise program after six months.

Both groups of patients received advice on lifestyle changes, or smoking cessation, eating a diet consistent with the level of severity of dyslipidemia, increased physical activity every day. In addition, for the study group patients was initiated an exercise program appropriate to their initial level of fitness. An aerobic workout was performed consisting of 5 minutes of warming-up followed by 30 minutes of aerobic exercise (cycling at cycloergometer) and 5 minutes cooling. Training was conducted over 24 weeks, with a periodicity of 3 sessions per week and took into account the principle of progressivity, starting at an intensity of 60% of the MHR, and reaching up to 75-80% of MHR.

Clinical evaluation has centralized the information collected by history, physical examination and laboratory investigations. We monitored following parameters: body weight, body mass index (BMI), waist circumference, waist-hip ratio, body composition.

Paraclinical evaluation included: lipidologic analysis, investigation of carbohydrate metabolism, exploration to assess associations or morbid complications: ECG, echocardiography, fundoscopy, oscillometrics, alkaline phosphatase, urea, creatinine, ultrasound abdomen - pelvis, ultrasound Doppler investigations completed, if needed, by subtle investigations in order to detect subclinical atherosclerosis: carotid ultrasound to establish intimate index / average exercise testing. They followed the evolution lipid profile (total cholesterol, LDL cholesterol, HDL cholesterol, trigiceridele), a series of derivative cardiovascular risk indices: index Reaven, Castelli index, cardiovascular risk score, hs CRP, peak aerobic capacity (VO2 max).

In assessing the quality of life we used the MOS SF-36 questionnaire.

Cardiovascular fitness testing used the submaximal exercise test, at the cycloergometer, up to a heart rate 85% of theoretical maximal heart rate.

To assess the cardiovascular risk we used SCORE charts both the classical format and theelectronic version known as HeartScore (www.escardio.org).

The participants in the study. Analysis of patients lots.

For data processing we used the module of Microsoft Excel Data Analysis, together with XLSTAT for MS Excel.

The analysis of data collected from selected subjects revealed the following aspects concerning the structure of groups of patients with dyslipidemia, differentiated into two categories according to the type of treatment in which they were implied: the group that performed aerobic exercise and the control group, without exercise.

Lot distribution by age groups reveals a proportion of the age group 45-49 years (24.24%) and 50-54 years (21.21%) in the patients with dyslipidaemia who performed aerobic training; the average age of the participants in aerobic training was 48,70 and for those in the control group was 50, 15. In both groups there was a slight female predominance (54.38% in the study group and 53% in the control group). The average BMI for the entire group was 28 kg/m², a value corresponding to the category of overweight, such patients being better represented in the group that performed aerobic exercise (72.73%). Most dyslipidaemic patients came from borderline hypercholesterolemia group (60.61% in the aerobic group and 55% in the control group), being followed by the group with moderate hypercholesterolemia and mixed moderate hyperlipidemia.

The distribution in the study groups of the lipid profile was consistent regarding the amount of HDL cholesterol in patients with cardiovascular risk due to hipoHDL-my (an HDL cholesterol less than 40 mg / dl) being divided almost equally in the control group (20%) and in the group with aerobic training (24.24%). This could ensure the objectivity of the experiment, taking into account that HDL cholesterol is the most sensitive the parameter to physical exercise.

HDL colesterol distribution plots

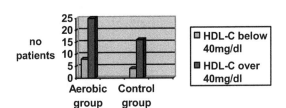

Figure no.1

HDL-Col (40mg/dl)	Average	Standard deviation	C.V.(%)
Aerobic group	44.71	8.64	19.32%
Control group	49.85	12.11	24.29%
Total group	46.65	10.29	22.05%

Table no.1

Further, cardiovascular risk markers will be presented, from Castelli index-the ratio of total cholesterol and HDL cholesterol whose values are correlated with cardiovascular risk [10]. Patients with high CVR (Castelli index over 11) were underrepresented both in the group with aerobic exercise (18.18%) and in the control group (15%). Usually these patients had already presented cardiovascular disease, or other conditions that give them a high CVR, which represented one of the exclusion criteria for patients under study.

Reaven index (ratio of TG / HDL cholesterol) is correlated with the number of LDL particles and small dense HDL and insulin resistance [10, 11]. A value of this index ≥ 3 is designated as atherogenic marker. From this point of view, the percentage of those with increased Reaven index was slightly higher in the group with aerobic training (57.58%).

SCORE cardiovascular risk showed the existence in the group of all categories of patients with low , moderate, high and very high risk, the best represented being the first two categories in both groups, relatively homogeneous distributed.

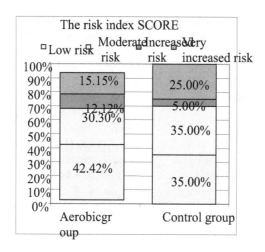

Figure no.2

Results

The results showed ,inside the aerobic group, variations of somatomethric clinical parameters, and of the laboratory parameters monitored, the improvement of cardiovascular risk score and SCORE SF 36 for assessing functional capacity, an increase in aerobic capacity. The patients in the control group showed improvement in clinical and biological somatosensory parameters but not as significant as in the study group. Among the somatometric parameters with the best development are waist circumference and body composition (by decreasing fat percentage).

Thus, the body composition of the study group evolved from an average value of 26.63% to 18.56%; the improvement was of 8.07 percent, this influencing positively the abdominal circumference which decreased from an average of 87.26 cm to 82 cm (6.02%). In the control group, the only beneficiary of the diet, there were less improvements of these parameters: 3% for fat percentage and 2.67% for waist circumference.

The evolution of the waist circumference

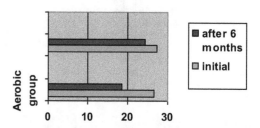

Figure no.3

Regarding the evolution of biochemical constants mentioned above, the values were significantly higher in the 33 patients of the study group compared to the control group. Thus, an increase in HDL cholesterol by 6.8%, from an average of 44.71 mg / dl to 47.83 mg / dl proved to be a beneficial consequence of performing the aerobic exercise; meanwhile, in patients of the control group the HDL cholesterol was constant and the average value of these parameter was slightly low at the end of the 24 weeks of treatment, from 49,85 mg/dl to 46,90 mg/dl
.

HDL cholesterol dynamics

Figure no.4

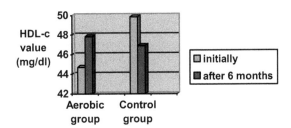

The impact of exercise on LDL cholesterol was a medium one. For the group of patients with exercise was a decrease in LDL cholesterol from an 163.75 mg / dl at 155.89 mg / dl, which represents a average of rate of 4.8%. It is encouraging that this decrease occurred only due to diet and exercise. Control group decreased more modest, in 1.8% LDL cholesterol from 172 mg / dl to 168.91 mg / dl
.

LDL cholesterol dynamics

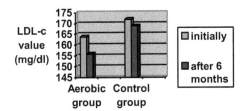

Figure no.5

Triglycerides have undergone significant improvement consequent to aerobic exercise, their average value decreasing from 147.85 mg / dl to 142.38 (down 3.7%) for aerobics group, while for the control group there was a much smaller decline: from an average of 138.65 mg / dl to 136.57 mg / dl (1.5%).

The calculated coefficients for cardiovascular risk, Reaven and Castelli index ranged in both groups as follows: the percentage of those with increased Reaven index was similar to those observed with aerobic exercise and in the control group (57.58% and 55%) the latter succeeding to fall below the value that designates it as atherogenic marker in more than half of the patients who increased values of Reaven index, within the aerobic group. For the control group, after six months, the percentage of patients with potential atherogenic Reaven index increased by 36%.

Castelli index underwent a favourable modulation in patients of aerobic group; the percentage of patients with moderate and normal risk increased while , within the control group, the percentage of patients with medium and high risk increased.

Under aerobic training we observed an increase in peak aerobic capacity with 18% while for the control group there was a decrease by 6%.

Discussions

We can notice a favourable action of aerobic exercise especially on HDL cholesterol, an aspect in concordance with the studies in the literature and the increase percentage observed during our study was 6.8%, a result within the limits of many studies (there was reported an increase between 5 and 15% [12-15]).

Positive correlations were established, statistically significant (p <0.001) between body composition changes and increased HDL cholesterol in patients from aerobic group.

A variable closely connected to increased HDL cholesterol was the lowering serum triglycerides (p <0.001).

The decrease in body weight was poorly correlated to increase in HDL cholesterol but there was a significant correlation between the change in body composition and HDL cholesterol. This is due to metabolic consequences of physical exercise that make weight loss influence differently the hoemostasis of somatic and biological parameters in aerobic group compared to control (sedentary) group.

Cardiovascular risk indices were significantly correlated (p <0.01) to increasing HDL cholesterol due to aerobic exercise, a fact with positive consequences in cardiovascular disease prevention.

Conclusions

1.The study was aimed to assess the impact of aerobic exercise on modified lipid profile and to give the optimal training parameters that can lead to favorable results. For this, there were 53 patients under study, with varying degrees of dyslipidemia which, after clinical, laboratory and functional investigation were classified into two groups.

2.The monitoring of the treatment effects was done by tracking the dynamics of several anthropometric, biological and functional parameters (BMI, waist circumference, body composition, direct and derivative components of the lipid profile, aerobic capacity of effort) and the impact on quality of life was reflected in the improvement of SF 36 scores (physical and mental component) and in the favorable results obtained from a questionnaire assessing self-esteem. From all the results the increasing of HDL cholesterol (6.8%)was the most obvious, a parameter poorly influenced by other therapeutic interventions.

3.Another very important parameter for proving therapeutic efficacy and for motivating the patient was considered in our opinion, the assessment of cardiovascular risk using the SCORE charts for high risk countries (where our country classifies too). According to this assessment, in the initial group, the dominating patients were those with medium risk (score above 5%) of getting a cardiovascular disease in 10-year time. We chose the diagram using total cholesterol / HDL cholesterol to highlight the importance of HDL cholesterol in quantifying risk and to emphasize once again the contribution of exercise to modulate this parameter. We found a decrease in cardiovascular risk score after six months of treatment, when SCORE risk decreased due to an improvement of the two terms of the report.

4.The study took into consideration the development of a gentle, progressive algorithm for changing the lifestyle and adopting the proposed exercise programs, so that the patient can easily accept and assimilate these measures to a normal life, according with their needs. The patient was constantly motivated in his healthcare approach and this reflected in the high rates of adherence to treatment.

5.In comparison with the control group, the results of the patients performing aerobic exercise were superior. In addition, patients had significantly improved anthropometric parameters, especially waist circumference and body composition, essential in lowering cardiovascular risk. We found that in the control group that received only diet there was a favorable evolution of G body in BMI, without excessive echo on body composition and lipid parameters.

6. There should not be neglected the influence of physical exercise on life quality of dyslipidemic male,

an observation reflected in the improvement of scale SF 36 scores concerning both physical and mental components. There was an improvement of self-esteem, fact that could not be observed for the patients who did not benefit form exercise.

References

1.Dorobantu M, Badila E Ghiorghe S RO Darabont, Olteanu I, Flondor P. *Total cardiovascular risk estimation in Romania. Data from the SEPHAR study.*Rom J Intern Med. 2008, 46 (1), 29-37

2.Leon AS, Sanchez OA. Response of blood lipids to exercise training alone or combined with dietary Intervention. Med Sci Sports Exercise 2001, 33 (suppl 6): S502-S15

3.Fourth Joint Task Force of the European Society of Cardiology and Other Societies on Cardiovascular Disease Prevention in Clinical Practice. *European Guidelines on cardiovascular disease prevention in clinical practice: full text.* Eur J Cardiovasc Prev Rehab of 2007, 14 (suppl 2): S1-S113

4.Sbenghe T. Aerobic exercise and with exercise training, theoretical and practical bases of kinesiology; 1999; Ed Medical, Bucharest, 312-366.

5.Slentz CA, Duscha BD, Johnson JL et al. Effects of the amount of exercise on body weight, body composition, and Measures of central obesity: randomized controlled study has STRRIDE. Arch Intern Med 2004; 164:31-9.

6.Davis J, Murphy M, Trinick T et al. Acute effects of walking on inflammatory and cardiovascular risk in sedentary post-menopausal women. J Sports Sci 2008, 26: 303-9

7.Roberts CK, Hama S, Eliseo AJ, Barnard RJ. Effect of a Short-term Diet and Exercise Intervention on inflammatory / anti-inflammatory properties of HDL in overweight / Obese Men with Cardiovascular Risk Factors, cardiopulmonary Physical Therapy Journal, 2007, Reprinted with permission from Journal of Applied Physiology. 2006, 101:1727-32

8.Michael A, Chet D Lifestyle modification in the treatment of metabolic syndrome, Mod Med 2009, 16 (5) :227-31

9.National Cholesterol Education Program-Adult Treatment Panel III-2003, amended 2004, Guidelines

10. European Atherosclerosis Society. New recommendations from the European Atherosclerosis Society Consensus Panel resolve Controversy about lipoprotein (a) and cardiovascular risk. Press release 23 June 2010.

11. N.Hâncu, Gabriela Roman, IAVereşiu: *Diabetes, Nutrition and Metabolic Diseases*, treated 2, Cluj Equinox Publishing, 2010, 231-656

12. Cooney MT, Dudin A, Bacquer D et al. HDL cholesterol protects against cardiovascular disease in both genders, at all ages and at all levels of risk. Atherosclerosis 2009, 206: 611

13. Satoh N, Wada H, Ono K, Yamakage H, Yamada K, Nakano T, Hattori M, Shimatsu A, Kuzuya H, Hasegawa K Small dense LDL-cholesterol relative to LDL-cholesterol is a strong independent determinant of hypoadiponectinemia in metabolic syndrome. Circ J. 2008, 72 (6) :932-9 (ISSN: 1346-9843)

14. Savage DB, Petersen KF, Shulman GI. *Disordered Lipid Metabolism of Insulin Resistance and the pathogenesis.* Physiol Rev 2007, 87: 507-20

15. Millan J, Pinto X, Munoz A et al. Lipoprotein ratios: *Physiological significance and Clinical Usefulness in cardiovascular prevention.* Mistletoe Health Risk Manag 2009; 5:757-65

39

The impact of differentiated sportprograms over the social - professional integration of technical universities students

Constantinescu AnaMaria

Motor and Sport Activities Department, Petroleum and Gas University of Ploieşti, Romania

Abstract Sport activity represents an efficient way of establishing an identity based on capacities already known, through which the subjects multiply their reintegration options in the provenance environment and the quality of life improvement options. They give to the individual the opportunity to reward, rebalance, release, improve physical and psycho-social condition, to engage in group activities, a strong position in relation to one self and others. It is known that exercise positively influences mental health, reduces the incidence and severity of diseases and pathological conditions, such as cancer, diabetes, cardiovascular disease, lung disease, obesity, all of which contribute to an improvement of the quality of life. Movement, physical exercises, competitive sport and mass activities contribute to the development of a positive image of oneself, to the implementation in everyday work of certain psychological states of self-regulation of the psycho- behavioral states.

Key words: *physical activities, students, quality of life, motility.*

Introduction

Physical education and sports lesson is the basic form of organizing the instructive-educational activities of the university, held with a group of students in a specific period and under a teacher guidance according to the analytical curriculum. Physical education is one of the oldest forms of exercise of the formative action comprising a plurality of activities that contribute to the formation and development of the human personality. Physical education and sport is, above all, a national social phenomenon with a specific strong practical content, a hyper complex social phenomenon and dynamic with an objective existence that can be influenced only through an interdisciplinary approach as the only way to obtain objective information necessary to the processes and activities specific of all structures.

Sport activity represents an efficient way of establishing an identity based on capacities already known, through which the subjects multiply their reintegration options in the provenance environment and the quality of life improvement options. They give to the individual the opportunity to reward, rebalance, release, improve physical and psycho-social condition, to engage in group activities, a strong position in relation to one self and others. It is known that exercise positively influences mental health, reduces the incidence and severity of diseases and pathological conditions, such as cancer, diabetes, cardiovascular disease, lung disease, obesity, all of which contribute to an improvement of the quality of life. (1)

Movement, physical exercises, competitive sport and mass activities contribute to the development of a positive image of oneself, to the implementation in everyday work of certain psychological states of self-regulation of the psycho- behavioral states.

According to certain studies conducted by Sporting Goods Association (2), physical inactivity is a real health hazard, being the main cause of death. The vast majority of people do not practice physical activities because they are not informed about the benefits they have on the human body, unaware that their systematic and moderate practice leads to the improvement of the quality of life.

Methods

Considering the fact that currently physical education takes place in technical faculties during a module of 100 minutes / every two weeks, drafting the project to improve the quality of life of the students demanded to answer the following questions:

➤ What will students need to know or to be able to do to improve their health, their bio-psycho-social potential, corresponding to an active life?

➤ What changes need to be made for the programs that we are trying to implement to improve the quality of lives of students for them to cope with everyday requirements?

➤ If we use structured training programs based on training models from sports games that match students' preferences, then it would be obtained the sum of immediate bio-psycho-motor effects and the creation of the habits of systematic practice of physical exercise in their active leisure activities as a factor to counteract the sedentariness and social integration and their family.

➤ **Purpose.** Our research is based on the finding that the physical development of students of technical faculties is not addressed yet at a level at which we to can say that physical education contributes to improving the quality of life for students. That is why the preliminary study and experimental approach presume that the development and use of certain programs based on physical education and sport specific means is strictly necessary, especially if we consider the relationship between the quality of life and the content of physical education and sports activities taught to students. In the operational support we started from the following assumptions:

➤ health state represents the key factor in improving the quality of students' lives from petroleum university and not only;

➤ practicing physical exercises systematically lead to a wellbeing state and to an improvement of the living conditions of the individual in order to cope with everyday social requirements.

In order to achieve the purpose of the paper we chose as study subjects the students from 5 the faculties of Petroleum and Gas University of Ploiesti. Specifically, after studying the issue and the context in which the teaching of physical education is made, it was considered that the experimental approach must be preceded by a preliminary study to track students' preferences for a particular sporting activity. This preliminary study was based on questionnaires with 15 items, where questions touched many crucial points for our research, namely: satisfaction / dissatisfaction with current curriculum, if there are sufficient hours for physical education, if they would like more / if there are sufficient the existing ones, what activities they would like to practice, etc.. The questionnaire was applied to determine student's opinion on the improvement of quality of life by specific means to physical education. With the help of this recording protocol sport activities were identified that influence the quality of life for students from Petroleum-Gas University of Ploiesti.

Starting also from the fact that physical activity is somewhat neglected, 100 minutes conducted in two weeks are totally insufficient, it is desired to offer to each student the possibility to independently develop physical skills, mental and moral ones by practicing physical activities, for an efficiency economic and social productivity. The need to review the specific instructional objectives of physical education is felt more and more, to establish certain priorities within them or even to renewal the training strategies aimed at achieving the finalities claimed by the social control, that lead to the improvement of the quality of life for students. It should be considered also the permanent maintaining of an optimal health state.

The experiment began in the academic year 2011/2012, ending in early June 2012. There were tested students, boys and girls, divided into preference groups (a control group and an experimental group). The research was conducted on the sports base from the Petroleum-Gas University of Ploiesti. In doing so, the groups submitted to the experiment developed their activity as follows:

The control group worked on the traditional curriculum developed and approved in the University Senate at the beginning of the academic year 2011/2012. The training was conducted under the direction of professional teachers, who conducted fairly activities on the schedule established at the beginning of each semester.

The experimental group worked in their spare time, after a series of sports programs developed by us, in which are better captured the specific means of physical education and sport and they are mainly teaching targets or instructional objectives on which we focused our attention. Thus, according to our findings, an important role was held by the fitness programs, aerobics, stretching, pilates, jogging, applied

throughout the academic year 2011/2012 and continued in the first half of 2012/2013, as well as in sports games such as soccer, handball and basketball.

The experiment pattern consists of 4 groups as follows:
➤ the experimental pattern 1 is represented by students participating in the program consisting of stretching, pilates, jogging and zumba.
➤ the experimental pattern 2 is composed of students participating in group sports programs such as sports games (football, handball, basketball).
➤ the experimental pattern 3 is represented of students participating in competitions organized as eliminatory system, or roundtrip system.
➤ the experimental pattern 4 consists of students participating in initiation programs and practicing gymnastics.

In this research we used as measurements and assessment tests:
➤ Anthropometric parameters: size, weight, bust, chest perimeter at rest, chest perimeter in deep inspiration.
➤ Functional parameters: heart rate, systolic blood pressure, diastolic blood pressure, vital capacity.
➤ Parameters and physical development indices: Quetelet index, Adrian Ionescu index, Amar index, the index of nutrition.
➤ Assessing the motor potential through the Eurofit tests, a battery of physical fitness tests are applied to test flexibility, speed, endurance and strength. This battery of standardized tests was developed by the Council of Europe for the school children and has been used in several European schools from 1988. The tests are designed so that they can be made within 35 - 40 minutes, using a simple equipment. (3) Eurofit test battery consists of: 6 anthropometric measurements (height, weight), 8 motor tests and 1 cardio respiratory endurance test. The order of administration of the tests is the following: the Flamingo balance test, Touch panels, trunk flexion forward from a sitting position, long jump without momentum (on site), hand dynamometer, lift the trunk from a sitting position, Maintained hung, run to and fro 10 x 5 meters (must be taken last). The endurance test: The run to and fro test. (4). Anthropometric measurements were carried out in collaboration with the medical staff inside Petroleum-Gas University of Ploiesti and specialist teachers of the Department of Physical Education and Sport, which gave me great support in the data collection. In general, these measurements was sought to be made with appropriate assessment tools: metric tape, technical installations, apparatus and under identical conditions. The measurement activity was made to allow the search of a great group in the shortest time possible.

Results. In the following we present the most conclusive results.

Explosive force of inferior limbs on horizontal (standing long jump)

Table 1 – Statistical indicators at the standing long jump -
Witness group

Statistic indicators	Verification	
	Initial	Final
Arithmetic mean	189.75	192.00
Median	195.00	197.50
Module	170.00	170.00
Standard deviation	23.59	23.42
Medium deviation	20.28	20.30
Amplitude	75.00	75.00
Variation coefficient	12.4%	12.2%
Standard error of the mean	5.28	5.24
Means difference		2.25
Effect dimension (Cohen)		0.88

Table 2 – The t test bilateral dependent – witness group – long jump from standing test

The set coefficient threshold - α	$\alpha = 0.05$
Null hypothesis H_0	$m_1 - m_2 = 0$
Alternative hypothesis H_1	$m_1 - m_2 \# 0$
Liberty degree - df	19
Number of subjects	20
t reference (from t tables)	2.093
t calculated	3.943
Trust interval	(1.13 , 3.37)
The determined trust threshold - P	< 0.05

Tables 1-2 At the standing long jump through which were tested the explosive force of inferior limbs on horizontal, the results increased on average by 2.25 cm after the training, from 189.75 to 192.00 cm. The data dispersion maintained its homogeneous structure also at the final testing. After verifying the statistical hypothesis with the bilateral t-test resulted that the mean difference is statistically significant, p <0.05. Cohen index value (0.88) shows that there is a big difference between the arithmetic means corresponding to the two tests. The null hypothesis (H_0) is rejected and the research hypothesis (H_1) is accepted. Graphical representation of the results is presented below.

Figure 1 – Long jump from standing – witness group

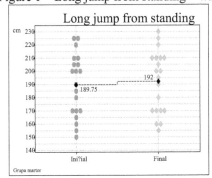 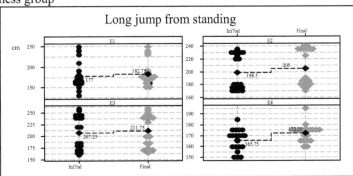

Figure 2 – Long jump from standing – experimental group

Table 3 –Statistical indicators at the long jump from standing – experimental groups

Group	Test	Mean	Median	Standard deviation	Maximum	Minimum	Amplitude-d	C.v. (%)	Difference (m F - m I)	Cohen Index
E_1	I	177.00	167.50	32.09	250	130	120	18.13%	5.75	0.94
	F	182.75	175.00	30.67	250	150	100	16.78%		
E_2	I	198.50	180.00	27.53	235	170	65	13.87%	6.50	1.00
	F	205.00	187.50	28.28	240	170	70	13.80%		
E_3	I	207.25	202.50	36.25	260	160	100	17.49%	4.50	0.58
	F	211.75	215.00	35.25	260	165	95	16.65%		
E_4	I	165.75	170.00	9.77	185	150	35	5.89%	6.50	1.20
	F	172.25	175.00	7.86	195	160	35	4.56%		

Table 4 –The results of the t test bilateral dependent at the long jump from standing – experimental groups

E_1		E_2		E_3		E_4	
t	P	t	P	t	P	t	P
4.20	< 0.05	4.47	< 0.05	2.59	< 0.05	5.38	< 0.05

Tables 3 and 4
• E_1 group: the mean increased with 5.75 cm, the Cohen Index (0.94) shows a difference between means high towards very high. The difference has reached the statistical threshold significance, p < 0.05.
• E_2 group: the mean increased with 6.50 cm, the Cohen Index (1.00) shows a difference between means high towards very high. The difference has reached the statistical threshold significance, p < 0.05.
• E_3 group: the mean increased with 4.50 cm, the Cohen Index (0.58) shows a difference between means medium towards high. The difference has reached the statistical threshold significance, p < 0.05.
• E_4 group: the mean increased with 6.50 cm, the Cohen Index (1.20) shows a difference between means high towards very high. The difference has reached the statistical threshold significance, p < 0.05.
Body weight

Table 5– Statistical indicators for weight– witness group

Statistic indicators	Verification	
	Initial	Final
Arithmetic mean	69.25	69.45
Median	67.00	69.50
Module	54.00	75.00
Standard deviation	11.00	9.94
Medium deviation	9.48	8.35
Amplitude	33.00	34.00
Variation coefficient	15.9%	14.3%
Standard error of the mean	2.46	2.22
Means difference		0.20
Effect dimension (Cohen)		0.07

Table 6 – The t test bilateral dependent – weight – witness group

The set coefficient threshold - α	α = 0.05
Null hypothesis H_0	$m_1 - m_2 = 0$
Alternative hypothesis H_1	$m_1 - m_2 \# 0$
Liberty degree - df	19
Number of subjects	20
t reference (from t tables)	2.093
t calculated	0.300
Trust interval	(-1.11 , 1.51)
The determined trust threshold - P	> 0.05

For the anthropometric parameters, body weight, the arithmetic mean increased by 0.20 kg, from 69.25 at the initial test to 69.45 kg at the final testing. The dispersion of data is relatively homogeneous respectively homogeneous. The bilateral t test shows that the mean difference did not reach the statistical significance threshold, p > 0.05. Although the differences are not significant, the Cohen index value (0.07) shows that there is a very little difference between the two means corresponding to the two tests. The null hypothesis (H_0) is rejected and the research hypothesis (H_1) is accepted. Graphical representation of the results is presented below.

Figure 3– Weight – witness group   Figure 4 – Weight – experimental group

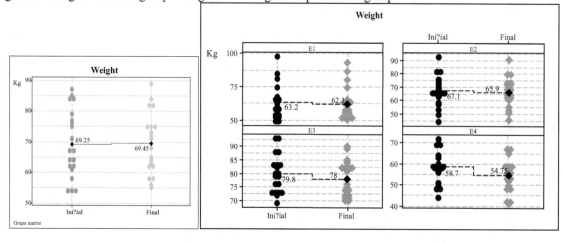

Table 7 – Statistic indicators – weight – experimental group

Group	Test	Statistical indicators								
		Mean	Median	Standard deviation	Maximum	Minimum	Amplitude-d	C.v. (%)	Difference (m_F - m_I)	Cohen Index
E₁	I	63.20	60.50	12.92	98	49	49	20.44%	-1.10	0.42
	F	62.10	57.50	12.34	93	50	43	19.87%		
E₂	I	67.10	65.00	11.75	93	44	49	17.51%	-1.20	0.67
	F	65.90	65.00	11.03	91	45	46	16.73%		
E₃	I	79.80	79.50	6.93	93	69	24	8.68%	-1.80	0.92
	F	78.00	77.00	6.35	90	70	20	8.14%		
E₄	I	58.70	59.00	7.79	72	44	28	13.28%	-3.95	1.96
	F	54.75	55.50	8.06	67	41	26	14.73%		

Table 8 – The t test dependent bilateral – weight – experimental group

E₁		E₂		E₃		E₄	
t	P	t	P	t	P	t	P
1.87	> 0.05	2.99	< 0.05	4.10	< 0.05	8.78	< 0.05

• E_1 group: the mean decreased with 1.10 kg, the Cohen Index (0.42) shows a difference between the means low towards medium. The difference did not reach the statistic significance threshold, $p > 0.05$

• E_2 group: the mean decreased with 1.20 kg, the Cohen Index (0.67) shows a difference between the means medium towards high. The difference is statistically significant, $p < 0.05$.

• E_3 group: the mean decreased with 1.80 kg, the Cohen Index (0.92) shows a difference between the means high towards very high. The difference has reached the statistical significant threshold, $p < 0.05$.

• E_4 group: the mean decreased with 3.95 kg, the Cohen Index (1.96) shows a difference between the means high towards very high. The difference has reached the statistical significant threshold, $p < 0.05$.

Conclusions.

1. Sports competitions should be in a number as large as possible because it is human nature to like to compete with the one next to you, or to be better than him. Students are supporters of competitions held during physical education lessons, especially outside the classroom, among the preferences being football, handball and basketball, girls preferring stretching exercises and aerobics more.

2. Current programs do not satisfy entirely the students' options and needs for training and socio-professional integration.

3. A special emphasis should be placed on maintaining and continuously improving health, body shaping by adopting rational activities and sport life programs.

4. The material base should be improved by arranging as many spaces as possible for sport activities and especially refurbishing the existing ones.

5. Regarding the forms of activity that may interfere with the quality of life in all 4 components, especially in the side covering the biological, psychological and social parts, we can draw the following conclusions:

➤ preferences for leisure activities, pilates, aerobics, zumba, stretching, kango jump.

➤ students' preferences for sports, especially as competition.

➤ preferences for jogging and athletic exercises.

References.

1.Constantinescu, A. 2012, Îmbunătătirea calitătii vieții studentilor din campusurile universitare prin activități specifice educației fizice şi sportului, teză de doctorat, Universitatea din Piteşti.

2.Sport Goods Asociation, 2004.

3.Eurofit, (1993), *Eurofit Tests of Physical Fitness*, 2nd edition, Strasbourg.

4.Epuran, M., (2005), *Metodologia cercetării activităţilor corporale*, Editura FEST, Bucureşti, pg. 384

5. Finichiu, M. (2010). *Optimizing physical condition of students oilman by use specific lesson athletics in physical education and sport*, Bucharest: PhD thesis, ANEFS.

6. Friedman, P. and Eisen, G. (2005). *Pilates method of physical and mental conditioning,* SUA: Studio Viking, p. 13-14.

Sport Goods Association, (2004). online sports - www.csga.ca

40

Study on the Developing of a Model Syllabus on Physical Education and Sports within the Curriculum on School's Decision for Pre-University Education

Chivu Daniel[1], Orţănescu Dorina[2], Nanu Marian Costin[2]

[1] *National University of Physical Education and Sport, Bucharest, Romania*
[2] *Department of Theory and Methodology of Motricity Activities, University of Craiova, Romania*

Abstract. This study is a questionnaire survey aimed to obtain information about teachers' view of activities within the school curriculum. A percentage of 60% of teachers consider obligatory the presence of students in such activities and the remaining percentages were directed to the optional participation in these activities. Physical education and sport are considered indispensable for the development of the individual personality, being an integral part of the overall education program for each student.
Key words: *curriculum, questionnaire, physical education.*

Introduction

The curricular reform of Romanian education has come halfway. This means that they have developed and published centrally in an integrated vision, documents that form the National Curriculum, appointed in the specialized literature as official curriculum or intended curriculum. The other half is the implementation, evaluation and revision of the National Curriculum, so what we call accomplished curriculum be made as close to the spirit and letter of the official curriculum. Part of this process is the publication of the National Council for Curriculum guides for the application of the new curricula. These guidelines are meant to provide a suitable route of personalized reading of the new curriculum in accordance with the actual situation at school and classroom level and the teaching experience of each teacher. (1). One of the central ideas behind the concept of educational reform as a whole, is the structuring of the curriculum on cycles, each of them having their specific objectives and periods of time allotted, estimated as targeting biological and psychological development of students and the fluency of the action of developing in accordance with the educational ideal. Each subject provided in the curriculum had to redefine objectives and to stagger them on years of schooling in line with the overall objectives of the curriculum cycle, to restructure content and, especially, to adopt methodologies meant to equip students with the capacities, skills and attitudes in personal and social domain in current and in future activities. The structuring of the educational framework on curriculum areas, the setting of the compulsory subjects and of the minimum and maximum number of hours that may be affected, the setting of a minimum and maximum number of hours for the optional subjects (without being named) and also the minimum and maximum number of hours per week for each class, requires from the teacher to develop a timetable, which may be special compared to any parallel class by the number of hours required by the subjects affected by the number of optional subjects studied and the amount of hours allotted to them as well as by the total number of hours specified in the weekly schedule. Through the right to make decisions given to school, the curriculum on school's decision (CDS) is actually the emblem of its real power. Derived from the freedom - provided by the educational framework - to decide on a segment of the national curriculum, this power allows defining individual learning paths for students. The freedom of decision at school level is consistent with a democratic society and is an opportunity for alignment to an open system with multiple options. CDS is a reality of today's schools, reality that has gained a number of followers (the important fact is that most of them are students) and that reveals normality through the acceptance of difference. In other words, CDS - as power of schools - allows an own ethos which makes the difference in the proximate genus "Romanian school at the beginning of the third millennium .(2)

Material and Method

In order to establish the need to introduce new subjects within students' activity, we applied a questionnaire to obtain information about teachers' view of activities within the school curriculum. The questionnaire involves a direct interaction between researcher and the subject, but it is mediated by a set of items related to knowledge, skills and attitudes relevant to the subject of the research.

The sociological survey conducted by us can provide important information on favorite sports disciplines preffered by teachers, disciplines that are not in the current curriculum, to its reassessment within CDS. This survey involved 30 teachers (including 28 permanent teachers), all having a teaching experience of more than 4 years. The questionnaire included a set of 15 questions

Analyzing the obtained answers we observe, without much surprise, that the first question (Are you familiar with the concept and content of curriculum on school's decision?) All respondents answered affirmatively.

For the next question, teachers ranked firstly the interest of students (40%) and then the material resources and school's interest

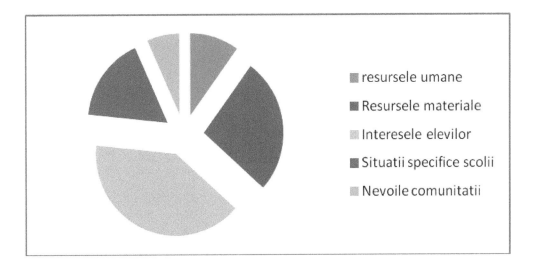

Figure 1. The order of the landmarks that teachers deemed to be an integral part of designing a curriculum on school's decision (human resources, material resources, students' interest, school specific situations, community needs)

To the question of assessing physical education and sports activities within the curriculum on school's decision, they obtained the following responses:

Question	How do you assess the physical education and sports activities within the curriculum on school's decision?			
Answer	Very important	Important	Relatively useful	Insignificant
Teachers	20	8	2	0

Thus, 66.6% of the teachers appreciate physical education and sports activities within the curriculum on school's decision as very important. Interestingly, none of the respondents considers these activities as worthless, which is a good thing.

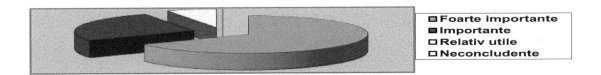

Figure 2. The assessment of physical education and sports activities within the curriculum on school's decision by teachers

Interestingly, more than half of the teachers surveyed (53.34%) see the curriculum on school's decision as an opportunity to prepare teams representing the school for competition, and another percentage, equally significant (43, 34%), sees these activities as an extension of the curriculum. Given the social and economic climate in which we live, we were not surprised at all by the answer of one teacher who believes the CDS to be a way of ensuring the number of hours for teachers.

The question on physical education and sports activities within the curriculum on school's decision, 83.3% of teachers said they have organized such events.

Regarding the top on sports subjects necessary to be introduced in the curriculum on school's decision, we have the following results. The top 3-4 disciplines were somewhat predictable (I - dance II - tae-bo, III - pilates, IV - gymnastics), considering that the majority of teachers surveyed have gym as specialization, it is natural to focus on subjects whose content is more familiar.

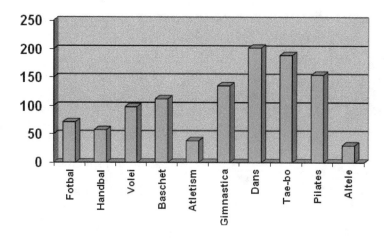

Fig. 3. The top of sports subjects necessary to be introduced in the curriculum on school's decision

Linked to students' interest in physical education and sports activities on school's decision in the curriculum, we found that only 33.3% appreciate that they have a great interest for physical education and sports activities in the curriculum on school's decision, and a slightly higher percentage 46.6% consider students' interest in these activities as great. What is important for our study is that all respondents openly acknowledge students' interest in such activities as long as the last two answers were not taken into consideration

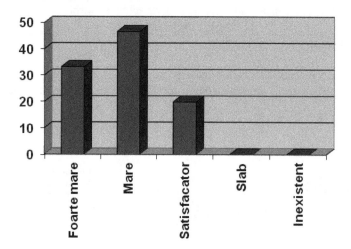

Fig. 4. Students' interest for physical education and sports activities in the curriculum on school's decision
In addition to this question, teachers were interviewed regarding the main difficulties encountered in the organization of physical education activities in the curriculum on school's decision. More than half (53.34%) draw attention to the already loaded program for students, but does not neglect the lack of material (23.33%) or, sometimes, a lack of interest from students (20%) .

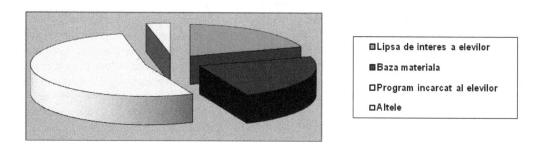

Fig. 5. The main difficulties encountered by teachers in the organization of physical education activities in the curriculum on school's decision (students' lack of interest/Material basis/Students' Loaded programme/ Others)

Another question was related to organizing the classes in the curriculum on school's decision. Almost half of the teachers (43.34%) think that the organization at two levels (V-VI VII-VIII) would be the most effective option. The next option would be the following response was to organize classes for each class in part (25.66%).

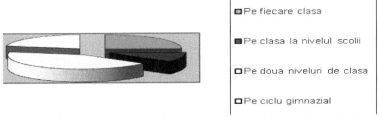

Fig. 6. Organizing the classes in the curriculum on school's decision (students and teachers) (for each class in part/ for each class at school level/on two levels of class/ on secondary school level)

As expected, the question on the number of hours in the curriculum on school's decision, brought expected results, rather high percentage 70% for the variant 2 hours / week, saying more about their options.

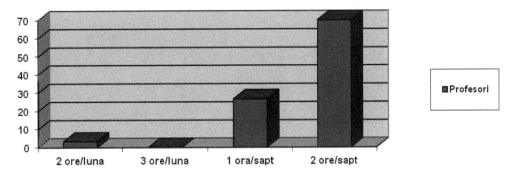

Fig. 7. The distribution of hours allotted within the curriculum on school's decision (2 hours/monthly, 3 hours/ month, 1 hour/ week, 2 hours/ a week)

Another question that obtained the expected results was that regarding students' participation in physical education and sports activities within the curriculum on school's decision. A percentage of 60% of teachers consider obligatory the presence of students in such activities and the remaining percentages were directed to the optional participation in these activities.

The questionnaire ended with a question that will come as a conclusion to all the other questions and confirm the purposes of this investigation. Thus, when asked: Would you need a syllabus for the physical education classes within the curriculum on school's decision?, 80% of the teachers surveyed responded affirmatively.

Conclusion

1. Physical education and sport are considered indispensable for the development of the individual personality, being an integral part of the overall education program for each student.
2. The investigation conducted by the questionnaire we noticed the interest of students as well as of teachers for physical education and sports activities within CDS.
3. The subjects for which teachers were mostly opted are Dance, Tae-Bo and Pilates. We note that these subjects were located in the first position and the

consideration that most of the teachers interviewed have as specialization gym, so they are familiar with the concepts and specifics of these disciplines.
4. Following the feedback from the respondents, the elaboration of a syllabus for the three subjects preferred by the respondents is clearly needed.

References
1. http://administraresite.edu.ro/index.php/articles/7337 - acces on 3.03.2013
2. http://www.docstoc.com/docs/27523421/Order-No-344915031999regarding--the-regime-of optional-subjects

41

Assessment of foot inbalance using biomechanical measurements

Rusu Ligia[1], Rusu P.F.[2],Dragomir Mihai.[1]

[1] *Sport Medicine and rehabilitation Department, University of Craiova, Romania*
[2] *Mechanic Department, University of Craiova, Romania*

Abstract: This study presents the role of biomechanical assessment of foot at soccer players for predict the foot instability and injuries. By this type of assessment is possible to build a specific training focused on improvement muscle strength and coordination. We study two lots of athletes: lot 1- soccer players (15 subjects, mean age 16years) and lot 2 field tennis players (15subjects, mean age 16years). We use for biomechanic assessment RSscan system, platform plate. We assess loading response at midfoot level during gait. Our recording use 300 frame/sec. The assessment include force and pressure parameters during a gait cycle and also few morphologic parameters like subtalar angle. The results show to us that risk of ankle foot injuries are high in field tennis then football, that can be corelate with high loading respond existed in tennis. If we see the graphics we observe that for left side, lot1, range –45+20 and for right side 0+59.For lot2, left side 0+15, right side +7+35. In conclusion we consider that a good assessment of biomechanic aspect of ankle foot is important not only for prevent or treatment and monitoring rehabilitation programm, but also for a good selection for each sport activity.
Key words: *assessment, foot, force, loading, pressure*

Introduction

In sport activity performance means to have a well structure and function of musculoskeletal system. This aspect is important for create a specific prophylactic training program and also rehabilitation program. The aim of this study is to present a comparative study of biomechanical parameters (1) of foot in two different sport activity, soccer player sand field tennis players. The role of this study is to create an image regarding functional parameters of foot specific for each sport activity, football and field tennis. The results of this study help us to assess the risk of a possible injury and to prevent it (2). So after this study is possible to: prevent foot injury, prevent ankle foot instability, improvement of training methods, prescribe a good orthotic system, improvement of diagnostic methods (3) in sport activity, development and monitoring of rehabilitation program.

Material and Method

We study two lots of athletes: lot 1- soccer players (15 subjects, mean age 16years) and lot 2 field tennis players(15subjects, mean age 16years). We use for biomechanic assessment RSscan system, platform plate. We assess loading response at midfoot level during gait. Our recording use 300 frame/sec. Parameters(5) that we assess are: %contact(%of contact time compared to the complete stance phase), load rate(N/cms) (the speed of loading in the midfoot region), maxP(N/cm) (the maxim pressure measured in midfoot region), maxF(N) (the maxim force measured in midfoot region), %surface(an overview on the load contact surface under the midfoot), foot axis angle (related movement direction), subtalar joint angle(related to the foot axes). Regarding two lasts parameters negative values means endorotation and positive values means exorotation (6). Our assessment is made during three phases of gait cycle: heel contact, midstance and propulsion. All these parameters help us to estimate foot balance and meta loading during gait to both lots of athletes.

Results and Discussions

We present the range of values for each parameters on both sides, left and right and two lots.

Parameters	Soccers		Field tenis	
	Left	Right	Left	Right
%contact	70-30	63-37	75-63	66-38
maxP	8,5-6,9	4,2-13,1	6-11,6	3,1-14,9
load rate	0,04-0,10	0,03-0,13	0,06-0,08	0,02-0,12

Table 1: Pressure parameters

Parameters	Soccers		Field tenis	
	Left	Right	Left	Right
%contact	73-30	74-73,7	78-70	69-40
maxF	321,4-315,8	191,2-275,5	277,4-902,4	145,2-620,3
load rate	1,32-0,16	1,40-0,20	2,45-6,15	0,87-46,52

Table 2: Force parameters

%surface for soccers player are 23,4-29,2% and for field tenis players 25,3-56,9%. Also we observe negative values for foot axis angle and subtalar joint angle, range –7,37° -2,11° for lot1and positive values for lot 2, means for lot1 endorotation and for lot2 exorotation. If we see all dates we can observe that in lot 2 load responding is higher then lot 1, also maxF are higher to lot2 , even if both lot have very closely values for %contact. From these dates we can to assess the prediction of an injury risk related to foot stability and balance.So we observe that at lot 1 lower risk for injury is present during heel contact and maxim intsability at left and right feet during propulsion phase(graphic1,2,3,4). For lot2 we see lower risk for injury during heel contact and midstance, foot stability during midstance phase at left side and left side intsability during propulsion phase. For right side we see to entire lot2, a high instability(graphics 5,6,7,8).

These results show to us that risk of ankle foot injuries are high in field tennis then football (7), that can be corelate with high loading respond existed in tennis. If we see the graphics we observe that for left side, lot1, range –45+20 and for right side 0+59.For lot2, left side 0+15, right side +7+35.

These can be corelate with high values of maxF (8) on right side and load rate also on right side and explain instability during propulsion phase. All these results are in accord with abnormal position of foot, to exo or endorotation, that involve a high risk of instability (9). So we can say, in according with literature (10) that high loading and extrem foot positions have been associated with a variety of injuries (11).

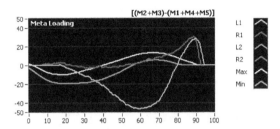

Graphic 1-metaloading and zone of lower injury risk
(soccer, 18years)

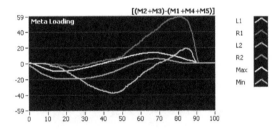

Graphic 2-metaloading and zone of lower injury risk
(soccer, 16,5years)

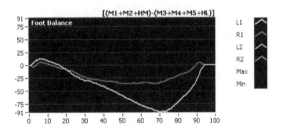

Graphic 3- foot balance
(soccer, 18years)

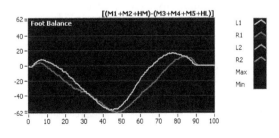

Graphic 4- foot balance
(soccer, 16,5years)

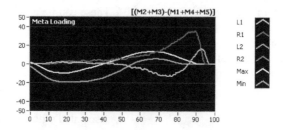

Graphic 5-metaloading and zone of lower injury risk
(tenis, 17years)

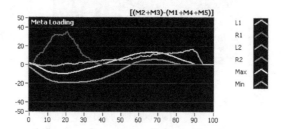

Graphic 6-metaloading and zone of lower injury risk
(tenis, 18years)

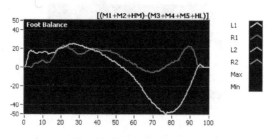

Graphic 7- foot balance
(tenis, 17years)

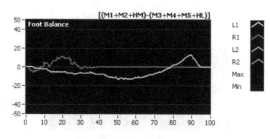

Graphic 8- foot balance
(tenis, 18years)

Conclusion

In conclusion we consdier that a good assessment of biomechanic aspect of ankle foot is important not only for prevent or treatment and monitoring rehabilitation programm, but also for a good selection for each sport activity. Also is important to know the load response because that help to prepare the entire muscle chain(12) for both side because how we see muscle inbalance between left and right, increase the possibility of injuries. All informations from force plate and biomechanical evaluation show that is possible to estimate the risk of injuries and explain these based on proprioceptive disorders that involve an increase of foot inbalanace and also postural control.

References

1. Hamill J., Knutzen Kathleen, *Biomechanical Basis of Human Movement*, Thrid edition, Lippincott and Wilkins, 2009
2. Andrews A, and Bohannon, R (2000), Distribution of muscle strength impairments following stroke. *Clinical Rehab 14:79*
3. Benedetti, M.G, Simoncini, L., Bonato, P., Tonini, A., Giannini, S. (1999), Gait abnormalities in minimally impaired multiple sclerosis patients, *Multiple Sclerosis*, 5(5): 363-8.
4. Vennila Krishnan; Neeta Kanekar; Alexander S Aruin (2012) Feedforward postural control in individuals with multiple sclerosis during load release. *Gait & posture* ;36(2):225-30.

5.C. Donze, O. Agnani, S. Demaille, P. Hautecoeur, P. Gallois (2009) Posturography and proprioceptive disorders in multiple sclerosis with low level of disability: clinical and electrophysiological correlations *25th Congress of the European Committee for the Treatment and Research in Multiple Sclerosis (ECTRIMS)* 09.09.2009 - 12.09.2009

6. Chaudry H., Bukiet B., Ji Zhmimg, Findley T., (2011) Measurement of balance in computer posturography: Comparison of methods—*A brief review, Journal of Bodyworkand Movement Therapies* , 15 (1)**:** 82-91.

6. Nutt J, Marsden C, Thompson P: Human walking and higher-level gait disorders, particularly in the elderly, Neurology 43:268-279, 1993.

7.Winter DA- *The Biomechanics and Motor Control of Human Gait*, University of Waterloo Press, Waterloo, Ontario, . 1991

8.Kim CM, Eng JJ.(2003), Symmetry in vertical ground reaction force is accompanied by symmetry in temporal but not distance variables of gait in persons with stroke. *Gait Posture* ;18:23-8.

9.Chen C, Patten C, Kothari DH.(2005), Gait differences between individuals with post-stroke hemiparesis and non-disabled controls at matched speeds. *Gait Posture* ;22:51-6.

10. RR Holt, D Simpson, JR Jenner, SGB Kirker, AM Wing (2000),Ground reaction force after a sideways push as a measure of balance in recovery from stroke , *Clinical Rehabilitation* ; 14: 88–95.

11. Kim CM, Eng JJ(2003),. Symmetry in vertical ground reaction force is accompanied by symmetry in temporal but not distance variables of gait in persons with stroke. *Gait Posture* ;18:23-8.

42

The impact of socio-cultural environment on the development management of sports activities

Barbu Mihai Constantin Răzvan, Barbu Dumitru, Stoica Doru, Ciocanescu Daniel
Department of Theory and Methodology of Motricity Activities, University of Craiova, ROMANIA

Abstract. Human social life involves a series of activities and concerns on a regular basis and an optional or necessary characteristic which in turn involve motric effort. Even if these activities are not what we define as a *social* concern, no doubt they are in a tight interdependence with the individual and global economic life by their conditioning and effects on this dimension. In other words, a life without motor activity will lead to the emergence of certain diseases, such as obesity, degenerative effect on the muscular system and disorders of the cardiovascular system which will have repercussions on the work efficiency at individual level and, eventually, at macro level. Thus, the human individual has to count on the balancing of the natural *social* evolution with the anthropo-physical needs characteristic to humans, such as movement, physical exercise and physical culture, in general terms. Here starts also the attempt, transformed during the last decades in economic phenomenon, to promote, to operate and to manage the physical culture and the benefits it provides globally, and to include it into the educational system. The remarkable economic evolution, largely due to the quick processes of mechanization and automation of the human society, has led to a reassessment of the needs of effort and physical behaviour of the individual, and of the degree of satisfying them in daily life.

Key words: *socio-cultural environment, management, sport*

Social life in our country maintains many of the shortcomings of the past. There is a certain reluctance to embrace the lifestyle of Western countries, on the background of a low purchasing power.

As long as there isn't an inner consciousness, a motivation for the implementation of new habits, the introduction of new mentalities of capitalist inspiration will be generating additional costs. The new rules of the game are not met: the system continues to function by a logic known only by local actors. Harmonious human development cannot be sustained as long as the causes of inefficiencies at the mental level are not removed: generalized corruption, switching from a short-term perspective to a long-term perspective, orientation towards employment and not towards a rentier-type behavior.

Human social life involves a series of activities and concerns on a regular basis and an optional or necessary characteristic which in turn involve motric effort. Even if these activities are not what we define as a *social* concern, no doubt they are in a tight interdependence with the individual and global economic life by their conditioning and effects on this dimension. In other words, a life without motor activity will lead to the emergence of certain diseases, such as obesity, degenerative effect on the muscular system and disorders of the cardiovascular system which will have repercussions on the work efficiency at individual level and, eventually, at macro level.

Thus, the human individual has to count on the balancing of the natural *social* evolution with the anthropo-physical needs characteristic to humans, such as movement, physical exercise and physical culture, in general terms. Here starts also the attempt, transformed during the last decades in economic phenomenon, to promote, to operate and to manage the physical culture and the benefits it provides globally, and to include it into the educational system.

The remarkable economic evolution, largely due to the quick processes of mechanization and automation of the human society, has led to a reassessment of the needs of effort and physical behaviour of the individual, and of the degree of satisfying them in daily life. Although hard to believe, most of the activities which materialize into motricity during the daily activity of the individual do not appropriately meet the needs of biological exercise, therefore it is necessary to promote and implement a physical culture as a method of fighting the immobility which threatens the society of the third millennium.

On the other hand, the physical effort is facing unfavorable associations, namely the sign of an unsophisticated life, of a low standard of living and of non-elitist preoccupations. On the other hand, however, we are witnessing the coming to the spotlight of the idea of a harmonious body, a healthy lifestyle, including a longer life.

On this backgrounds a new form of exercise develops at a high pace - sport as a social phenomenon. The sport is currently recognized and promoted as a real pylon of the fundamental human values: freedom, health, culture and association. Structured and boosted following the general rules of management, eventually enriched with specific provisions, sport has evolved into a profitable commercial activity.

Sport promptly responds to the needs of a society in constant metamorphosis, going beyond any of language, ethnic or racial barriers. This ability is likely to confer a dynamic and innovative aura adaptive to social and cultural trends.

Sport as a socio-cultural phenomenon practices and advocates the change, thus stimulating the individuals' need for novelty and helping by its international manifestation form to the integration into the globalization process.

Without making a mistake, sports can be considered, on the one hand a globalizing factor, and on the other hand a democratizing factor. Physical culture is in a close relationship with social life as an integral part of it and, of course, receives its same course of evolution. The fact that sport constantly interacts with the other subsystems of the social life, makes it a particularly comprehensive phenomenon, bringing together under the scope of its concerns billions of individuals with different cultural and historical background.

Sport encompasses not only individuals, but also efforts of organization, operations, physical resources, research, laws systems, etc. Thus, sport shows itself as expression of an impressive diversity, perhaps even unique, which denies barriers of any kind.

The fact that its coverage is so vast could not remain without an echo, thus sport benefits or it should benefit, where it still doesn't happen this way, from the aggregate support from both the society and the political system, both on regional and local level, and on international level.. Sport, in every of its forms (school sports, recreational sports, performance sports, etc.)is the common element of over 2.5 billion people around the world, a justifying argument of his character argument of globalizing factor. At the same time, sport is a democratizing factor, as it promotes libertarianism, every individual's personal expression without any relation with his/her socio-political orientation, color, age or sex. This ease of access has made the number of lovers and practitioners of sport to constantly multiply.

Quality of sports products and services. Typically, given a choice between two products or sporting experiences with similar prices, the customer will almost always choose the best quality. But quality can be defined in many ways. In November 2005, the USOC chose New York to present the special offer to host the 2012 Summer Games. The stakes for a successful bid to win the Games was really high because the USOC members have decided that hosting the Olympic Games in the United States will significantly contribute to the increasing of public interest. It was believed that New York would provide sponsors with maximum visibility and activation opportunities, and thus a strong comeback of investments that would help the U.S. offer at the time of the competition against foreign competitors (1).

In November 2002, the USOC has chosen New York City to enter the race for the 2012 Summer Olympic Games. The USOC's question was which of the finalists' bids will be considered by the IOC voters in July 2005 as one qualitative enough to equal Paris, London, Moscow and Madrid. But the competition for New York will be much tougher against those international cities, notably London and Paris. It was estimated that New York City 2012 will have to collect $ 7 billion ($ 3 billion for the development of the proposed Olympic Stadium and the surrounding area in Lower Manhattan and $ 1.5 billion for the Olympic Village in Queens). But the stadium, which will be used by the New York Jets of the NFL after the Olympics are over, it will be the biggest obstacle in New York offer.When representatives of the IOC officially chose the place in March 2005, the message was that the stadium plan was completed for the offer to succeed (2). When the representatives of the IOC officially chose the place in March 2005, the message was that the stadium plan had to be completed for the offer to succeed (3).

When the time came to vote in July of that year, in Singapore, each of the bidding cities were making sustained efforts to convince voters and the public of the merits of their tender, spending in total an amount estimated at $ 150 million, the highest amount ever

spent. The voting process runs as follows: in the first round, all the five bidding cities are eligible and the members vote their choice. After this official number, who gets the fewest votes is eliminated. The process continues until a city gets the simple majority of votes. As many experts predicted, Moscow was eliminated in the first round; New York was eliminated in the second round, also as predicted, surprisingly leaving London as winner after surpassing Paris in the fourth round, by 54-50. The reasons for the success of the London have been the soundness of the plan of jurisdiction, with three agglomerations at less than half an hour from the proposed Olympic village; the fact that much of the development will revitalize East London (one of the poorest areas of England); and the striving efforts of President Sebastian Coe (himself winner of two Olympic medals in races) and former Prime Minister Tony Blair. The result of the problem of the stadium which has condemned New York bid was that the USOC decided to continue with any future offer, the city will have to have a built stadium or a fully approved construction plan (4).

Achieving the quality and its continuous raising is now one of the most important responsibilities of the sports manager. IOC members are responsible with providing athletes and spectators with the best possible facilities and jurisdictions available and supposedly London bid had the most constrained circumstances in achieving this goal.

Speed and *flexibility* are other dimensions that became more and more important in order to progress in the competition when added to quality. The organizations, too large to be flexible or too rigid in terms of policies or procedures, are unable to take advantage of the advantages that come and go so quickly in all segments of the sports industry. In terms of the Olympic movement and hosting the Olympic Games, the terrorist attacks of September 11 have determined the organizers to worry that the games will become a target of this type of actions. Indeed they have been the target of such violence in 1972, during the 8th edition of the summer Olympic Games in Munich, Germany, when the terrorists took hostage nine Israeli athletes and coaches demanding the release of Palestinian prisoners held in Israel. The siege, broadcast live during the ABC broadcast of the games, ended after an attack by German police at a nearby airfield. In total, nine hostages and five terrorists were killed (5).

This was an assurance that all hosting of the Olympic Games should take place in the world after 9/11. Organizers in Salt Lake City had to make this insurance with just a few months before the opening of the ceremonies. Athens OCOG (ATHOC) too had countless challenges to face in preparing for the Olympic Games, such as incorporating some of their centuries-old locations (Panathinaikos stadium near the Acropolis), numerous protests on various issues but also Greece's infrastructure full of issues along with the usual delays of transportation to locations for the game determined the former President of the IOC, Juan

Antonio Samaranch, to name the preparations for that edition of the OG as the worst organizational crisis in his career, and, more than that, it determined him to propose that the games be moved somewhere else. To all of these setbacks are added the preparation of nearly 50,000 people who provided security, a negligence of the control system, a local history of bombings of November 17, a local terrorist group and the location of Athens, so close to the unstable Middle East, meaning that nearly $ 1 billion will be spent in insuring the safety of the Olympic Games. Athens officials have involved staff from the FBI and CIA along with troops from US Special Forces and similar staff from outside the US (6).

Despite worries about security and other preparations, the Athens Games began on time and did not encounter serious problems. Part of the success can be attributed to the fact that the security of most events was extremely expensive (it is estimated that the games have left the Organizing Committee with a debt of nearly $ 2 billion). However, having in view the limited time the organizational committees had to prepare the Games, *speed and flexibility have contributed to the successful management of the Games*.

Continuous development. The concept of continuous development means that organizations do not want to be as big as they could be, nor to grow as fast as possible, although they could. Constant development means that organizations must grow only to a certain degree and at a size that can be sustained over the long term (7). Of course, with so many sports organizations that compete for the money and attention of potential consumers, each sports organization must undergo a process of constant development.

In recent years, the IOC has observed that in terms of size and range of the Summer Olympics, bigger is not necessarily better and decided to remove a few sports. Summer Olympics became increasingly larger and difficult to host. At the Los Angeles Games in 1984, there were fewer than 7,000 athletes; in Athens in 2004, there were more than 11,000. Seven sports were added during the last two decades. There have been motivated concerns from the IOC President Jacques Rogge (himself a former Olympic rower) that the size and range of the Games made it impossible for smaller and poorer countries to host them. An official IOC report coincides with this information, concluding that "bigger doesn't necessarily mean better and higher expenditure does not necessarily guarantee the quality of the games" (Powers, 2003, p. D3). The result of the olympic elimination will be costly for the potential prominent sports because a large percentage of the the IOC's proceeds from television ($ 256 million between 2004 and 2008) finances the international federations that lead each of the sports in the Summer Games, money used to put into service the organizations and to internationally promote their sports (8).

In 2005, for example, at the same session where members have decided the host of 2012 Summer Games, the IOC decided the removal of baseball and softball (which were added in 1992 and 1996 respectively) starting with the London Games, the first time since 1936, when the total number of sports offered decreased. IOC members were asked to vote on each of the 28 sports (a simple majority should remain). Not only baseball and softball have been eliminated but also none of the five sports that wanted to be accepted (golf, karate, roller sports, rugby sevens and squash) did not receive enough votes to be included. However, there were some subterfuge in the voting process, sports often mocked such as synchronized swimming, rhythmic gymnastics and trampoline have never been voted on separately, but rather included within the category of aquatics and gymnastics, sports that will never be removed from the games due to well known competitions in other regions.

There are multiple reasons to explain why these two sports were eliminated. Softball has been dominated by the United States (winning all three gold medals since it was included), Major League of Baseball (MLB) has fallen by allowing the best players to leave their teams in the middle of the session, steroid scandals within the MLB, and the fact that 40% of the votes of the IOC belong to Europe. According to Carlos Rodrigues, President of the Cuban Federation of Baseball (whose team won three of the four gold medals since the game was included), "those who bear the greatest blame are the owners of the professional leagues who refuse to allow players to compete," while Mike Candera, coach of the US softball team in 2004, summed up the situation of his sport saying: "I think this is a matter of Europe against US" (6). Candera's comments have some legitimacy as none of these sports is not really practiced in Europe (10).

In this respect it should be noted that in 2004 the Olympic baseball team of Greece was composed almost entirely of Americans of Greek descent, only a few with MLB experience, and the financial support came from the owner of the Baltimore Orioles baseball team, Peter Angelos, an American of Greek origin.

The IOC has taken a decision that perhaps angered the American athletes, coaches and managers, but the decision had the purpose to make the games less expensive and easier to manage for the future OCOG.

Integrity. The decisive standard of performance is different than quality, speed and flexibility, innovation and sustained development. It is, in a way, the framework for the others. Integrity serves as the guiding principle by which all organizational decisions and actions are combined and activated. Like the vision and goals, the mission and goals of conduct, the integrity serves alot in helping sports managers to determine the direction of their organizations and to take decisions similar to the corresponding conditions of operation.

Any sports organization from any segment of sport industry meets challenges that put into question its sense of duty in the processes it carries on. In recent years, USOC had to question about the proper use of funds in the management, the IOC had to fight in the continuing battle to prevent and detect the use of illegal substances that increase performance and, in the case of the offers to host the Games, to face a scandal involving bribes given by members of the OCOG to the IOC members to win their favor in the voting rounds. After they lost to Nagano, Japan the offer for the 1998 Games, the members of the Organizing Committee of Salt Lake offered bribes in cash and other gifts including weekends to ski with all expenses paid, snowmobile rides and walks in on Christmas Eve, totalling $ 7 million to the IOC members in exchange for favorable votes for granting the Games in 2002. After the scandal broke, 10 members of the 126 members with voting rights have been removed or resigned, and fraud, conspiracy and blackmail proceedings were initiated against some in the leadership of the Salt Lake Organizing Committee. The fact that bribes from many major cities took place for several years, was blamed on the automatic adjustment and on the closed manner of the CIO, and also former President Juan Antonio Samaranch was widely regarded as responsible for "allowing a trade mark of corruption that threatens to disturb the entire Olympic movement." However, after the scandal, the IOC adopted a more transparent managerial and collegial process and instituted reforms based on ethics. Samaranch said about changes that "It was not easy to convince the members that it is time for change. Our organization was not updated. I have convinced them after the Salt Lake City crisis. The new revised procedures of tenders were incorporated before granting the 2010 Winter Games to Vancouver. The new guidelines do not allow IOC members to visit the cities nor to be visited by the OCOG persons who make lobby (11).

Conclusion

The examination of the environment of sports activities in the context of the Olympics or other sporting events helps to emphasize the importance of increased focus on quality, speed and flexibility, innovation, sustainable development and integrity. Fundamentally, all sports managers will be judged by those standards and sports organizations who have success are already attentive to them and are watching them continuously. Long-term viability, for example, of the Olympic Games will depend on how managers and the decision-makers will recognize these factors and will use them as the consumers will appreciate their products and services if the organizations are honest and fair.

References

1. Michaelis, V, (2005), *U.S. Games boost bottom line*, USA Today
2. Powers, J, (2003), *IOC takes games out of bidding*, Boston Globe
3. Powers, J, (2002), *NY: High hurdles*. Boston Globe
4. Zinser, L, (2005), *I.O.C. drops baseball and softball*. The New York Times.
5. Zinser, L, and Cardwell, D, (2006), *U.S.O.C. to visit 5 cities, seeking bids for the 2016 Games*, The New York Times
6. Zinser, L, (2005), *London wins '12 Olympics; New York lags*. The New York Times
7. Byrne, J,A, (1992, October 23), *Postmodern Paradigms for managers*. Business Week/Renewing America
8. Cazeneuve, B, (2003, September 8), *One Hellenic situation*, Sports Illustrated
9. Garfield, C, (1992), *Second to none, Homewood*. IL: Business One Irwin
10. Caple, J, (2004, April 19). *Give'em Hellas*, ESPN Magazine
11. Barlett, D.L, Steele, J,B, Karmatz, L, and J, Levinstein, (2001, December 10), *Snow job*. Sports Illustrated

43

The contribution of kinetic in hypertension

Trăilă Liviu-Alexandru, Mircea Dănoiu

University of Craiova, Faculty of Physical Education and Sport, România

Abstract: Introduction: High blood pressure (HBP) is a clinical syndrome characterized by an increase in systolic blood pressure, diastolic dysfunction or diastolic sistolo – over the values considered normal in the presence or absence of detectable organic cause. Objective: Balancing the nervous system and influence of positive vasomotors; promote vasodilatation and decongestion of peripheral parts of the body; achieving and maintaining optimum body weights; prevention of atherosclerosis ; getting vasodilataţion and decreasing peripheral resistance. Material and Method: It was a random group, comprising 20 patients at diagnosis and were specified in the medication for hypertension . In the studied for 3 months were patients with hypertension stage I and stage II disease without severe forms or organic disease. Physical therapy in hypertension: leg exercises, exercises for the trunk in the form of circumductions, upper limb exercises for derivation of the thoracic mobilization exercises all segments analytical, Results: 19 patients were considered useful programs followed, leading to a better mental condition and reduce associated symptoms; at 17 of the cases studied were obtained, on average, decreases with 25 mm Hg to TAS and with 20 mm Hg to TAD; 1 person dropped out of the study; 2 people have maintained the same values of yours. TA. Discussion and conlusions: Frequency of hypertension increases with age, with the maximum incidence in people over the age of 60 years. The incidence of the disease is higher in urban areas (65%) than rural (35%, due to the multitude of endogenous risk factors. The risk factors most encounter were: heredity, obesity, psychosocial stress, improper diet. Measures for prevention of hypetension, health education of the population can result in lowering the incidence of this disease. The study showed the importance of kinetoterapeutic treatment with drug treatment and igienodietetic

Key words: hypertension, pressure, factors, vasodilatation

Introduction

High blood pressure (HBP) is a clinical syndrome characterized by an increase in systolic blood pressure, diastolic dysfunction or diastolic sistolo – over the values considered normal in the presence or absence of detectable organic cause.

A Committee of experts, OMS(1959,1962), proposed that the values below 140\90 mm Hg is considered normal blood pressure, and level or above 160\95 mmHg are considered high blood pressure. The young subjects, interim values ranging between 140\90 – 160\95 mmHg arouse the suspicion of "young predisposed" and require periodic supervision (1).

The HTA is encountered at about 10% of the population over 50 years of age, and around 20% of the population over 65 years (2).

Blood pressure is determined by cardiac, peripheral vascular resistance. Cardiac flow is assured, muscular organ located in the hollow lower floor of mediastinum with pump (3). The disease can be asymptomatic for a long period . Symptoms of the disease may express variations in blood pressure values, or the suffering of the various organs and tissues, which occurs in chronic form.. Sick accused headache in the form of a pressure in the occipital region, dizziness, sounds in ears, undefined in precordial region of sensations (4).

HTA results from the interaction of numerous factors endogenous and exogenous.

Exogenous factors are heredity, age, sex, race, obesity, blood group .

Endogenic are: stress, salt intake, excessive caloric intake, height, smoking, alcohol intake, drinking coffee in excess (2).

The main change of heart in Hypertension is left ventricular hypertrophy .

Disease prevention is very important and is achieved through monitoring, avoiding exogenous factors.

After thorough research the treatment starts the etiology of essential hypertension . Drug treatment is individualized by age, stage of disease, complications associated with the binding associated with a dietary igieno (5).

Application of cinethotherapy in HTA differ depending on the stage of evolution of the disease, the patient's age, the reaction to the effort and associated diseases (6).

Objectives

Physical therapy has the following objectives (7):
- balancing the nervous system and influence of positive vasomotors;
- promote vasodilatation and decongestion of peripheral parts of the body;
- achieving and maintaining optimum body weights;
- prevention of atherosclerosis ;
- getting vasodilataţion and decreasing peripheral resistance;
- muscle relaxation and neuro-psychic .

Material and method

It was a random group, comprising 20 patients at diagnosis and were specified in the medication for hypertension . In the studied for 3 months were patients with hypertension stage I and stage II disease without severe forms or organic disease.

Evaluation of epidemiological data.

➢ Gender distribution in the studied cases

Table 1 Distribution by sex

Sex	Number cases	%
Male	12	60
Female	8	40
Total	20	100%

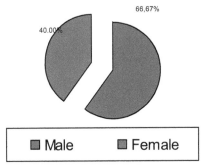

Fig. 1 Distribution by sex of the group to be studied

The data in fig.1 and table 1, highlight the fact that the HTA appears in men in the proportion of 60%, while in women the percentage was 40%.

➢ The origin of patients in the studied group.

Table 2 The origin of patients from the studied group

The origin	Number cases	%
Urban	13	65
Rural	7	35
Total	20	100

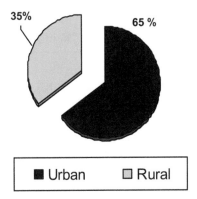

Fig. 2 Percentage distribution of patients according to the origin

Fig. 2 and table 2 is observed in the incidence of the patients studied, that is dominant in the urban environment (65%) compared to rural (35%). An increased incidence in urban areas was due to exogenous factors: psychosocial stress, salt intake and excessive caloric intake, reducing the physical effort.

➢ Group components studied fit the following age groups:

Table No. 3 Cases studied by age group

Age Groups (years)	Number cases	%
31 – 40	2	10
41 – 50	3	15
51 – 60	6	30
61 - 70	9	45
TOTAL	20	100

Fig. 3 Distribution by age group

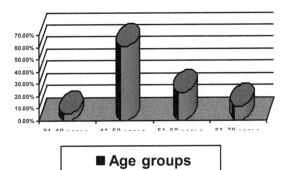

The study of the fig. 3 and table 3 it is observed that the incidence of the disease increases with age, the highest percentage by registering it with patients over the age of 60 years..

➤ The risk factors studied in patients experiencing the lot.

Table 4 Studied cases by age group

Risk factors	Number cases	%	Obs.
Heredity	15	75	
Age	15	75	over 50 years
Obesity	14	70	
Psychosocial stress	12	60	
Excessive salt intake	14	70	
Consumption of alcohol, coffee, cigarettes	12	60	

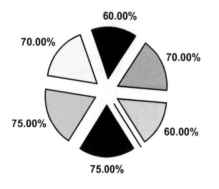

Legend:
- Heredity
- Age
- Obesity
- Psychosocial stress
- Excessive salt
- Alcool, cafea, tigari
- Alcohol, coffee, cigarettes

Fig. 4 The influence of risk factors

Action: it is proposed to patients from the studied further treatment and dietetic (fighting obesity, reducing the consumption of salt and convulsive).

In the treatment of hypertension has an important role physical supply, isotonic, aerobic exercise, moderate loudness have hipotensoare, because vasodilatation action produced during muscle contraction, which causes decreased peripheral resistance. However, patients should avoid physical efforts static (isometric), carried out in conditions of anaerobioza (lifting weights pushups).

In the first 2 weeks, because the subjects of the study were not physical efforts outside of everyday activities, have been recommended for beginning the most affordable treatment methods to the effort, the HTA:
- walking, dosed gradually made for riding to work, shopping, a stroll ,
- avoid short car journeys;
- progressive gymnastics in the morning;
- climbing stairs and slopes .
- progressive increase in physical activity (cleaning, gardening);
- sport therapy (pin-pong, volleyball, cycling, etc);
- respiratory exercises-Tirala-deep inhalation technique for training coastal and diaphragmatic breathing for 5-10 sec, followed by a prolonged, lasting about 45 sec.

Still, for two and a half months gradually intensified actions above, and physical therapy in hypertension: leg exercises, exercises for the trunk in the form of circumductions, upper limb exercises for derivation of the thoracic mobilization exercises all segments analytical, analytical isometric muscle contractions or "intermediate" relaxation exercises: balancing of the limbs, snatches shall occur by the patient or member of the snatches shall occur conducted by passive physical therapist, twisting trunk or some positions with twisting the torso.

Training, controlled and sustained, reduce your values with 10-20 mm Hg hypertension. Training for endurance effort achieves the most significant decrease, both in value and in time. Subjects performed 3 weekly sessions of 20 minutes It started with simple exercises, and after reaching a certain capacity of effort have introduced exercises analytical outreach to all segments, running, cycling and treadmill ergometrical determination of accurate and tracking patient effort during exercise. Before and after training sessions to your FC and blood pressure measured.

Results

In the study conducted for 3 months, have achieved the following results:
- 19 patients were considered useful programs followed, leading to a better mental condition and reduce associated symptoms;
- at 17 of the cases studied were obtained, on average, decreases with 25 mm Hg to TAS and with 20 mm Hg to TAD;
- 1 person dropped out of the study;
- 2 people have maintained the same values of blood pressure.

Conclusions

Frequency of hypertension increases with age, with the maximum incidence in people over the age of 60 years. The incidence of the disease is higher in urban areas (65%) than rural (35%, due to the multitude of endogenous risk factors.

The risk factors most encounter were: heredity, obesity, psychosocial stress, improper diet.

Measures for prevention of hypetension, health education of the population can result in lowering the incidence of this disease.

precocious detection of the disease is very important to prevent serious complications of hypertension.

Drug treatment and dietetic igieno-must be monitored continually .

The study showed the importance of kinetoterapeutic treatment with drug treatment and igienodietetic.

The life of the patient must be ordered HTAE with avoiding stress somatic (physical exhaustion moods, cold, heat, noise) and the psychic (anxiety, fear, assaults).

References

1. Voiculescu, M., (1990), Medicină generală, Editura Medicală, Bucureşti

2. Avramescu, E., T., s.a., (2007), Kinetoterapia în afecţiuni cardiovasculare, Editura Universitaria Craiova

3. Traşcă, E., Traşcă, E.T., Pătraşcu, M., ş.a., (2007), Clinical Anatomy, Medical University Publishing House Craiova.

4. Branea, I., Mancaş, S., (1989), Exerciţiile fizice şi rolul lor în programul complex de recuperare al bolnavilor coronarieni, Timişoara Medicală, Timişoara, XXXIV, 4

5. Trăilă, L., A., (2008), Exerciţiul şi controlul greutăţii, Conferinţa ştiinţifică naţională cu participare internaţională „Exerciţiul fizic mijloc complex şi modern de promovare a sănătăţii", Craiova

6. Marza, D., (1996), Kinetoterapia în afecţiunile aparatului cardio-vascular, Caiet de lucrări practice, Universitatea din Bacau

7. Vlaicu, R., Achimaş, A., Ilea, V., (1988), Controlul şi recuperarea bolnavilor cu hipertensiune arterială esenţială prin exerciţii respiratorii, Ed. Dacia, Cluj-Napoca

44

The role of the muscular toner methods in fitness pilates

Lupu Stănică Gabriel, Cristuță Alina Mihaela

"Vasile Alecsandri"University from Bacău, Bacau, Roumania

Abstract. By monitoring permanent the last news in the field of fitness and the movement sciences in the last decade I have found that there are two complementary concepts of which the notorious increase exponentially – muscular toner and the method of Pilates exercises, both controversial and which also make the purpose of this research. Both, the method Pilates as well as the methods of de muscular toners are highly publicized and intensely promoted as being the key to obtaining an ideal physical conditions without too much effort. Sure, an intense media coverage and exposure of society to activities involving various forms of motion is beneficial, but a old method of almost a hundred years, as is the method Pilates can respond to the needs,but also needs as expected on which modern man has from. Despite its popularity Pilates method, in Romania but also at world level, clinical studies and research which has as a subject of identification and scientific demonstration of the effects in application of Pilates exercises are not enough present, fact what conditioned our research to reporting and account on the results obtained from its own procedure to check exposed theme for the purpose of research.

Key words: *muscular toners, activity, fitness pilates*

Introduction

We always question what expectations we have to be from a workout and in particular how caliber that method that allows us obtaining a good physical conditions? On the whole evolution of the primitive movement up until the present time answers come so natural - the movement, the acquisition of good physical conditions are closely related to mind and body regarded as a whole,that's why maybe we should turn our attention to those methods of exercise to restore correlation between mind and body, and which guides you step-by-step in achieving a good physical conditions.

By monitoring permanent the last news in the field of fitness and the movement sciences in the last decade I have found that there are two complementary concepts of which the notorious increase exponentially – muscular toner and the method of Pilates exercises, both controversial and which also make the purpose of this research. Both, the method Pilates as well as the methods of de muscular toners are highly publicized and intensely promoted as being the key to obtaining an ideal physical conditions without too much effort. Sure, an intense media coverage and exposure of society to activities involving various forms of motion is beneficial, but a old method of almost a hundred years, as is the method Pilates can respond to the needs, but also needs as expected on which modern man has the physical exercise.The answer comes naturally, the Pilates method handed over in our days differ by more than the one built by Joseph Pilates over a hundred years. To enter in the "goodpublic graces " this has lowered bar, has adapted to the century speed, he promised those ideals as regards provided physical searches for de man muscle fast, body remodeling, decrease in weight (1).

Material and methods

As too genuine method of Pilatesexercises is based on the belief that between physical activity and mental control of movements there is a interdependence, and effects are observable Pilates exercises and visible in so far as to establish this interdependences, we decided to rely on our of experimental observationmethod and autoobservation. We believe that this approach,

through experimentalself-observation is relevant in this case, because this is the method by which Joseph Pilates himself verified efficiency of physical exercisesmethod bearing his name.

Our research proposes verification of the following hypotheses, we believe that the consequence that a program structured and controlled by Pilates exercises can have a direct impact on muscular toners of thebody because of the exercises influence specify which request the main types of muscle contractions, eccentric contractions, concentric and isometric; if they are running a program of Pilates exercises systematically and settled it should be possible to make both a good muscle energy as well as visible and to improve the physical condition of subjects observed?

As methods of research i used: Thetheoretical documentation method, biographical method, the observation method, the method of measuring and evaluation (antropometry, body composition, tests for the assessment of physical condition- Ruffier test, the method of recording data, processing data and graphic recording.

Research took place during the period January 2012 - July 2012, on a sample of 2 subjects, within the framework of the fitness gym Junona. Training programs have included types of Pilates exercises which had an impact on tonnig the abdominal muscles, but they have been alternately and other sets of Pilates exercises aimed at various groups of muscles to achieve a harmonious development of the body(2).

Stages of work consisted in the scan field research both in consultation with the specialized literature as well as by the approach of specialists in the area of research in the study (comparative of Pilates, coaches the fitness, bodybuilders); establishing the sample of subjects, in the place of progress of the study, it was comparative and purchased logistics required research purposes (equipment and measurement instrumentation); it has been exploring and evaluating subjects research, have been drawn up the record sheets (required observation evolution of the subjects), have been completed the forms for anamnesis to each subject, have been made pretest measurements and it has been compared Pilates training plan (selecting Pilates exercises with potential impact on muscular toners and drawing up routine of exercises); communication and train each topic on the working routine; the last stage in the table of contents the final measurement posttest (exploration and evaluation) ,and on the basis of the data recorded and processed has been passed on to their interpretation comparativewith the prettest data, (2).

RUTINA DE EXERCITII	EXERCITIUL EFECTUAT	LUNA 1												
		Saptamana 1			Saptamana 2			Saptamana 3				Saptamana 4		
		Mi	V	D	Ma	J	S	L	Mi	V	D	Ma	J	S
BAZA	#1 The Standing Roll Down	5R	5R	5R	5R	6R	6R	6R	8R	8R	10R	10R	10R	10R
BAZA	#2 The Start Stretches	5R	5R	5R	5R	6R	6R	6R	8R	8R	10R	10R	10R	10R
BAZA	#3 The Spine Stretch	5R	5R	5R	5R	6R	6R	6R	8R	8R	10R	10R	10R	10R
BAZA	#4 The Side Leg Lifts	5R	5R	5R	5R	6R	6R	6R	8R	8R	10R	10R	10R	10R
BAZA	#5 The Hundreds: Basic	5R	5R	5R	5R	6R	6R	6R	8R	8R	10R	10R	10R	10R
BAZA	#6 The Perfect Abdominal Curl	5R	5R	5R	5R	6R	6R	6R	8R	8R	10R	10R	10R	10R
BAZA	#7 The Lumbar Stretch	5R	5R	5R	5R	6R	6R	6R	8R	8R	10R	10R	10R	10R
BAZA	#8 Arm Swings - Alternating	5R	5R	5R	5R	6R	6R	6R	8R	8R	10R	10R	10R	10R
BAZA	#9 Resting Position (Baby Pose)	1R	1R	1R	1R	1R	1R	1R	1R	1R	1R	1R	1R	1R
Durata estimativa a esiuni de exercitii (min)		10'	10'	10'	10'	15'	15'	15'	20'	20'	25'	25'	25'	25'
DURATA TOTALA A RUTINEI DE EXERCITII/ZI		10'	10'	10'	10'	15'	15'	15'	20'	20'	25'	25'	25'	25'

Figure 1. The basic training routine

RUTINA DE EXERCITII	EXERCITIUL EFECTUAT	LUNA 2												LUNA 3											
		Saptamana 5			Saptamana 6			Saptamana 7			Saptamana 8			Saptamana 9			Saptamana 10			Saptamana 11			Saptamana 12		
		L	Mi	V	Ma	J	S	L	Mi	V	Ma	J	S	L	Mi	V	Ma	J	S	Ma	J	S	L	Mi	V
BAZA	#1 The Standing Roll Down																								
BAZA	#2 The Start Stretches	5R	5R	5R	5R	5R	5R	8R	8R	8R	8R	8R	8R	8R	8R	8R	8R	8R	8R	8R	8R	8R	8R	8R	8R
BAZA	#3 The Spine Stretch	5R	5R	5R	5R	5R	5R	8R	8R	8R	8R	8R	8R	8R	8R	8R	8R	8R	8R	8R	8R	8R	8R	8R	8R
BAZA	#4 The Side Leg Lifts																								
BAZA	#5 The Hundreds: Basic																								
BAZA	#6 The Perfect Abdominal Curl	5R	5R	5R	5R	5R	5R	8R	8R	8R	8R	8R	8R	8R	8R	8R	8R	8R	8R	8R	8R	8R	8R	8R	8R
BAZA	#7 The Lumbar Stretch	5R	5R	5R	5R	5R	5R	8R	8R	8R	8R	8R	8R	8R	8R	8R	8R	8R	8R	8R	8R	8R	8R	8R	8R
BAZA	#8 Arm Swings - Alternating																								
BAZA	#9 Resting Position (Baby Pose)	1	1R	1R	1R	1R	1R	1R	1R	1R	1R	1R	1R	1R	1R	1R	1R	1R	1R	1R	1R	1R	1R	1R	1R
Durata estimativa a esiuni de exercitii (min)		7'	7'	7'	7'	7'	7'	15'	15'	15'	15'	15'	15'	15'	15'	15'	15'	15'	15'	15'	15'	15'	15'	15'	15'
INTERMEDIAR	# 10 The Hamstring Stretch	5R	5R	6R	6R	6R	6R	8R	8R	8R				8R	8R	8R									
INTERMEDIAR	# 11 The Thigh Stretch: Kneeling	5R		6R		6R				8R	10R		10R			8R	10R		10R	10R		10R	10R		10R
INTERMEDIAR	# 12 The Spine Rotation		5R		6R		6R	8R	8R	8R	10R	10R	10R	8R	8R	8R	10R	10R	10R	10R	10R	10R	10R	10R	10R
INTERMEDIAR	# 13 The Hundreds: Intermediate	5R	5R	6R	6R	6R	6R	8R	8R	8R	10R	10R	10R	8R	8R	8R	10R	10R	10R	10R	10R	10R	10R	10R	10R
INTERMEDIAR	# 14 The Corkscrew		5R	6R	6R	6R	6R	8R				10R		8R				10R			10R			10R	
INTERMEDIAR	# 15 The Control Balance	5R							8R						8R										
INTERMEDIAR	# 16 The Pelvic Lift	5R	5R	6R	6R	6R	6R	8R	8R	8R	10R	10R	10R	8R	8R	8R	10R	10R	10R	10R	10R	10R	10R	10R	10R
Durata estimativa a esiuni de exercitii (min)		20'	20'	25'	25'	20'	25'	30'	30'	30'	40'	40'	40'	30'	30'	30'	40'	40'	40'	40'	40'	40'	40'	40'	40'
DURATA TOTALA A RUTINEI DE EXERCITII/ZI		27'	27'	32'	27'	27'	27'	45'	45'	45'	45'	45'	45'	45'	45'	45'	45'	45'	45'	45'	45'	45'	45'	45'	45'

Figure 2. Intermediate training routine

RUTINA DE EXERCITII	EXERCITIUL EFECTUAT	LUNA 4													
		Saptamana			Saptaman			Saptamana 16				Saptamana 17			
		L	Mi	V	Ma	J	S	L	Mi	V	D	Ma	J	S	D
BAZA	#1 The Standing Roll Down														
BAZA	#2 The Start Stretches	8R	8R	8R	5R	5R	5R	5R	5R	5R	5R	5R	5R	5R	5R
BAZA	#3 The Spine Stretch	8R	8R	8R	5R	5R	5R	5R	5R	5R	5R	5R	5R	5R	5R
BAZA	#4 The Side Leg Lifts														
BAZA	#5 The Hundreds: Basic														
BAZA	#6 The Perfect Abdominal	8R	8R	8R	5R	5R	5R	5R	5R	5R	5R	5R	5R	5R	5R
BAZA	#7 The Lumbar Stretch	8R	8R	8R	5R	5R	5R	5R	5R	5R	5R	5R	5R	5R	5R
BAZA	#8 Arm Swings -														
BAZA	#9 Resting Position (Baby	1R	1R	1R	1R	1R	1R	1R	1R	1R	1R	1R	1R	1R	1R
Durata estimativa a esiuni de exercitii (min)		15'	15'	15'	7'	7'	7'	7'	7'	7'	7'	7'	7'	7'	7'
INTERMEDIAR	# 10 The Hamstring Stretch														
INTERMEDIAR	# 11 The Thigh Stretch:														
INTERMEDIAR	# 12 The Spine Rotation	5R													
INTERMEDIAR	# 13 The Hundreds:	5R	5R	6R	6R	6R	6R	8R	8R	8R	8R	10	10	10	10
INTERMEDIAR	# 14 The Corkscrew		5R	6R	6R	6R	6R	8R	8R	8R	8R		10		
INTERMEDIAR	# 15 The Control Balance														
INTERMEDIAR	# 16 The Pelvic Lift														
Durata estimativa a esiuni de exercitii (min)		6'	6'	8'	8'	8'	8'	12'	12'	12'	12'	8'	16'	8'	8'
AVANSAT	# 17 The Hundreds:	5R	5R	5R	6R	6R	6R	6R	6R	8R	8R	10		10	10
AVANSAT	# 18 Pendulum				6R		6R		6R						
AVANSAT	# 19 Helicopter Hundreds					6R	6R			8R		10		10	
AVANSAT	# 20 Stamina Stretch		5R	5R				6R	6R		8R		10		
AVANSAT	# 21 Hip Circles				6R		6R					10			10
AVANSAT	# 22 Jackknife	5R		5R				6R		8R				10	
MODELARE	# 23 Teaser 2	5R	5R		6R	6R	6R	6R	6R	8R	8R	10	10	10	10
MODELARE	# 24 Lying Torso Stretch					6R									
MODELARE	# 25 Boomerang										8R		10		10
MODELARE	# 26 The Hundreds: Lower&	5R	5R	5R	6R	6R	6R	6R	6R	8R	8R	10	10	10	10
Durata estimativa a esiuni de exercitii		25'	25'	25'	30'	30'	40'	40'	40'	50'	50'	60'	50'	60'	60'
DURATA TOTALA A RUTINEI DE EXERCITII/ZI		46'	46'	46'	45'	45'	55'	59'	59'	69'	69'	75'	73'	75'	75'

RUTINA DE EXERCITII	EXERCITIUL EFECTUAT	LUNA 5													
		Saptaman			Saptaman			Saptamana 20				Saptamana 21			
		L	Mi	V	Ma	J	S	L	Mi	V	D	Ma	J	S	D
BAZA	#1 The Standing Roll Down														
BAZA	#2 The Start Stretches	8R	8R	8R	5R	5R	5R	5R	5R	5R	5R	5R	5R	5R	5R
BAZA	#3 The Spine Stretch	8R	8R	8R	5R	5R	5R	5R	5R	5R	5R	5R	5R	5R	5R
BAZA	#4 The Side Leg Lifts														
BAZA	#5 The Hundreds: Basic														
BAZA	#6 The Perfect Abdominal	8R	8R	8R	5R	5R	5R	5R	5R	5R	5R	5R	5R	5R	5R
BAZA	#7 The Lumbar Stretch	8R	8R	8R	5R	5R	5R	5R	5R	5R	5R	5R	5R	5R	5R
BAZA	#8 Arm Swings -														
BAZA	#9 Resting Position (Baby	1R	1R	1R	1R	1R	1R	1R	1R	1R	1R	1R	1R	1R	1R
Durata estimativa a esiuni de exercitii (min)		15'	15'	15'	7'	7'	7'	7'	7'	7'	7'	7'	7'	7'	7'
INTERMEDIAR	# 10 The Hamstring Stretch														
INTERMEDIAR	# 11 The Thigh Stretch:														
INTERMEDIAR	# 12 The Spine Rotation	5R													
INTERMEDIAR	# 13 The Hundreds:	5R	5R	6R	6R	6R	6R	8R	8R	8R	8R	10	10	10	10
INTERMEDIAR	# 14 The Corkscrew		5R	6R	6R	6R	6R	8R	8R	8R	8R		10		
INTERMEDIAR	# 15 The Control Balance														
INTERMEDIAR	# 16 The Pelvic Lift														
Durata estimativa a esiuni de exercitii (min)		6'	6'	8'	8'	8'	8'	12'	12'	12'	12'	8'	16'	8'	8'
AVANSAT	# 17 The Hundreds:	5R	5R	5R	6R	6R	6R	6R	6R	8R	8R	10		10	10
AVANSAT	# 18 Pendulum				6R		6R		6R						
AVANSAT	# 19 Helicopter Hundreds					6R	6R			8R		10		10	
AVANSAT	# 20 Stamina Stretch		5R	5R				6R	6R		8R		10		
AVANSAT	# 21 Hip Circles				6R		6R					10			10
AVANSAT	# 22 Jackknife	5R		5R				6R		8R				10	
MODELARE	# 23 Teaser 2	5R	5R		6R	6R	6R	6R	6R	8R	8R	10	10	10	10
MODELARE	# 24 Lying Torso Stretch					6R									
MODELARE	# 25 Boomerang										8R		10		10
MODELARE	# 26 The Hundreds: Lower&	5R	5R	5R	6R	6R	6R	6R	6R	8R	8R	10	10	10	10
Durata estimativa a esiuni de exercitii		25'	25'	25'	30'	30'	40'	40'	40'	50'	50'	60'	50'	60'	60'
DURATA TOTALA A RUTINEI DE EXERCITII/ZI		46'	46'	46'	45'	45'	55'	59'	59'	69'	69'	75'	73'	75'	75'

RUTINA DE EXERCITII	EXERCITIUL EFECTUAT	LUNA 6									
		Saptaman			Saptaman			Saptamana 24			
		L	Mi	V	Ma	J	S	L	Mi	V	D
BAZA	#1 The Standing Roll Down										
BAZA	#2 The Start Stretches	8R	8R	8R	5R	5R	5R	5R	5R	5R	5R
BAZA	#3 The Spine Stretch	8R	8R	8R	5R	5R	5R	5R	5R	5R	5R
BAZA	#4 The Side Leg Lifts										
BAZA	#5 The Hundreds: Basic										
BAZA	#6 The Perfect Abdominal	8R	8R	8R	5R	5R	5R	5R	5R	5R	5R
BAZA	#7 The Lumbar Stretch	8R	8R	8R	5R	5R	5R	5R	5R	5R	5R
BAZA	#8 Arm Swings -										
BAZA	#9 Resting Position (Baby	1R	1R	1R	1R	1R	1R	1R	1R	1R	1R
Durata estimativa a esiuni de exercitii (min)		15'	15'	15'	7'	7'	7'	7'	7'	7'	7'
INTERMEDIAR	# 10 The Hamstring Stretch										
INTERMEDIAR	# 11 The Thigh Stretch:										
INTERMEDIAR	# 12 The Spine Rotation	5R									
INTERMEDIAR	# 13 The Hundreds:	5R	5R	6R	6R	6R	6R	8R	8R	8R	8R
INTERMEDIAR	# 14 The Corkscrew		5R	6R	6R	6R	6R	8R	8R	8R	8R
INTERMEDIAR	# 15 The Control Balance										
INTERMEDIAR	# 16 The Pelvic Lift										
Durata estimativa a esiuni de exercitii (min)		6'	6'	8'	8'	8'	8'	12'	12'	12'	12'
AVANSAT	# 17 The Hundreds:	5R	5R	5R	6R	6R	6R	6R	6R	8R	8R
AVANSAT	# 18 Pendulum				6R		6R		6R		
AVANSAT	# 19 Helicopter Hundreds					6R	6R			8R	
AVANSAT	# 20 Stamina Stretch		5R	5R				6R	6R		8R
AVANSAT	# 21 Hip Circles				6R		6R				
AVANSAT	# 22 Jackknife	5R		5R				6R		8R	
MODELARE	# 23 Teaser 2	5R	5R		6R	6R	6R	6R	6R	8R	8R
MODELARE	# 24 Lying Torso Stretch					6R					
MODELARE	# 25 Boomerang										8R
MODELARE	# 26 The Hundreds: Lower&	5R	5R	5R	6R	6R	6R	6R	6R	8R	8R
Durata estimativa a esiuni de exercitii		25'	25'	25'	30'	30'	40'	40'	40'	50'	50'
DURATA TOTALA A RUTINEI DE EXERCITII/ZI		46'	46'	46'	45'	45'	55'	59'	59'	69'	69'

Figure 3. Final training routine

Results

By analysing dynamic values obtained from the measurements circumferences pretest and posttest is observed a decrease in average between 1-5cm (-1,04% vs pretest posttest) of boundary values body subject to measurement, the most significant change is observed around his waist Tinitiala 79 cm vs Tfinala 74cm in fact easy to predict because the Pilates exercises applied were based on stimulating "center of gravity". These values shall be translated into a production ascending growing muscle energy.

Regarding body composition and here it is observed significant changes of the values of Vs pretest posttest. Using the method of calculation Jackson Pollok of

measurement of the 7 plici using mechanic caliper were determined following parameters: percentage of adipose tissue, fatty tissue in kilograms and weight active.

Regarding to the rate of adipose tissue to subject 1 there has been a general decrease by approximately 1, 81% (Tinitial Tfinal 11,03 % vs 9.22 %) in such a way that active mass increased by 1.00 % (Tinitial Tfinal 71.18 vs 71.74) - we can infer from this clearly an enhancement to the body composition.

And as regards the index of Ruffier tissueit saw an improvement (Tinitial Tfinal 9.60 vs 8.65) even if results remain in the sphere mediocre results.

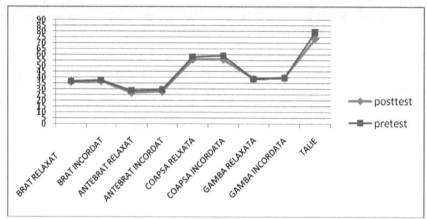

Graph no. 1 Variation In measurements circumferinte pretest-posttest (M. I.)

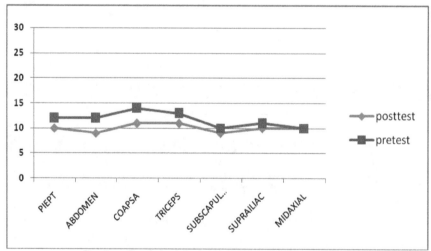

Graph no. 2 variation in body compozitie pretest-posttest (M. I.)

By analysing dynamic values obtained from the measurements circumferences pretest and posttest is observed a decrease in average between 1-3 cm (-1.06% vs pretest posttest) of boundary values body subject to measurement, the most significant change is observed in waist Tinitiala 68cm vs Tfinala 63 cm, these values could be translated in a production ascending growing muscle energy.

As regards the composition harm and here it is observed significant changes of the values of vs pretest posttest. Using the method of calculation Jackson Pollok of measurement of the 7 spalsh using mechanic caliper were determined following parameters:

procentege of adipose tissue, the tissue adipose mass in kilograms and active. With regard to the rate of adipose tissue to subject 2 s- has been a general decrease of approximately 1.82 % (Tinitial Tfinal 10.43% vs 8.61 %) in such a way that the active increased by 1.02 % (Tinitial Tfinal 73.45 vs 71.74) - we can infer from this clearly a upgrade to the composition, to the physical condition in general.

As regards the index Ruffier test its been seen a visible upgrade (Tinitiala Tfinala 9.60 vs 5.00) and may qualify the result as enhancement to physical condition by the exercises Pilates as a consequence of Pilates training.

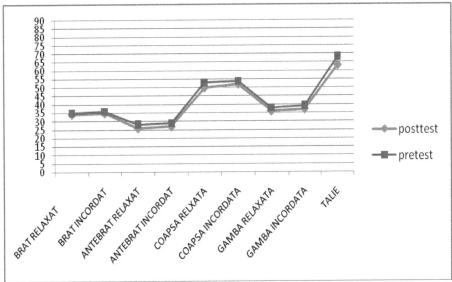

Graph no. 3 Variation in measurements circumferences pretest-posttest (D. S.)

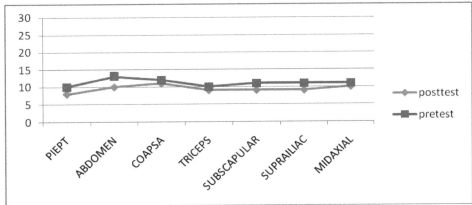

Graph no. 4 variation in body composition pretest-posttest (D. S.)

Discussions and conclusions

Fundamental characteristics of physical activities to ensure that physical condition are the following:

• to work large muscle groups,

• to impose a more load than usual

• impose a energy consumption substantially higher.

In practice this means carrying out frequent, (daily) of rhythmic exercises, supported, for at least 20-30 minutes.

Therefore, through this research they have watched impact confirmation application of the method of exercises authentic Pilates on the process of de muscular and highlighting changes observed in the elasticity and force level and as a consequence of the implementation of this method. A secondary purpose of the research was to identify the impact Pilates method of exercise on the improvement of physical condition in general(3,4).

Regarding the methods and measurement tools applied in this study in concordance with their relevance to achieve the aim of research and demonstration ofassumptions, they were laid down by following the steps process of measurement – assessment specified in science movements.

References

1.Anderson, B.D., (2001), Pushing for pilates:lack of scientific research holds the movement system back, but interest in its use remains high. RehabManagement: *The Interdisciplinary Journal of Rehabilitation*

2.Bernardo L., (2007), The effectiveness of Pilates training in healthy adults: an appraisal of the research literature. *J BodywMovTher;*

3.Donahoe B. si colab,(2007), The effects of a home Pilates program on muscle, Journal of Women's Health Physical Therapy:Summer - Volume 31;

4.Johnson E, si colab., (2007), The effects of Pilates-based exercise on dynamic balance in healthy adults. *J BodywMovTher.*

45

The Contribution of Skill to the Development of Motric Ability and the Appropriation of Technique For the Beginner Volleyball Players

Oprea Mihaela, Ion Gheorghe

Physical Education and Sport – University of Pitești, Romania

Abstract. The content and the methodology used in the training of beginner volleyball players do not suit the expectations. The initiation of the study starts from the premise of existing progress stores concerning the optimization of achieving the main goal of the beginner's training: the ABC appropriation by the volleyball players including the building of a motric, functional and technical-strategical basis. The decisive involvement in the technical appropriation and its possible development at this age have contoured and directed for me the experimental context of the hypothesis check according to which, by potentiating the development of skill behaviours one can influence both the level of the other qualities and the one of appropriating the technique of the actions and the game. The operational programmes of the foreseen instructive components and the structures of the means used for developing coordinative aptitudes (skill) proved, by test results, their adequation to the achievement of the pursued instructive goals, the operational value of the used means and the high efficiency of the methodology proposed for experimental check, thus validating the study hypothesis.
Key words: *Game action; Coordinative aptitudes; Development; Motricity; Technical-strategical component; Efficiency.*

Introduction

The level reached in practice by the training of the beginner volleyball players concerning both the content and the used methodologies, is not at the maximum parameters, possible to reach. Welcoming the desire of the ,beginner' to practise as quick as possible the volleyball game of the adults, many trainers forget that this is not a ,miniatural grown up' but a ,becoming one', who has to accumulate in sequences, the correlated content of all training components: physical development, skills and talents, motric qualities, technical-strategical content, the game ensemble, theoretical knowledge, etc. The minimization of the interest for motricity development and giving a major importance to the appropriation of the technical-strategical component proves to be on a long term a ,limitative option' for the final volleyball progress of the player. The rich content which the actual volleyball has reached can be valued only by the players that possess a rich luggage of game actions with a special level of efficiency , sustained by a biomotric support prepared at the highest parameters. Any motric action, simple or complex is the result of the multiple forms of combining motric qualities with elements of technique. The level of quality development has a major influence on the possibilities of technique apprehension. The motric aptitudes or the physical qualities, as Zațiorschi V.M. defined them (1), constitute the basic motric pre-request on which man builds his technical abilities'.
In any motric act all qualities express in a various percentage, ,the skill' recording the largest interconditioning with the other motric qualities. None develops independently from the others. The development of ,skill' includes the development of ,force' and ,speed', as the development of ,speed' and ,resistance' includes the development of ,force' and ,skill'."The multitude of these combining forms, the relations of interconditioning and the level of development of the dominant qualities specifically involved in every game action are major in the process of appropriation and enhancement of these:
- At serving – Skill and Force-Speed (Explosive force);

- Receiving the serve – Speed (reaction, execution) and Skill;
- At the attack hit – Speed-Force (expansion) inferior part, Skill and Force-Speed (explosive force) upper part;
- Receiving the attack – Speed (execution, reaction) and Skill;
- At blockage – Speed-Force (expansion) and Skill;
- At rising – Skill and Speed of execution" (2).
The skill (the coordinative ability, similar term (3) considered one of the most complex psycho-motric aptitude, in whose structure there are a multitude of distinct components (The space-time orientation, the accuracy of actions, the balance, the rythm, the ambidexterity, the kinesthetic differentiation, the motric reaction, the movement combination, etc) constitutes the main premise that makes possible to appropriate motric abilities, more complex and more well organized. A rich luggage of motric skills and abilities enables positive transformations in the technical-strategical field, by the coordinating capacity. The method of perfectioning the coordinative capacities is based on the increase of the number of general and specific motric skills and abilities. The relation between the general skill and the specific one has a special inportance, because the general skill creates premises for the specific one. The exercises for the general skill, in time, will transform into operational structures of a coordinative type, with specific features for each procedure and technical-strategical action. The main way in the methodics of educating general skill constitutes the continuous apprehension of new and various abilities. ,For the development of skill there are not special exercises and methods. Any exercise, no matter its complexity, develops skill in a larger or smaller degree.' (Firea, 1984)

The purpose and the goals of research

The necessity of increasing the efficiency for the instructive approach of the beginners must start from the fulfillment of the main strategical goals of the action directed to:
- Harmonious development;

- The correct appropriation and the enforcement of all game actions;
- The complex increase of the level of motric capacity indexes, both regarding basic skills and abilities, and the motric qualities ‚Skill' and ‚Speed'

Starting from the premise of an existing possibility of training optimization , the initiated study has fixed as a goal the experimental check of the possibilities of influencing the general motric capacity and the appropriation of the technical component of the game actions by coordinative aptitudes (skill) at the echelon of the beginner volleyball players.

In this context **the research goals** were directed to:
- The identification of the methodological resources concerning the possibilities of optimizing the development of the components of coordinative aptitudes adapted to the features and the psycho-somato-motric potential echelon;
- The evidentiation of specific involvement of coordinative aptitudes in the appropriation and valuing the execution of each game action;
- The contouring and applying of some "operational training programmes" which should harmonise the contents and goals of all components (motric, technical, psychological, theoretical) expected for the volleyball training of the beginners with those especially destined for the coordinative aptitudes subjected to experimental check;
- The selection and the creation of the structures of means used for influencing different components of the coordinative aptitudes;
- The choice of the measurement and accumulation evaluation system and of the expected instructive efficiency (initial tests, tests, date operations, etc);
- The choice of the experimental context for checking the degree in which the development of the coordinative aptitudes can increase the general efficiency of all the components in the beginners' training.

Premises and hypotheses
Premises:
- For the volleyball game, most of the questioned specialists consider that skill and its manifestation in regimes combined with ‚Speed' and ‚Force', is the motric quality with the highest rate of involvement;
- The main components of coordinative aptitudes (skill) which are necessary for acquiring and valuing game actions are: space-time orientation, movement coordination, ambidexterity, the kinesthetic sense, the precision, the sense of rythm and balance.
- As movement regulators, the coordinative aptitudes constitute the basic motric pre-request in order to appropriate the technique. Recording the largest rate of potentiation in the pre puberty period (7-12 years) their level of development has a major influence on the possibilities of technique appropriation.
- In the context of these premises we have drawn the **hypothesis** according to which by developing coordinative aptitudes, one can influence significantly both the level of the other motric qualities involved in the procedure execution and the level of efficiency regarding the appropriation of the technical-strategical component of game actions.

The research organisation
- For checking the instructive efficiency in experimental conditions experiment and check samples were chosen, after testing the somatic-motric and aptitude potential of the beginners from five sports institutions from the capital city. A significant battery of measurements, examinations and tests was conceived in order to note the level of somatic and motric development. Composed of 4 measurements and examinations of general motricity and 3 tests, each of them with 5 indicators, which should evidentiate the level of coordinative aptitudes specific to volleyball.
- A number of 16 beginners from S.S.C. Buftea were chosen as a sample of experiment, whose somatic and motric potential is compared with that of the value sample on national level and with that of the check sample S.S.C. 39.
- The experimental activity took place between September 2010 – August 2011, including an interval of 400 hours, shared in 230 trainings.
- According to the goals and the instructive content recommended by the specialised institutions, the experiment focused on structuring this content within some operational training programmes in which to integrate the goals of the coordinative aptitudes development, expected on the experimental check.

In order to influence the constitutive components of skill by involving in the game actions of volleyball, various categories of means were conceived, selected and used as action structures, as follows:
For orienting the body in space
- Versions of running associated with releases, pirouettes with various rotation degrees and landings in mentioned positions and areas, followed by other actions requested on-the-spot;
- Actions with balls of various sizes and weights (catch, pass, lead, hit, throw, etc.) associated to preceding or mixed movements (jumpings, turnovers, shifts, rollings);
- Simultaneous actions of body segments (arms, body, legs) associated to different versions of moving (specified fixed points, reduced areas, marked itineraries, restricted areas, obstacles).
For coordinating the movements
- Versions of moving with running, jumping, dancing steps etc.and the association of symmetric-non-symmetric arm movements;
- Executions "in mirror" and opposite to the received orders with action in plans, speeds, various and unknown rythms;
- Versions of jumpings with associating various movements and actions requested instantaneously during releases, flights or landings;
- Movements of arms, body and legs in various plans and rythms, with and without objects and changes on signals.

For analytical motricity

- Juggles with balls of different dimensions accomplished with arms, legs or body parts, staying or moving;
- Various sequels of game actions, mixed and associated, performed with segments or their portions;
- Sport games with changing the procedures of acting on the ball and the set of rules;
- Contests and adapted dynamic games, with combined performing of hitting, leading, saving, transport, with balls and different objects, involving all body segments.

For skill improving in the conditions of other existing motric qualities

- Sprints with starts in various poses and the association of preceding or ulterior actions;
- Ball performing simultaneously with actions for the other members (jumpings, genuflections, shifts, dribling, etc.)
- Adapted dynamic or sport games (tig with change of roles, challenging partners, cock fight, sitting football, basketball, handball with passing the ball with volleyball procedures, etc.).

Conclusions

The comparative value of the progress achieved after the experiment with the sample on which the content and the methodology regarding the development of skill components were applied, underlines the value superiority and their practical efficiency, reflected and evidentiated both by the higher level of development of the other motric qualities, and the one of appropriating the technical component of the game actions, comparing to the ones recorded by the check sample. The superiority of the final increases achieved at every test and especially the dimension of the progress marked between the initial test and the final one, constitute the most objective argument for the efficiency of the methodology used by the experimental sample, thus confirming the validity of the study hypothesis.

References

1.Zatiorschi, V. M., (1968), Calităţile fizice ale sportivului, CNEFS, Bucureşti
2.Lăzărescu D., (2006),Conţinutul instruirii voleivalistice îb unităţile de profil, Buletin Informativ, Nr.332, F.R.V., pag. 82 – 103

3.Epuran M, (2005), Metodologia Cercetarii Activitatilor Corporale, Editura FEST, pag.367
4.Firea E., (1984), Metodica educatiei fizice, Editura Sport Turism, Bucureşti, pag.65

TABLE NO.1 – THE QUANTIFICATION OF THE TRAINING COMPONENTS AT THE LEVEL OF THE LEVEL OF 1ST YEAR BEGINNERS

TRAINING YEAR / THE VALUE LEVEL OF GROUPS		BEGINNERS YEAR I	
OBJECTIVES	OF SELECTION	ACHIEVEMENT = 65%	
	OF PERFORMANCE	Participation in local competitions - reduced game 4:4	
THE DISTRIBUTION OF THE VOLUME IN TRAINING COMPONENTS	OFICIAL	340 hours = 85%	400 hours
	COMPLEMENTARY	60 hours = 15%	
COMPONENT	PHYSICAL		150 hours = 40%
	TECHNICAL-STRATEGICAL		220 hours = 55%
	THEORETICAL		20 hours = 5%
TECHNICAL-STRATEGICAL COMPONENT			220 hours = 55%
TECHNICAL-STRATEGICAL INDIVIDUAL ACTIONS	Global practice	35%	80 hours = 20%
	Analytical practice	140 hours	60 hours = 15%
COLLECTIVE STRATEGICAL ACTIONS	Sit.I - Personal service	5%	8 hours = 2%
	Sit.II - Opponent service	20 hours	12 hours = 3%
	SCHOOL (HOMEWORK)	15%, 60 hours	40 hours = 10%
INTEGRAL GAME	CHECK		20 hours = 5%
	OFFICIAL		
PHYSICAL COMPONENT	%		160 hours = 40%
Morfo-functional indexes			20 hours = 5%
Major importance segments			20 hours = 5%
Skills and aptitudes			40 hours = 10%
Metric qualities		V=80%, I=8%, F=2%, R=2%, TOTAL = 20% = 40 hours	20 hours = 5%
THEORETICAL COMPONENT			

QUALITY INDICATORS FOR GAME ACTIONS	TOTAL	TECH. ANALYTIC	TECH.-STRAT. GLOBAL	STRAT. GAME
SERVICE	33 hours = 15%	10 hours=30%	16 hours=50%	7 hours = 20%
SERVICE TAKE OVER	22 hours = 10%	5 hours = 25%	15 hours=70%	2 hours = 5%
RISING	120 hours=55%	18 hours=15%	96 hours=80%	6 hours = 5%
ATTACK	33 hours = 15%	10 hours=30%	23 hours=70%	.
BLOCKAGE				.
ATTACK TAKE OVER	12 hours = 5%	4 hours = 25%	7 hours = 70%	1 hours = 5%

OBJECTIVES

SELECTION:
- Constituting the groups after the morfo-functional and psychic criterion in a percentage over 70%.

PERFORMANCE:
- Participation at local competitions with stable teams 3:3 and 4:4, on reduced field, with a selection objective.

GAME ENSEMBLE:
- Learning the reduced game with taking over line-ups in 2 and 3 players and passing the ball over the net with 3 hits.

INDIVIDUAL TECHNICAL-STRATEGICAL ACTIONS:
- The consolidation of the dominant aspect from the technical component of TAKING OVER WITH TWO HANDS UPWARDS.

PHYSICAL COMPONENT:
- Developing the motric qualities Speed and Skill;
- Invigorating the extensors;
- Compensating defective attitudes.

NEW TECHNICAL-STRATEGICAL ACTIONS:
- Consolidating taking over actions with two hands upwards; service and taking over service with two hands upwards.

STRATEGICAL ACTIONS IN DEFENCE:
- Taking over from service and from game with two players and orientation to the right with medium-high trajectories.

PSYCHOLOGICAL COMPONENT:
- Educating love for game, wish for self-overtaking and team and competitiveness spirit.

INDIVIDUALIZATION:
- Depending on individual features open small value groups will be opened in a differentiated work.

STRATEGICAL ACTIONS IN ATTACK:
- Learning line-ups with 2 and 3 players at taking over and organising passing the ball over the net with 3 hits.

THEORETICAL TRAINING:
- Knowing the rules of the game with reduced field and number of players and evaluating the incorrect play of taking over (DOUBLE; HELD; LED).

COMPONENTS OF INSTRUCTIVE MODEL			MONTH: SEPT. OCT. NOV. DEC. JAN. FEB. MAR. APR. MAY JUNE JULY AUG. — WEEK 1.2.3.4.5.6.7.8.9.10.11.12.13.14.15.16.17.18.19.20.21.22.23.24.25.26.27.28.29.30.31.32.33.34.35.36.37.38.39
GAME ENSEMBLE 60 ore = 15%	SCHOOL (HOMEWORK)	10%=6h	22h
	CHECK	5%=3h	18h
STRATEGICAL COMPONENT 20 hours = 5%	Personal Service Situation	2%=1h	5h
	Opponent Service Situation	3%=1h	9h
INDIVIDUAL TECHNICAL STRATEGICAL ACTIONS 140 hours = 35%	SERVICE	15%=33h	1000
	SERVICE TAKE OVER	10%=22h	1000
	RISING	55%=120h	12000
	ATTACK	5%=33h	3300
	ATTACK TAKE OVER	5%=12h	2000
	BLOCKAGE	-	-
PHYSICAL COMPONENT 160 hours = 40%	MORFO-FUNCTIONAL	5%=8h	26h
	IMPORTANT SEGM.	5%=8h	26h
	SKILLS AND APTITUDE	10%=16h	53h
	MOTRIC QUALITIES	10%=16h	53h

TABLE NO. 2 – THE PROGRESS RECORDED AT TESTING THE GENERAL MOTRICITY OF THE EXPERIMENTAL GROUP

TESTS	1	2	3	4	5	6	7	8	9	10	11	12	13	14	15	16	17
GROUP INITIAL EXPERIMENT	18,62	9,95	10,72	11,93	7,56	23,2	32,4	15,29	8,78	4,33	155,06	24,13	19	13	15,53	33	34
INTERMEDIATE	17,76	9,59	10,36	14,73	8,24	25,46	34,86	16,2	8,41	4,27	161	28,4	23,06	17,8	18,66	36,2	24,46
INTERMEDIATE INCREASE YEAR I	0,86	0,36	0,36	2,8	0,68	2,26	2,46	0,91	0,37	0,06	5,94	4,27	4,06	4,8	3,13	3,2	9,54
END YEAR I	17,28	9,22	9,70	18,26	8,90	30,86	36,33	17,52	8,09	3,43	172,53	33,66	25,33	22,53	24,26	38,86	10,46
INCREASE YEAR I	0,48	0,37	0,66	3,53	0,66	5,4	1,47	1,32	0,32	0,84	11,53	5,26	2,27	4,73	5,6	2,66	14
TOTAL INCREASE	1,34	0,73	1,02	6,33	1,34	7,66	3,93	2,23	0,69	0,9	17,47	9,53	6,33	9,53	8,73	5,86	23,54

TESTS:

1	COMBINED TEST	7	BALANCE SHIFT
2	JAG RUNNING	8	SHIFT REACTION 5"
3	SHUTTLE SHIFT	9	SPEED RUNNING
4	SUPPORT PASSING	10	RESISTANCE RUNNING
5	VOLLEYBALL THROW	11	BROAD JUMP ON SPOT
6	PUSH-PULL PASSING	12	BODY RAISING
13	BACK EXTENSIONS		
14	ARM CHIN-UPS		
15	ROUNDERS BALL TOSSING		
16	HIGH JUMP		
17	THE MATORIN TEST		

GENERAL MOTRICITY TESTS – THE EXPERIMENT GROUP – CHART

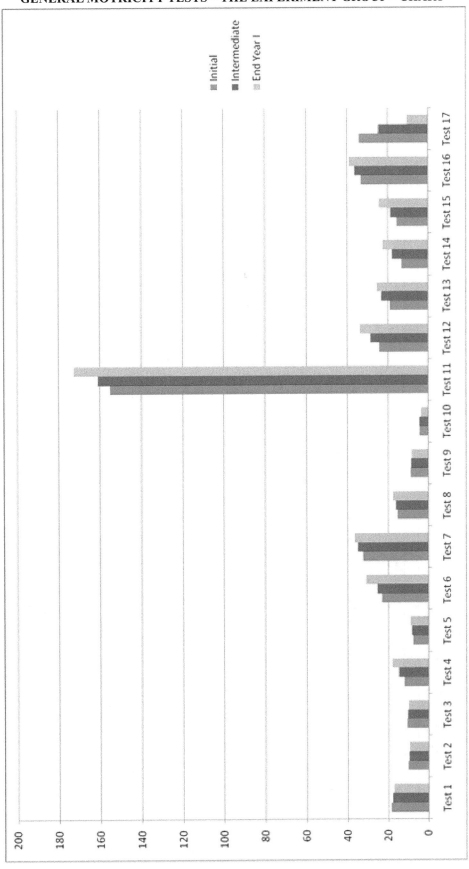

TABLE NO. 3 – THE PROGRESS RECORDED AT TESTING SPECIFIC APTITUDES AT THE EXPERIMENTAL SAMPLE

CONTINUOUS SELF-TAKING OVER																		
	TOTAL NO. OF HITS			TOTAL NO. OF CYCLES			NO. CYCLES 5-15 HITS			NO. CYCLES OVER 15 HITS			MAXIMUM NO. OF HITS/ CYCLE			EFFECTIVE TIME		
	1			2			3			4			5			6		
MED.	40,93	49,06	65,73	3,66	1,6	1,86	1,33	0,33	0,4	0,6	1	1,46	25,06	43,2	51,8	24,6	29,2	53,66
M	42	48	68	4	1	2	1	0	0	1	1	1	21	45	56	23	30	54
MOD.	43	48	68	4	1	2	2	0	0	1	1	1	21	45	60	22	30	60
AS	10,152	6,850	8,480	1,543	0,828	0,639	0,899	0,487	0,507	0,507	0,377	0,516	14,488	11,117	16,275	4,339	1,373	5,407
D	96,19	43,79	67,12	2,22	0,64	0,38	0,75	0,22	0,24	0,24	0,13	0,24	195,90	115,36	247,22	17,57	1,76	27,28
CV	6,66 %	6,66 %	6,66 %	6,65 %	6,66 %	6,62 %	6,61 %	6,59 %	6,66 %	6,66 %	6,5 %	6,42 %	6,66 %	6,66 %	6,66 %	6,66 %	6,66 %	6,66 %
TAKING OVER REBOUNDING BALL																		
	TOTAL NO. OF HITS			TOTAL NO. OF CYCLES			CYCLE NO. 5-15 HITS			CYCLE NO. OVER 15 HITS			MAXIMUM NO. OF HITS/ CYCLE			EFFECTIVE TIME		
	1			2			3			4			5			6		
MED.	33,33	46,4	60,13	3,73	1,6	1,6	1,33	0,86	0,4	0,66	1,26	1,26	19	41,06	50,53	19,93	24,46	28,13
M	33	46	60	3	1	2	1	0	0	1	1	1	17	44	50	20	24	28
MOD.	33	46	58	3	1	2	1	0	0	1	1	1	16	52	50	21	24	28
AS	5,498	7,208	5,208	1,624	0,910	0,507	1,046	1,407	0,507	0,487	0,457	0,457	9,710	11,615	9,859	1,533	1,995	1,552
D	28,22	46,50	25,31	2,46	0,77	0,24	1,02	1,84	0,24	0,22	0,19	0,19	88	125,92	90,72	2,19	3,71	2,24
CV	6,66 %	6,66 %	6,66 %	6,66 %	6,63 %	6,66 %	6,65 %	6,63 %	6,66 %	6,59 %	6,47 %	6,47 %	6,66 %	6,66 %	6,66 %	6,64 %	6,65 %	6,64 %
TAKING OVER THE NET																		
	TOTAL NO. OF HITS			TOTAL NO. OF CYCLES			CYCLE NO. 5-15 HITS			CYCLE NO. OVER 15 HITS			MAXIMUM NO. OF HITS/ CYCLE			EFFECTIVE TIME		
	1			2			3			4			5			6		
MED.	30,87	46,25	65	5,25	2	1,87	1,62	0,62	0,37	0,25	1,25	1,5	9,75	34,25	50,75	51,5	55,25	57,25
M	30	46	66	5	2	2	2	1	0	0	1	1	9	34	48	52	56	57
MOD.	30	48	66	6	2	2	2	1	0	0	1	1	9	38	48	52	56	57
AS	3,514	2,872	4,780	0,906	0,654	0,750	0,365	0,365	0,365	0,327	0,327	0,377	1,636	6,576	11,709	0,755	1,721	1,451
D	11,52	7,69	21,33	0,76	0,4	0,52	0,12	0,12	0,12	0,1	0,1	0,13	2,5	40,36	127,96	0,53	2,76	1,96
CV	6,66 %	6,65 %	6,66 %	6,60 %	6,66 %	6,60 %	6,39 %	6,39 %	6,39 %	6,66 %	6,66 %	6,5 %	6,66 %	6,66 %	6,66 %	6,62 %	6,65 %	6,64 %

46

Aspects of the rehabilitation management of the spastic upper limb for the child with cerebral palsy

Stănoiu Cosmina[1], Zăvăleanu Mihaela[2], Roșulescu Eugenia[2],

1. Children Residential Rehabilitation Center DGASPC Craiova
2. Faculty of Physical Education and Sports, University of Craiova, Romania

Abstract. Our article is based on two parts; one is the therapy for the spastic upper limb from cerebral palsy area presented by the clinicians. The other part presents the importance of evaluation, with the recommendations equally for clinicians and research from child cerebral palsy a neuromotor development area. For such a broad clinical signs and syndromes, the clinicians need to have a proper value of their works after applying the treatment; this value is given by a proper evaluation that can underline the positives effect, prognosis of complex therapy on subject's status.
Key words: *cerebral palsy, rehabilitation, spasticity, scales evaluation, management*

Introduction

Cerebral palsy (CP) **is** the most common cause of severe physical disability in children [1], approximately 80% of the children who are treated in our clinic present involvement of the upper spastic extremities. In our study, the extent of upper extremity involvement varies from mild clumsiness in fine motor control to fixed muscle contractures that limit active extension of the elbow, wrist or fingers, and supination of the forearm.

Cerebral palsy patients with upper limb involvement have difficulty in performing coordinated movements against spasticity [2] that is also the most important fact that we discover after the evaluation of our patients. Performances of hand tasks in these patients require gross and fine hand motion coordinated with visual perception and postural control to enable them to complete all the functionalities of the hand an upper limb: reach, grasp, release and manipulate objects. The management of the upper limb in CP is complex and new therapeutic approaches are continuously being developed for the management of variety impairment in individuals with CP [3]. Recent published works on cerebral palsy were focused on the management of upper extremity deformity and spasticity [4, 5].

The available symptomatic therapeutic options place cerebral palsy among the costliest chronic childhood conditions. [6] . The options for managing upper limb dysfunction in children with CP are varied and the goals of management must be individualized for each child and are usually determined by the severity and extent of CP involvement [7]. A multimodal rehabilitation team foremost *aim* is always the prevention of disability by diminishing the effects of impairments, preventing secondary and tertiary effects of the disability and maximizing motor function throughout the CP subject life. The *focus* of treatment can shifts over the years because many reasons (the child age or needs, clinical evolution) but the principles remain the same: to prevent contractures of the involved side, to strengthen the weak muscles, to enable functional use of the upper extremity and to establish the learning of a better functional pattern. Over the years, therapists have tried to implement a great variety of treatment interventions with different theoretical bases; they have studied their effects and benefices in elaborated studies.

Treatment of children with CP requires a long-term process during growth by a multidisciplinary team, focusing on all developmental aspects of the child and planning interventions in relation to the most urgent needs of the child and the family. [8] Currently there is no specific treatment for the brain insults leading to motor dysfunction in cerebral palsy. [6] The long-term goal is the optimal functioning in adulthood. [9]

Method of therapy for the spastic upper limb - tool description

Neurodevelopmental Treatment (NDT) is one of the best known and applied from all interventions addressing the movement and posture of children with CP since 1940 when it was invented and applied by the Bobath spouses. Their idea for the therapeutic Bobath Method were to promote the use of handling techniques to inhibit abnormal tone and primitive reflexes and to facilitate normal movement [10] in order that the child, even if we talk about CP, he should experience the normal movement. These tonic reflexes, such as the tonic labyrinthine reflex, symmetrical tonic neck reflexes and asymmetrical tonic neck reflexes, have to be inhibited. The theory is that if the body is prepared through aligning the joints, normalizing tone in the muscles, and facilitating stability then optimal performance can occur and atypical activity can be avoided by establishing more normal movement patterns [11]

There is controversy about whether the principles of NDT treatment influenced initially by the reflex and hierarchical models of motor control are still valid in light of current models which do not focus exclusively on neural explanations of motor performance.[12]

Constraint induced movement therapy known like **CIMT** or **CI** has been receiving increasing attention in pediatric rehabilitation [13]. Because many research studies have indicated the effectiveness of this intervention with adults post stroke in improving upper extremity function [14] constraint induced movement therapy (CIMT) [15] is a promising approach for rehabilitation of the upper limb in hemiparetic type of CP. Based on the already demonstrate fact that brain can reorganize itself after the damage of the motor area for example, Charles underline in her article [13] that so far, the evidence suggests that practice associated with CI therapy may improve impaired unimanual hand function in some children with hemiplegic CP.

The two CIMT treatment principles are: (1) extensive affected upper-limb training, and (2) constraining the unaffected limb. The movements are made in a certain pattern, which helps to the brain reorganization. The intervention encourages brain reorganization to increase its motor capacities [16] and the cortical space devoted to the affected upper limb [17].

Is based on a theory proposed by E. Taub [18] who notes that individual with upper limb motor dysfunction learns to depend increasingly unaffected member for usual activities, whereas the use of affected often cause failure and frustration. A randomized controlled trial found that CIMT therapy seems to be effective in improving the efficient movement of the affected limb, and another study of 4 patients with stroke showed induction of cortical reorganization measured by MRI. [19]

Sensory integration therapy refers both to a theory proposed by A. Jean Ayres in the 70s. to the neurological process that allows the individual to take, analyse, integrate and use spatial and temporal aspects of sensory information from the body and from the environment in order to plan an organized his motor behaviour. Ayres explored the association between sensory processing and the behavior of children with learning, developmental, emotional, and other disabilities in scientific journals and later in her groundbreaking book, *Sensory Integration and Learning Disorders* [20]. Some children with cerebral palsy may have dysfunction in sensorimotor integration field because of the absence of normal motor control. PCI employs occupational therapists child in activities such as climbing, ball games, puzzle games and more growing body sensory stimuli by sensitizing stimuli vestibular system, superficial and deep sensitivity and fine motor skills [21].

The Hare method was develop and used with the aims to exercise the trunk and central core of the body in order to establish a viable base for the primary positions of lying, sitting, and standing. The approach is applicable for all ages [22], the balance and maintaining the postures being like we already know important issues for the cerebral palsy patient. Treatment techniques aim to develop the pattern to control movement of the trunk by the use of arm and legs, below-knee plaster boots, aids and adapted furniture. [22] Treatment techniques aim to encourage a child's ability to control movement of the trunk by the use of arm and leg gaiters, below-knee plaster boots, aids and adapted furniture.

Cognitive approach. Cognitive or learning approaches is a combined educational and therapeutic task-oriented approach for children with CP as a method with focus on learning control of movement for function rather than emphasizing quality of movement. Motor learning or training programs use task analysis to breakdown functional tasks into basic motor components or patterns. These components are then practised and learned as a motor skill for functional use [23]. The tasks are the activities of daily living, motor skills

including hand function, balance and locomotion.

Conductive education (CE) or the Peto method is a type of cognitive approach which utilizes rhythm, music and counting to initiate and moderate movements [24]. A study comparing individual PT or OT with CE, showed that CE improved coordinative hand functions and activities of daily living. [25]

Strength training. In PC management, increasing muscle strength by the rehabilitation technics has been controversial because in theory it would increase muscle tone and abnormal movements. While spasticity was once thought to be the primary contributor to the motor dysfunction noted in CP, many have challenged this perspective and now consider _negative' signs such as muscle weakness to be more harmful to function.[26] Several studies conducted by Damiano showed clear benefits of exercise to enhance muscle strength [27]. American Physical Therapy Association (APTA) published in 2007 recommendations regarding strength training in children with PC arguing that should be an important component of the rehabilitation program [28]. Children with CP also appear to gain strength at the same rate as persons with weakness who have no CNS pathology in programs of similar intensity and duration. [27] It has been shown that even highly functional children with spastic CP are likely to have considerable weakness in their involved extremities compared to age-related peers, with the degree of weakness increasing with the level of neurologic involvement [29]. To participate in a strength-training program, the child must be able to comprehend and to consistently produce a maximal or near-maximal effort.

Orthotic therapy. Orthoses are based upon two widely used approaches for the spasticity managements: the biomechanical approach, which aims to prevent deformity by aligning, mobilizing and stabilizing joints, and the neurophysiological approach, which aims to reduce spasticity by sustained stretch and reflex-inhibiting positions [30, 31]. The most common use of upper extremity orthotics is in children with quadriplegic pattern involvement who develop significant wrist and elbow flexion contractures. The exact amount of time an orthotic should be worn in order to be beneficial is unknown, but 4 to 8 hours of brace wear a day are probably required [32].

Serial casting in spastic upper extremity is based on the premise that shortened muscles maintain the plasticity for lengthening. Yasukawa et al [33] examined the use of serial casting to obtain gains of 15-20° in passive range, followed by the use of a custom orthosis. In all six subjects the serial casting was successful in gaining the required passive range, however maintaining range using the orthosis was dependent on wearing compliance. The conclusion of a review led by Autti-Ramo and colleagues [34] including articles on children and adults with brain injury is that the devices improve upper extremity, diminishes the amplitude of movement and muscle tone. The effect on quality of arm movement and the hand function remains unclear, although there is the suggestion that short term increases the quality movement [34].

Electrostimulation is usually used for more than 50 years in medicine, with multiple applications, from heart disease to treat certain complex treatments in neurology. Is a treatment option proposed regimen of PCI is less invasive technique compared with neuro-pharmacological agents or surgery, providing better clinical outcomes in studies. The goal is to stimulate trophicity of stimulation and muscle strength, and is believed to work by increasing blood flow and muscle mass. [35] The stimulus is often applied to the antagonist of the spastic muscle on the grounds that this will decrease spasticity by reciprocal inhibition. Medical research concerning the electrostimulation use and this method beneficence in PCI is dominated by case studies or uncontrolled not standardized studies. The evidence in children is still controversial and poor, especially for Carmick's studies [15], but there is increasing interest in this therapy option.There is a wide variety of devices and a bewildering range of regimes for pulse frequency, duration, and stimulus intensity. However optimistic results of these studies demonstrate reasons to support electro therapeutic value.

Evaluation of Therapy

After Minear, in 1956, Cerebral palsy comprises the motor and other symptom complexes caused by a non-progressive brain lesion (or lesions).[36] and then he also said that is a general lack of agreement on the various terms used in cerebral palsy. With that he underline in his article some need, for the point of view of pioneer therapist and researcher not having yet all the evaluation and assessment possibilities existing today. After our opinion the importance and the development of multiples evaluation technics available today help to the understanding, classification and finding new principles and methods of therapy in cerebral palsy and neuro-motor development area.

Evaluation of a child with cerebral palsy requires a multidisciplinary approach [37] The assessment is necessary to confirm the diagnosis, determine the cause, assess the motor function and associated problems. [37] The evaluation of a child with CP is an ongoing process and should be a part of continuing care as the child grows from infancy to adolescence [37]

Once the treatment is completed, it should be critically evaluated to improve the outcome and plan for future treatment. Any therapy, whether complementary or allopathic, should be evaluated in terms of its effects on targeted body functions and structures, activities, and participation [38].

In practice, the positive score of the therapy and clinical status evaluation from the beginning and then periodically is the only way to prove that the rehabilitation team and the patient are doing what is necessary and are going in a desired direction. A good evaluation process, offer time and concrete data referring to the cerebral palsy child status. One CP case is not affected in the same way that the next one, the evaluation instrument can be used for systematic evaluation of the needs of the children and parents, the total development and evaluation of the goals of rehabilitation on the level of activities [8], the patterns of movement are discussed by many therapist before and after therapy.

Result of therapy must be evaluated in order to demonstrate the clinical status and other characteristic of life of the child/adolescent/adult person with CP and also the effective efficacy of all methods of rehabilitation the evolution, to come across the needs of children with neuromotor delays.

In order to do these, in our rehabilitation clinics we use some scales that can meet our purposes. Our purposes, like clinicians in the face of the child with cerebral palsy or with neuro-motor development are:

- *evaluation of the clinical facts that are presented for any case for an early diagnosis*
- *periodic surveillance of the clinical status or therapy effects*
- *revising of diagnosis, in case of neuro-motor disabilities that can change after*
- *evaluation of accompanying problems of CP and neuro-motor disabilities*
- *proper differential diagnosis with other diseases.*

Development of a treatment plan begins with the definition of objections and consideration of the effects of growth and development on the patient's abilities. [39]

Centres of Excellence for cerebral palsy at Gillette [www.gillettechildrens.org] propose a classification of CP effects in three area: primary, secondary and tertiary, that shape in a certain way the body and his functions. This classification can help the clinician understand the all the situation of CP child, can make easier the clinical approach.

Table 1. Main principals form of cerebral palsy by localization of the lesion to the brain

		MAIN PRINCIPALS FORM OF CEREBRAL PALSY		
Primary Effects ↓	Varying degrees of injury/damage of the central nervous system ↳ *slightly affected or* ↳ *severely disabled*	**Spastic CP**	**Athetoid CP**	**Ataxic CP**
		Lesion of different area of central cortex	Lesion of basal ganglia	Lesion of cerebelum
Secondary Effects ↓	Inadequate Muscle Growth Malformed/rotated bones and joints	- spasticity muscle tone being hypertonia - decreased range of movement - difficulties with speech or continence	- uncontrolled, involuntary, sustained or intermittent muscle contractions - tone of the muscle can change from hypotonia to tight with slow,	- affects the whole body - difficult to balance - poor spatial awareness - can walk, probably with unsteady, shaky movements - speech/language can

			rhythmic twisting movements.	be affected
Tertiary Effects	Stiff knees Use more energy and tire more easily	**Coping response to primary and secondary effect** ↳ When medical treatment reduces the severity of cerebral palsy's primary and secondary effects,		

A careful physical examination and analysis of the postural deformities and functional deficits follows. Varieties of scales are used to assess the functional status of patients with CP. We use in our practice few evaluation scales like:

- Manual Ability Classification System for children with cerebral palsy 4-18 years – MACS [40], designed to highlight the importance of hand function for independences in daily life, from 2012 available also in romanian at http://www.macs.nu/files/MACS_Roman_2010.pdf

- Gross Motor Function Classification System (GMFCS) is a 5 level classification instrument for early classification the severity of the motor disorder [41] the translation in romanian is available at http://motorgrowth.canchild.ca/en/GMFCS/resources/GMFCS_Romanian.pdf

Emphasis is on usual **performance** in home, school, and community settings (i.e., what they do), rather than what they are known to be able to do at their best (capability). It is therefore important to classify current performance in gross motor function and not to include judgments about the quality of movement or prognosis for improvement. [41]

Discussions

Tests of motor development should be selected carefully to meet the needs of each child. [42] A functional analysis of simple motor skills may yield more information regarding a child's level of neuromotor development, particularly as it relates to treatment planning. [43] From our point of view, is important to apply other scales, more comprehensive and more detailed, that can also evaluate the secondary or tertiary effects of the disease and also of therapy.

The availability of validated new scales in the native language may permit to the clinicians to better understand what are the effects of the work with the CP subject, sometimes to meet his needs and resources also. We start to use, a new scale, SED-PCI [44], with an easy design, in order to compare the result from already mentioned validated scale. Using his scale, our purpose was to cultivate a good developmental screening and monitoring for the child with neuro-motor development problems in order to enhance the early intervention therapy and management.

New instrument adapt easily to evaluation program needs that are culturally sensitive in a particular region and ethnic group, and are intended to be useful in community-based programs which usually have limited resources and depend on the efforts of parents and personnel who have little formal training. [44]

Conclusions

The article is based on two parts. The first part present different therapy modalities used in the rehabilitation of spastic upper limb from cerebral palsy area presented by the clinicians. The other part presents the importance of evaluation, with the recommendations equally for clinicians and research from child cerebral palsy and neuromotor development area.

For such a broad clinical signs and syndromes, like those presented to CP subject, the clinicians need to have a proper value of their works after applying a treatment; this value is given by a proper evaluation that can underline the positives effect, prognosis of complex therapy on subject's status.

Acknowledgements. This work was supported by the strategic grant POSDR/89/1.5/S/61968, Project ID 61968 (2009), co-financed by the European Social Fund within the Sectorial Operational Program Human Resources Development 2007-2013

References
1. Ryan M. McAdams, Sandra E. Juul (2011) Cerebral Palsy: Prevalence, Predictability, and Parental Counseling, *Neoreviews*;12;e564, http://neoreviews.aappublications.org/content/12/10/e564,
2. Flett PJ (2003) Rehabilitation of spasticity and related problems in childhood cerebral palsy. *J Paediatr Child Health*, 39:6-14
3. Patrick JH, Roberts AP, Cole GF. (2001) Therapeutic choices in the locomotormanagement of the child with cerebral palsy-more luck than judgment? Arch Dis Child; 85: 275–279.
4. House JH, Gwathmey FW, Fidler MO: A dynamic approach to the thumb-in-palm deformity in cerebral palsy. *J Bone Joint Surg* 1981, 63(2):216-25.
5. Van Heest E, House H: Upper extremity surgical treatment of cerebral palsy. *J Hand Surg* 1999, 24A(2):323-330.
6. Papavasiliou A.S., (2009) Management of motor problems in cerebral palsy: A critical update for the clinician, European Journal of Paediatric Neurology Volume 13, Issue 5, September, Pages 387–396
7. Peter Rosenbaum (2003) Cerebral palsy: what parents and doctors want to know, *BMJ*;326:970–4
8. Becher, J. G., (2002) Pediatric Rehabilitation in Children with Cerebral Palsy: General Management, Classification of Motor Disorders JPO Journal of Prosthetics & Orthotics Volume 14, Issue 4, p 143: 149
9. van der Dussen DL, Nieuwstraten W, Roebroeck M, Stam HJ. (2001) Functional level of young adults with cerebral palsy. *Clin Rehabil.*;15:84-91
10. Bobath K; Bobath B. (1984) The neurodevelopmental treatment In: Scrotton D, ed. Management of the motor disorders of children with cerebral palsy. Oxford: Blackwell Scientific Publications Ltd;
11. Kramer, P., & Hinojosa, J. (2010). *Frames of Reference for Pediatric Occupational Therapy.* (3rd ed.). Philadelphia: Wolters Kluwer/Lippincott Williams & Wilkins
12. Boyd RN, Morris ME, Graham HK. Management of upper limb dysfunction in children with cerebral palsy: a systematic review. *Eur J Neurol.* 2001;8(suppl 5):150-166
13. Charles J., A. M Gordon (2006) Development of hand–arm bimanual intensive training (HABIT) for improving bimanual coordination in children with

hemiplegic cerebral palsy Developmental Medicine & Child Neurology , Volume 48, Issue 11, November, pp 931-936

14. Levine, P., & Page, S. J. (2004). Modified constraint-induced therapy: A promising restorative outpatient therapy. *Topics in Stroke Rehabilitation, 11,* 1-10.

15. Siebes, R.e., Wijnroks, L. & Vermeer, A. (2002) Qualitative analysis of therapeutic motor intervention programmes for children with cerebral palsy: an update. *Dev. Med. Child Neurol.,* 44, 593-603.

16. Kim, Y.H., Park, J.W., Ko, M.H., Jang, S.H., Lee, P.K. (2004) . Plastic changes of motor network after constraint-induced movement therapy Yonsei Med J , 45 (2) , 241 – 246

17. Liepert, J., Bauder, H., Wolfgang, H.R., Miltner, W.H., Taub, E., Weiller C. (2000). Treatment-induced cortical reorganization after stroke in humans . Stroke , 31 (6) , 1210 – 1216 .

18. Taub, E., Uswatte, G., King , D.K., Morris, D., Crago, J.E., and Chatterjee, A. (2006) . A placebo controlled trial of constraint-induced movement therapy for upper extremity after stroke . Stroke , 37 (4) , 1045 – 1049 .

19. Jerzy P Szaflarski, Stephen J. Page, Brett M. Kissela, Jing-Huei Lee, Peter Levine and Stephen M. Strakowski: (2006) Cortical Reorganization Following Modified Constraint-Induced Movement Therapy: A Study of 4 Patients with Chronic Stroke, Archives of physical medicine and rehabilitation, volume 87, issue 8, 1052-1058.

20. Ayres, A. J. (1972). *Sensory integration and learning disorders.* Los Angeles: Western Psychological Services.

21. Schaaf R, Miller LJ. (2005) Occupational therapy using a sensory integrative approach for children with developmental disabilities. Mental Retardation and Developmental Disabilities Research Reviews; 11: 143-148.

22. Hare NS, Durham S, Green EM, 1998, The cerebral palsies and motor learning disorders In : Stokes M(ed), Neurological Physiotherapy London : Mosby, P 320

23. Shepherd RB. (1995) Physiotherapy in paediatrics. 3rd ed. Oxford: Butterworth Heinemann;.

24. Reddihough DS, King J, Coleman G, Catanese T. (1998) Efficiency of programs based on conductive education for young children with cerebral palsy. Dev Med Child Neurol; 40:763–770

25. Blank R, von Kries R, Hesse S, von Voss H. (2008) Conductive education for children with cerebral palsy: effects on hand motor functions relevant to activities of daily living. Arch Phys Med Rehabil;89(2):251–9.

26. Sahrmann SA, Norton BJ. (1977) The relationship of voluntary movement to spasticity in the upper motor neuron syndrome. *Annals of Neurology* 2: 460–5.

27. Damiano DL, Vaughan CL, Abel MF. (1995) Muscle response to heavy resistance exercise in children with spastic cerebral palsy. Dev Med Child Neurol; 37:731–9.

28. Boyd, R. N., Morris, M. E., & Graham, H. K. (2001). Management of upper limb dysfunction in children with cerebral palsy: a systematic review. *European Journal of Neurology, 8,* 150-166.

29. Wiley ME, Damiano DL. (1998) Lower-extremity strength profiles in spastic cerebral palsy. Dev Med Child Neurol;40:100–7

30 Wilton JC. (1997) Hand Splinting: Principles of Design and Fabrication. London: WB Saunders.

31. Hogan L, Uditsky T. (1998) Pediatric Splinting: Selection, Fabrication and Clinical Application of Upper Extremity Splints. San Antonio, Texas: The Psychological Corporation.

32. Tyson SF, Kent RM. (2011) The effect of upper limb orthotics after stroke: a systematic review. *NeuroRehabilitation.*;28(1):29-36.

33. Yasukawa A., Lulinski J., Thornton L., & Jaudes P. (2008). Improving elbow and wrist range of motion using a dynamic and static combination of orthosis. *Journal of Prosthetics & Orthotics*, 20: 41-48.

34. Autti-Rämö, I., Suoranta, J., Anttila, H., Malmivaara, A, & Mäkelä, M. (2006). Effectiveness of upper and lower limb casting and orthoses in children with cerebral palsy: An overview of review articles. *American Journal of Physical Medicine & Rehabilitation*, 85:89-103.

35. Kamper DG, Yasukawa AM, Barrett KM, Gaebler-Spira DJ. Effects of neuromuscular electrical stimulation treatment of cerebral palsy on potential impairment mechanisms: a pilot study. Pediatr Phys Ther 2006; 18: 31–8.

36. Minear W. L. (1956) Special Article : A Classification Of Cerebral Palsy, Pediatrics Vol. 18 No. 5 November 1, pp. 841 -852

37. Aneja S. (2004) Evaluation of a Child with Cerebral Palsy The Indian Journal of Pediatrics, Volume 71, Issue 7, pp 627-634

38. World Health Organization (WHO). International Classification of Functioning, Disability and Health ICF. Geneva, Switzerland: WHO

39. Russman, B. S., Tilton, A. and Gormley, M. E. (1997), Cerebral palsy: A rational approach to a treatment protocol, and the role of botulinum toxin in treatment. Muscle Nerve, 20: 181–193.

40. Eliasson AC, Krumlinde Sundholm L, Rösblad B, Beckung E, Arner M, Öhrvall AM , Rosenbaum P. (2006) The Manual Ability Classification System (MACS) for children with cerebral palsy: scale development and evidence of validity and reliability Developmental Medicine and Child Neurology 48:549-554

41. Palisano, R., Rosenbaum, P., Walter, S., Russell, D., Wood, E., & Galuppi, B. (1997). Development and reliability of a system to classify gross motor function in children with cerebral palsy. *Developmental Medicine & Child Neurology,* 39, 214-223.

42. Montgomery PC (1981)Assessment and Treatment of the Child with Mental Retardation : Guidelines for the Public School Therapist *PHYS THER.*; 61:1265-1272. Downloaded from http://ptjournal.apta.org/

43. Montgomery PC, Richter EW. (1977) Sensorimotor Integration for Developmentally Disabled Children: A Handbook. Los Angeles, CA, Western Psychological Services, pp 1-83

44. Zavaleanu M.; Rosulescu E.; Vasilescu M; Ilinca I; Stanoiu C (2012) Development of a new Motor Development Evaluation Scale for CP diagnosed children (SED-PCI): Phase I-Development of New Items. Sports Medicine Journal Vol. 8 Issue 1, p1784

47

Study concerning the optimization of physical training of junior handball players

Chepea Bogdan[1], Orţănescu Dorina[2], Shaao Mirela[2]

U.N.E.F.S Bucharest[1], University of Craiova[2]

Abstract. In the complex process of optimizing physical training process of handball players, according to the new features of competitive effort from the analysis of elite handball teams play all over the world, there is a particular importance as a starting point to identify concrete strategies (the factual basis necessary to achieve them) and their realization and application.

In this study we followed to obtain information on the importance given to physical training, weight and content - data collected through the questionnaire survey applied to the specialists. The data analysis reflects, in essence, that there is a medium degree of identification between the coordinates of the training of junior handball players in our country compared with those observed in large-scale competitions. Factors that need to be further developed are tactical and physical preparation. So, coaches opt for higher weights assigned to these components in the training, to professional model recommended by the federation. For physical training is reflected in expanding it to 35-40% to 30%. It also assigns an important general physical training, covering all driving skills, their share recommendations ranging from literature: speed (+5%), strength (+10%), power (± 10%), capacity coordination (-10%), intermediate skills (10%). In the means used to solve general physical preparedness objectives, we believe that the share allocated specific funds basic gymnastics is too low, and their choice is made apparent by reference to their Structure of.

Keywords: *handball, physical training, motor skills.*

Introduction

The fact that handball shows a higher development is no longer a novelty. Observation and analysis of elite handball teams constantly confirms this (Hantau, 2000). On top of that, these analyzes is the source of new directions detachment and development trends of modern handball.

Adapting to the new training methodology, seeking solutions for maximizing performance entails simultaneously pursuing game development, adjustment training models, usually based on extensive research (Colibaba-Evulet, 1998).

In this complex process, the challenge is addressed to both researchers and coaches, and begin to analyze existing models, a concrete starting point, then goes on to identify trends and ways to solve new situations that will materialize at some point, the development and implementation of a new training course, which means the drive to be used both to improve the driving ability of the general and specific, will be selected in a pyramidal system with maximum fidelity to the target.

Purpose

This approach is a study on the importance of the place, the weight and content of physical training junior handball training - indicators relevant questionnaire survey results.

Methods

Assessing the current level of physical training and of importance, weight, content, and its evaluation was performed using survey-questionnaire. This was done with support by 36 specialists who responded to our requests. Those interviewed included acting as coaches teams in the National Hockey Championships - Junior II Edition from 2011 to 2012.

The questionnaire included 12 questions and was administered during April-May 2012.

The first question that asks for information on the current level of preparation handball player compared to our country identified in major international competitions, most coaches 22 (61.11%) believe that these coordinates are identified in a proportion of 35 - 50% and 14 (38.89%) of specialists claim that only 50-75% of the landmarks of the two models are identical.

On the positive and negative aspects that motivate previous answer, coaches were asked to indicate "which of the components of the preparation, and to what extent, are responsible for matters relating to the current level of preparation handball player", respectively, at what level is currently preparing components (fig. 1).

In conclusion, for technical training, 19 (52.78%) specialists have found that it is within the range of 75 - 100%, 14 (38.89%) think that this level is in the range 50-75% and 3 (8.33%) specialists consider that the technical level of athletes is in the range 35-50%.

If tactical training, 4 (11.11%) specialists consider that it is at an optimum level in the range of 75 to 100%, 13 (36.11%) coaches appreciate the tactical level are in the range 50-75% and 19 (52.78%) of those interviewed is within the range of 35-50%. Physical training was seen by 3 (8.33%) coaches at a level of 75 to 100% by 12 (33.33%) coaches - between 50 to 75%, and 21 (58.34%) coaches believe that its level is in the range 35-50%. On psychological preparation, 7 (19.44%) coaches believes that its level is in the range 75 to 100%, 16 (44.45%) triggered a fall in the range of 50-75%, while 13 (36.11 %) coaches believes that psychological preparation has achieved its objectives in a proportion of 35-50%. If theoretical training 28 (77.78%) of specialists consider the level is between 75 - 100%, 7 (19.44%) the specific coaches between 50 - 75%, and 1 (2.78%) specialist considers that the theoretical training within the range 35-50%.

In conclusion, most experts believe the main components of training are located at an optimal level theoretical and technical. At a critical level appear to be located tactics and physical training. Regarding weight training components (fig. 2) experts consider optimal following combinations: 40% physical training, 40% technical and 20% tactical - 15 (41.67%) coaches, 35% physical training, 40% training 25% technical and tactical training - 12 (33.33%) coaches and 35% physical training, 35% technical and 30% tactical - 9 (25.00%) coaches.

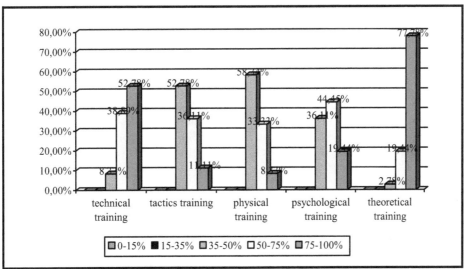

Fig.1. The weight attached to the components of training process

Regarding the share allocated to physical training preparatory period, of a total of 36 coaches, most 21 (58.34%) prefer to provide this type of training 50-75% of the total hours of training and 15 (41.66%) allocate between 35-50%. Regarding the share of physical training during the competitive largest number of

responses 30 (83.33%) was oriented between 15-35% of the total, and 6 (16.67%) of specialists argue that given the physical over 35% of the total hours of training. For the transition period, all specialists opted to range from 0 to 15%.

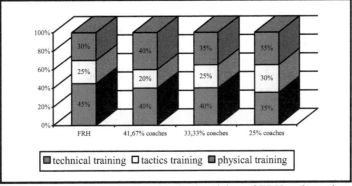

Fig.2. Components of preparation in the vision of FRH and coaches

When asked "Which of the following driving skills, and to what extent, do you think need to be addressed in training junior handball?", 36 (100%) experts have considered speed (with a contribution of 30%) and strength (with a 30%) as primary qualities necessary player. Regarding force 22 (61.11%) of specialists consider that it should represent 20% of all qualities, 9 (25.00%) experts believe that labor representation should be 30%, and 5 (13.89%) specialists consider that 10% is the proportion representative of this quality. For coordinative abilities (found in practice as "skill") responses showed the following distribution: 21 (58.33%) of specialists consider this as required 20%, and 15 (41.67%) specialists - 10 %. Of the total of 36 experts, 15 (41.67%) believe that flexibility is a quality that must be addressed in preparing handball at a rate of 10%. Combinations on motor skills considered essential specialists handball player, be aware of the following forms: speed under stress - 35 specialists (97.22%), the skill under stress - 28 specialists (77.78%) skill and speed under - 26 specialists (72.22%). Coaches also mentioned: force under stress (18 specialists, 50%), speed force under (16 specialists, 44.44%) and speed under force (13 specialists,

36.11%).

Question that specialists were asked to list, in order of importance, which considers that specific motor skills stations were obtained following content and distribution of responses:

▪ The goalkeeper: (I) speed - 36 (100%), (II) skill regime speed - 26 (72.22%), skill - 10 (27.78%), (III) flexibility - 15 (41 67%), speed under power - 14 (38.89%), mobility - 7 (19.44%).

▪ For extreme: (I) speed under power - 21 (58.33%), speed - 8 (22.22%), power - 7 (19.45%), (II) skill - 11 (30, 55%), skill in speed mode - 10 (27.78%), power - 8 (22.22%), speed 7 - (19.45%), (III) resistance - 36 (100%).

▪ For inter: (I) speed - 20 (55.56%) speed under skill - 9 (25%), speed strength under 7 (19.45), (II) power - 20 (55.56 %), strength under stress - 16 (44.44%), (III) skill - 16 (44.45%), skill under stress - 12 (33.33%), resistance - 8 (22, 22%).

▪ For pivot: (I) speed under power - 24 (66.67%), power - 12 (33.33%), (II) skill - 25 (69.44%) skill regime of power - 11 (30.56%), (III) resistance - 32 (88.89%), speed endurance mode - 3 (8.33%), flexibility 1 (2.78%).

■ The center: (I) power - 29 (80.55%), speed - 7 (19.45%), (II) speed - 29 (80.55%), force 7 (19.45%) (III) skill under stress - 19 (52.78%), skill - 10 (27.78%), resistance 7 (19.45%).

Regarding the question of adapting the content according to job physical training (specialization in line positions), most coaches 32 (88.89%) specified that in terms of general physical preparation means not considered necessary to adapt and 4 (11.11%) said means for adapts and general physical training requirements jobs - difference between goalkeeper and other players, but not on line posts. Regarding specific training, all 36 states that adopted criteria required to

the job - through physical content designed to prepare technical and tactical means.

Regarding the question "what kind of means used to solve general physical preparedness goals? Please specify their share", specialists responses (fig.3) were directed to: specific athletics (which they devote majority share decreasing from 40%, 50%, 60% or 10%), specific means game handball (weighted majority, in descending order, 20%, 40%, 30% or 10%), other sports (10% and 20%), other branches / sporting events (athletics, with 10% and 20 %), basic gymnastics (10% and 20%), other (10% movement games).

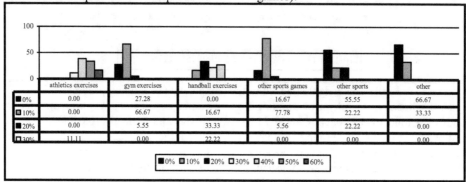

	athletics exercises	gym exercises	handball exercises	other sports games	other sports	other
■ 0%	0.00	27.28	0.00	16.67	55.55	66.67
□ 10%	0.00	66.67	16.67	77.78	22.22	33.33
■ 20%	0.00	5.55	33.33	5.56	22.22	0.00
□ 30%	11.11	0.00	22.22	0.00	0.00	0.00

■0% □10% ■20% □30% □40% ■50% ■60%

Fig.3. Means used by coaches in general physical preparation

If the question "using the selection criteria means? If your answer is positive, please specify", most specialists (86.11%) indicated that the means chosen according to the objectives set without specifying another criterion, while 13.89% responded negatively.

On "methods for checking the effectiveness of selected media", 5 (13.89%) coaches did not pronounce themselves, 4 (11.11%) responded negatively, 19 (52.78%) specified that they use samples control (without understanding the meaning of the question), 5 (13.89%) responded positively but did not specify, 3 (8.33%) responded positively, saying that occasionally they record the heart rate of athletes.

When asked the coaches control samples used for checking the physical training, 24 specialists (66.66%) prefer the evidence specified by F.R.H, 9 specialists (25.00%) use their control samples and 3 specialists (8.33%) replied that they use specific control samples. On its own evidence, the coaches indicated that they consist of tactical and technical structures checking games.

Conclusions

The analysis of the responses revealed the following:
There is an average of identifying coordinates the training of junior handball players in our country to those observed in large-scale competitions and improving tactical and physical training could help to increase the training of our athletes. The coaches opt for higher weights assigned to these components in the training, to the model recommended by the federation of specialized, resulting in the expansion of 35% - 40% compared to 30% for physical training and the continuation or expansion of 30% of 25% for tactical training. The annual training cycle allocates most important share general physical preparation, covering all driving skills, speed and endurance conditional

capacity ratio is higher than literature recommendations by 5% (speed) and 10% (resistance), and the force per unit varying opinions are not recommended around with (+) or (-) 10% for coordination capabilities specified percentage of specialists is lower (20%, 10%) of the recommended (25%) and for intermediate capacities opinions converge to a value of 10%. While adhering to the idea of "the specific content of the post motric" which will focus at a time players (junior), consider that coaches do not put enough since its foundation pre (junior II) statement is justified by (answers on questions No.8 and No.12) indiscriminate application of general physical training content to players specializing on the 9m line (profile: power - 50% Speed - 30% coordinative capacity - 20%) and those specialized on the semicircle line (profile: Speed - 40% coordinative capacity - 40% power - 20%). With regard to the means used to solve general physical preparedness goals, the highest place is held by specific means of athletics and handball game, consider that the share of resources allocated to specific basic gymnastics is too low.

Also, there is the choice of orientation exercises after the lesson objective, using the apparent structure of them (after the outlines: "I learned from coach", "as seen" and so on) without deep knowledge of their substrate and especially effects on their players (most coaches not using methods to verify the efficiency of the means applied).

Reference

1. Hantau, C., 2000, Handball, Alpha Publishing House, Buzau.
2. Colibaba-evuleț, D., Bota, I., 1998, Sports Games - Theory and Methodology, Aldin Publishing House, Bucharest.
3. Orțănescu, C., 2001, Handball Performance - Theory and Practice, Universitaria Publishing House, Craiova.

48

Study on the Developing of a Model Syllabus on Physical Education and Sports within the Curriculum on School's Decision for Pre-University Education

Chivu Daniel[1], Orţănescu Dorina[2], Nanu Marian Costin[2]

[1] *National University of Physical Education and Sport, Bucharest, Romania*
[2] *Department of Theory and Methodology of Motricity Activities, University of Craiova, Romania*

Abstract. This study is a questionnaire survey aimed to obtain information about teachers' view of activities within the school curriculum. A percentage of 60% of teachers consider obligatory the presence of students in such activities and the remaining percentages were directed to the optional participation in these activities. Physical education and sport are considered indispensable for the development of the individual personality, being an integral part of the overall education program for each student.
Key words: *curriculum, questionnaire, physical education.*

Introduction

The curricular reform of Romanian education has come halfway. This means that they have developed and published centrally in an integrated vision, documents that form the National Curriculum, appointed in the specialized literature as official curriculum or intended curriculum. The other half is the implementation, evaluation and revision of the National Curriculum, so what we call accomplished curriculum be made as close to the spirit and letter of the official curriculum. Part of this process is the publication of the National Council for Curriculum guides for the application of the new curricula. These guidelines are meant to provide a suitable route of personalized reading of the new curriculum in accordance with the actual situation at school and classroom level and the teaching experience of each teacher. (1). One of the central ideas behind the concept of educational reform as a whole, is the structuring of the curriculum on cycles, each of them having their specific objectives and periods of time allotted, estimated as targeting biological and psychological development of students and the fluency of the action of developing in accordance with the educational ideal. Each subject provided in the curriculum had to redefine objectives and to stagger them on years of schooling in line with the overall objectives of the curriculum cycle, to restructure content and, especially, to adopt methodologies meant to equip students with the capacities, skills and attitudes in personal and social domain in current and in future activities. The structuring of the educational framework on curriculum areas, the setting of the compulsory subjects and of the minimum and maximum number of hours that may be affected, the setting of a minimum and maximum number of hours for the optional subjects (without being named) and also the minimum and maximum number of hours per week for each class, requires from the teacher to develop a timetable, which may be special compared to any parallel class by the number of hours required by the subjects affected by the number of optional subjects studied and the amount of hours allotted to them as well as by the total number of hours specified in the weekly schedule. Through the right to make decisions given to school, the curriculum on school's decision (CDS) is actually the emblem of its real power. Derived from the freedom - provided by the educational framework - to decide on a segment of the national curriculum, this power allows defining individual learning paths for students. The freedom of decision at school level is consistent with a democratic society and is an opportunity for alignment to an open system with multiple options. CDS is a reality of today's schools, reality that has gained a number of followers (the important fact is that most of them are students) and that reveals normality through the acceptance of difference. In other words, CDS - as power of schools - allows an own ethos which makes the difference in the proximate genus "Romanian school at the beginning of the third millennium .(2)

Material and Method

In order to establish the need to introduce new subjects within students' activity, we applied a questionnaire to obtain information about teachers' view of activities within the school curriculum. The questionnaire involves a direct interaction between researcher and the subject, but it is mediated by a set of items related to knowledge, skills and attitudes relevant to the subject of the research.

The sociological survey conducted by us can provide important information on favorite sports disciplines preffered by teachers, disciplines that are not in the current curriculum, to its reassessment within CDS. This survey involved 30 teachers (including 28 permanent teachers), all having a teaching experience of more than 4 years. The questionnaire included a set of 15 questions

Analyzing the obtained answers we observe, without much surprise, that the first question (Are you familiar with the concept and content of curriculum on school's decision?) All respondents answered affirmatively.

For the next question, teachers ranked firstly the interest of students (40%) and then the material resources and school's interest

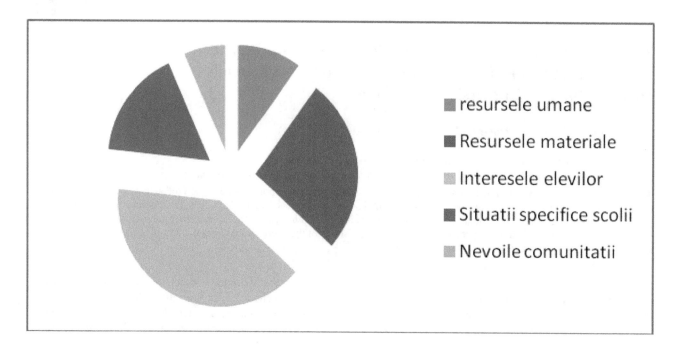

Figure 1. The order of the landmarks that teachers deemed to be an integral part of designing a curriculum on school's decision (human resources, material resources, students' interest, school specific situations, community needs)

To the question of assessing physical education and sports activities within the curriculum on school's decision, they obtained the following responses:

Question	How do you assess the physical education and sports activities within the curriculum on school's decision?			
Answer	Very important	Important	Relatively useful	Insignificant
Teachers	20	8	2	0

Thus, 66.6% of the teachers appreciate physical education and sports activities within the curriculum on school's decision as very important. Interestingly, none of the respondents considers these activities as worthless, which is a good thing.

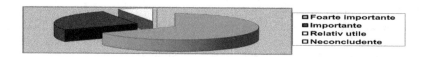

Figure 2. The assessment of physical education and sports activities within the curriculum on school's decision by teachers

Interestingly, more than half of the teachers surveyed (53.34%) see the curriculum on school's decision as an opportunity to prepare teams representing the school for competition, and another percentage, equally significant (43, 34%), sees these activities as an extension of the curriculum. Given the social and economic climate in which we live, we were not surprised at all by the answer of one teacher who believes the CDS to be a way of ensuring the number of hours for teachers.

The question on physical education and sports activities within the curriculum on school's decision,

83.3% of teachers said they have organized such events.

Regarding the top on sports subjects necessary to be introduced in the curriculum on school's decision, we have the following results. The top 3-4 disciplines were somewhat predictable (I - dance II - tae-bo, III - pilates, IV - gymnastics), considering that the majority of teachers surveyed have gym as specialization, it is natural to focus on subjects whose content is more familiar.

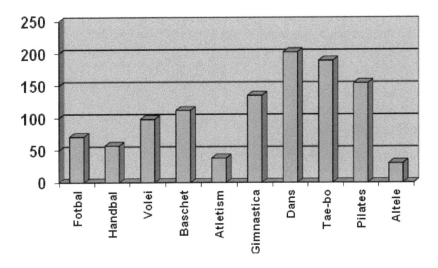

Fig. 3. The top of sports subjects necessary to be introduced in the curriculum on school's decision

Linked to students' interest in physical education and sports activities on school's decision in the curriculum, we found that only 33.3% appreciate that they have a great interest for physical education and sports activities in the curriculum on school's decision, and a slightly higher percentage 46.6% consider students' interest in these activities as great. What is important for our study is that all respondents openly acknowledge students' interest in such activities as long as the last two answers were not taken into consideration

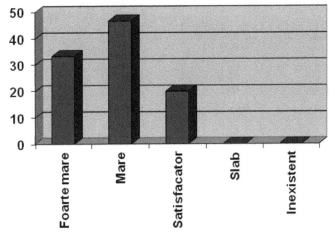

Fig. 4. Students' interest for physical education and sports activities in the curriculum on school's decision

In addition to this question, teachers were interviewed regarding the main difficulties encountered in the organization of physical education activities in the curriculum on school's decision. More than half (53.34%) draw attention to the already loaded program for students, but does not neglect the lack of material (23.33%) or, sometimes, a lack of interest from students (20%) .

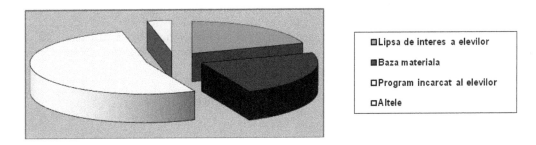

Fig. 5. The main difficulties encountered by teachers in the organization of physical education activities in the curriculum on school's decision (students' lack of interest/Material basis/Students' Loaded programme/ Others)

Another question was related to organizing the classes in the curriculum on school's decision. Almost half of the teachers (43.34%) think that the organization at two levels (V-VI VII-VIII) would be the most effective option. The next option would be the following response was to organize classes for each class in part (25.66%).

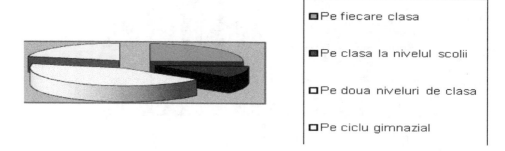

Fig. 6. Organizing the classes in the curriculum on school's decision (students and teachers) (for each class in part/ for each class at school level/on two levels of class/ on secondary school level)

As expected, the question on the number of hours in the curriculum on school's decision, brought expected results, rather high percentage 70% for the variant 2 hours / week, saying more about their options.

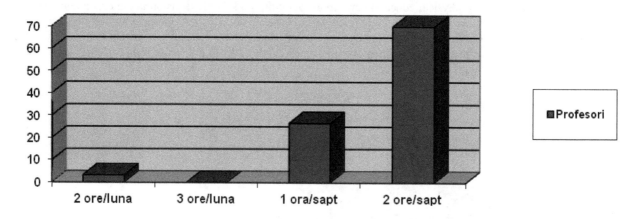

Fig. 7. The distribution of hours allotted within the curriculum on school's decision (2 hours/monthly, 3 hours/ month, 1 hour/ week, 2 hours/ a week)

Another question that obtained the expected results was that regarding students' participation in physical education and sports activities within the curriculum on school's decision. A percentage of 60% of teachers consider obligatory the presence of students in such activities and the remaining percentages were directed to the optional participation in these activities.

The questionnaire ended with a question that will come as a conclusion to all the other questions and confirm the purposes of this investigation. Thus, when asked: Would you need a syllabus for the physical education classes within the curriculum on school's decision?, 80% of the teachers surveyed responded affirmatively.

Conclusion
1. Physical education and sport are considered indispensable for the development of the individual personality, being an integral part of the overall education program for each student.
2. The investigation conducted by the questionnaire we noticed the interest of students as well as of teachers for physical education and sports activities within CDS.
3. The subjects for which teachers were mostly opted are Dance, Tae-Bo and Pilates. We note that these subjects were located in the first position and the consideration that most of the teachers interviewed

have as specialization gym, so they are familiar with the concepts and specifics of these disciplines.
4. Following the feedback from the respondents, the elaboration of a syllabus for the three subjects preferred by the respondents is clearly needed.

References
1. http://administraresite.edu.ro/index.php/articles/7337   -
acces on 3.03.2013
2. http://www.docstoc.com/docs/27523421/Order-
No-344915031999regarding--the-regime-of   optional-
subjects

Permissions

List of Contributors

Ghețu Roberta Georgiana, Călinescu Brăbiescu Luminița and Burcea George Bogdan
University of Craiova

Stoica Doru, Barbu Dumitru, Barbu Mihai Constantin Răzvan and Ciocanescu Daniel
University of Craiova – Faculty of Physical Education and Sport

Babolea Oana Bianca
Scoala Gimnazială Specială „Sf. Vasile",Craiova, Romania, Universitatea de Educație Fizică și Sport București - Școala Doctorală I.O.S.U.D

Ionescu George and Avramescu Elena Taina
University of Craiova, Faculty of Physical Education and Sport, Department of Sport Medicine and Kinesitherapy

Luminita Georgescu
University of Pitesti, Faculty of Science

Marius Cristian Neamtu
University of Medicine and Pharmacy, Craiova

Ciuvăț Dragoș
Medicine and Farmacy University of Craiova

Georgescu Luminita
University of Pitesti

Ciocănescu Daniel, Stoica Doru, Barbu Dumitru and Barbu Răzvan Mihai
University of Craiova, Faculty of Physical Education and Sport

Danciulescu Daniel and Stuparu Gabriela-Lia
University of Craiova

Mitricof Anamaria Bianca
Faculty of Physical Education and Sport, University of Craiova, Romania

Dăian Gligheria, Shaao Mirela and Ilona Ilinca1
University of Craiova

Dăian Ioan
Petrache Triscu Sports High School

Pițigoi Gabriel
UMF „Carol Davila" Bucharest

Ungureanu Aurora
University of Craiova , Faculty of Physical Education and Sports, Romania

Albina Constantin
University of Craiova, Faculty of Physical Education and Sport

Fita Ioana Gabriela and Gabriel Ioan Prada
"Carol Davila" University of Medicine and Pharmacy Bucharest, National Institute of Geriatrics and Gerontology "Ana Aslan" Bucharest National Institute of Geriatrics and Gerontology "Ana Aslan" Bucharest

Mihaela Macovei-Moraru and Luminita Diana Marinescu
University of Medicine and Pharmacy of Craiova, Romania

Albină Alina Elena
University of Craiova, Faculty of Physical Education and Sport

Cosma Germina and Orțănescu Dorina
Department of Theory and Methodology of Motricity Activities, University of Craiova, Romania

Paunescu Mihaela
National University of Physical Education and Sport, Bucharest, Romania

Zavaleanu Mihaela, Ilinca Ilona and Danoiu Mircea
Faculty of Physical Education and Sports, University of Craiova, Romania

Rosulescu Eugenia
Faculty of Physical Education and Sports, University of Craiova, Romania
Children Residential Rehabilitation Center DGASPC Craiova

Mârza-Dănilă Doina and Mârza-Dănilă Dănuț Nicu
"Vasile Alecsandri" University of Bacau, Faculty of Movement, Sports, and Health Sciences, Department of Physical Therapy and Occupational Therapy, Bacău, Romania

Popescu Sorin and Cosma Germina
University of Craiova

Forţan Cătălin, Popescu Cătălin, Mangra Gabrie and Popa Gabriel Marian
University of Craiova,

Podeanu Radu
L.P.S. Petrache Triscu

Păsărin Daniel
National University of Physical Education and Sport, Bucharest, Romania

Orţănescu Dorina
University of Craiova, Faculty of Physical Education and Sport, Romania

Chiriţescu Ileana Mihaela
Department of Foreign Languages, University of Craiova, Romania

Chivu Daniel
National University of Physical Education and Sport, Bucharest, Romania

Nanu Marian Costin and Cosma Germina
Department of Theory and Methodology of Motricity Activities, University of Craiova, Romania

Neferu Florin
University of Tg.Jiu, Romania

Stăncescu Camelia
University of Craiova, Faculty of Law "Nicolae Titulescu", Romania

Lică Marcelina Eliana and Dragomir Marian
University of Craiova, Faculty of Physical Education and Sport

Cosma Alexandru and Lică Eliana
National Colleges "Nicolae Titulescu" Craiova, Romania

Pascu Dănuţ
University of Craiova, Faculty of Physical Education and Sport, Romania

Anghel Mihaela
University "Vasile Alecsandri" FŞMSS, Bacau, Romania
National University of Physical Education and Sports PhD Student, Romania

Raţă Gloria
University "Vasile Alecsandri" FŞMSS, Bacau, Romania

Călina Mirela Lucia
Faculty of Physical Education and Sport, University of Craiova, Romania

Polyclinic of Sports Medicine, Emergency Clinical Hospital Craiova, Romania

Neamţu Marius Cristian
University of Medicine and Pharmacy Craiova, Romania

Cosma Alexandru
National University of Physical Education and Sport, Bucharest, Romania

Raţă Gloria, Raţă Bogdan Constantin, Raţă Marinela
"Vasile Alecsandri" University of Bacău

Popescu Marius Cătălin, Forţan Cătălin, Mangra Gabriel Ioan, Popa Gabriel Marian
University of Craiova, Faculty of Physical Education and Sport

Dumitru Roxana, Cosma Germina
University of Craiova, Faculty of Physical Education and Sport

Alexe Cristina Ioana
"Stiinta" Bacau Sports Club, Bacău, România

Alexe Dan Iulian
"Vasile Alecsandri" University Of Bacău,1 Department of Physical Therapy and Occupational Therapy

Cristuţă Alina Mihaela and Raţă Gloria
„Vasile Alecsandri" University from Bacău, Bacau, Romania

Lupu Gabriel
National University of Physical Education and Sport, Bucharest, Romania

Constantinescu AnaMaria
Motor Activities and University Sport Department, Petroleum and Gas University from Ploieşti

Barbu Dumitru, Stoica Doru, Barbu Mihai, Ciocănescu Daniel
University of Craiova, Faculty of Physical Education and Sport

Macovei-Moraru Mihaela, Luminiţa Diana Marinescu, Roxana Popescu
University of Medicine and Pharmacy of Craiova, Romania

Chivu Daniel
National University of Physical Education and Sport, Bucharest, Romania

Orțănescu Dorina and Nanu Marian Costin
Department of Theory and Methodology of Motricity
Activities, University of Craiova, Romania

**Barbu Mihai Constantin Răzvan, Barbu Dumitru,
Stoica Doru, Ciocanescu Daniel**
Department of Theory and Methodology of Motricity
Activities, University of Craiova, ROMANIA

Trăilă Liviu-Alexandru and Mircea Dănoiu
University of Craiova, Faculty of Physical Education
and Sport, Romania

Lupu Stănică Gabriel and Cristuță Alina Mihaela
„Vasile Alecsandri"University from Bacău, Bacau,
Roumania

Oprea Mihaela and Ion Gheorghe
Physical Education and Sport – University of Pitești,
Romania

Stănoiu Cosmina
Children Residential Rehabilitation Center DGASPC
Craiova

Zăvăleanu Mihaela and Roșulescu Eugenia
Faculty of Physical Education and Sports, University
of Craiova, Romania

Chepea Bogdan
U.N.E.F.S Bucharest

Orțănescu Dorina and Shaao Mirela
University of Craiova

Index

Printed in the USA
CPSIA information can be obtained
at www.ICGtesting.com
LVHW081119151124
796642LV00005B/467